Hoppenfeld's
TREATMENT AND REHABILITATION OF FRACTURES

Second Edition

Hoppenfeld's

TREATMENT AND REHABILITATION OF FRACTURES

Second Edition

Michael Suk, MD, JD, MPH, MBA

Professor and Chair, Department of Orthopaedic Surgery
Geisinger Commonwealth School of Medicine
Chair, Musculoskeletal Institute, Geisinger Health System
Chief Physician Officer, Geisinger System Services
Danville, Pennsylvania

Daniel S. Horwitz, MD

Professor of Orthopaedic Surgery
Geisinger Commonwealth School of Medicine
Chief, Orthopaedic Trauma Division
Geisinger Health System
Danville, Pennsylvania

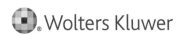
. Wolters Kluwer

Philadelphia • Baltimore • New York • London
Buenos Aires • Hong Kong • Sydney • Tokyo

Director, Medical Practice: Brian Brown
Senior Development Editor: Stacey Sebring
Editorial Coordinator: Sean Hanrahan/Emily Buccieri
Editorial Assistant: Maribeth Wood
Marketing Manager: Phyllis Hitner
Production Project Manager: Kirstin Johnson
Design Coordinator: Steve Druding
Manufacturing Coordinator: Beth Welsh
Prepress Vendor: TNQ Technologies

2nd edition

9 8 7 6 5 4 3 2 1

Printed in China

Library of Congress Cataloging-in-Publication Data

ISBN-13: 978-1-4511-8568-3

Cataloging in Publication data available on request from publisher.

shop.lww.com

Contributors

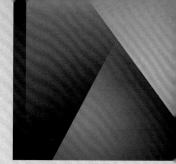

Michael T. Archdeacon, MD, MSE
Peter J. Stern Professor and Chairman
Department of Orthopaedic Surgery
University of Cincinnati
Cincinnati, Ohio

Basem Attum, MD, MS
Resident Physician
Department of Orthopaedics
University of California – San Diego
San Diego, California

Mirza Shahid Baig, MD
Orthopedic Trauma Research Fellow
Department of Orthopedics
Geisinger Medical Center
Danville, Pennsylvania

Amrut Borade, MBBS, MS, MCh
Hip and Knee Surgery Fellow
Department of Trauma & Orthopaedics
University Hospital of North Midlands
Stoke-on-Trent, England, United Kingdom

Michael P. Campbell, MD
Resident Physician
Department of Orthopaedic Surgery
Virginia Commonwealth University
Richmond, Virginia

Lisa K. Cannada, MD, FAAOS, FAOA
Orthopaedic Trauma Surgeon
Hughston Clinic
Novanr Health
Jacksonville, Florida

Laurence Cook, MD
Orthopaedic Surgeon
Fremont Medical Center
Sacramento, California

Robert M. Corey, MD
Resident, Department of Orthopedic Surgery
Saint Louis University
Saint Louis, Missouri

Brett D. Crist, MD, FAAOS, FACS, FAOA
Associate Professor
Vice Chairman of Business Development
Director Orthopaedic Trauma Service
Co-Director Orthopaedic Trauma Fellowship
Surgery of the Hip and Orthopaedic Trauma
Department of Orthopaedic Surgery
University of Missouri
One Hospital Dr.
Columbia, Missouri

Diarmuid De Faoite, MBS, BBS, BA
PhD in Public Health Candidate
Lancaster University
England, United Kingdom

Andrew Dodd, MD, FRCSC
Clinical Assistant Professor
Department of Surgery
University of Calgary
Calgary, Alberta, Canada

Jennifer T. Dodson, OTD, OTR/L, CHT
Occupational Therapist/Certified Hand Therapist
Randolph Hand Therapy
OrthoCarolina
Charlotte, North Carolina

Mary Kate Erdman, MD
Resident Physician
Department of Orthopaedic Surgery
Los Angeles County+University of Southern California
    Medical Center
Los Angeles, California

Lisa G.M. Friedman, MD, MA
Orthopaedic Trauma Research Fellow
Department of Orthopaedic Surgery
Geisinger Medical Center
Danville, Pennsylvania

Kenneth W. Graf, MD
Director, Orthopaedic Trauma Program, Cooper Bone and
    Joint Institute
Attending Orthopaedic Surgeon, Cooper University
    Hospital
Assistant Professor of Orthopaedic Surgery
Cooper University Hospital
Camden, New Jersey

Renée Genova, MD
Assistant Professor, Department of Orthopaedic Surgery &
    Rehabilitation
University of Florida- Jacksonville
Jacksonville, Florida

David J. Hak, MD, MBA
Professor of Orthopedic Surgery
University of Central Florida
Hughston Clinic Orthopedic Trauma
    Surgeons
Central Florida Regional Hospital
Sanford, Florida

Beate Hanson, MD, MPH
Clinical Assistant Professor
University of Washington, Seattle
Department of Public Health
Seattle, Washington

A. Michael Harris, MD
Orthopaedic Trauma Surgeon
Hughston Clinic Orthopaedic Trauma Surgeons
Memorial Hospital
Jacksonville, Florida

David L. Helfet, MD
Chief Emeritus
Orthopaedic Trauma Service
Hospital for Special Surgery and New York Presbyterian
    Hospital
Professor of Orthopaedic Surgery
Weill Cornell School of Medicine
New York, New York

Paul Henkel, DO
Assistant Professor
Associate Program Director
Orthopaedic Surgery Residency Program
Orthopaedic Trauma Surgery
Sports Traumatology
East Tennessee State University
Johnson City Medical Center
Johnson City, Tennessee

Dolfi Herscovici Jr, DO, FAAOS
Attending, Foot and Ankle Surgery
Center for Bone and Joint Disease
Hudson, Florida

Lindsay E. Hickerson, MD
Orthopaedic Trauma Surgeon
Health First Medical Group
Melbourne, Florida

Matthew S. Hoehn, MS, OTR/L, CHT
Occupational Therapist
Musculoskeletal Institute
Geisinger Medical Center
Danville, Pennsylvania

Daniel S. Horwitz, MD
Professor of Orthopaedic Surgery
Geisinger Commonwealth School of Medicine
Chief, Orthopaedic Trauma Division
Geisinger Health System
Danville, Pennsylvania

L. Jared Hudspeth, MD
Orthopaedic Surgeon
Sports Medicine and Shoulder Reconstruction
Piedmont Ortho
Macon, Georgia

A. Alex Jahangir, MD, MMHC
Professor of Orthopaedic Surgery
Director, Division of Orthopaedic Trauma
Vanderbilt University Medical Center
Nashville, Tennessee

Stephen L. Kates, MD
Chairman
Department of Orthopaedic Surgery
Virginia Commonwealth University
Richmond, Virginia

Deborah Kegelmeyer, PT, DPT, MS, GCS
Professor Clinical Health and Rehabilitation Sciences
Department of Physical Therapy
The Ohio State University Wexner Medical Center
Columbus, Ohio

Harish Kempegowda, MD
Attending Physician
Orthopaedic and Spine Surgery
Heartland Regional Medical Center
Marion, Illinois

Bruce A. Kraemer, MD
President and Lead Physician, Oberle Institute
SSM Health Saint Louis University Hospital
Chief, Plastic and Reconstructive Surgery
Saint Louis University School of Medicine
Saint Louis, Missouri

James R. Lachman, MD
Assistant Professor
Department of Orthopaedic Surgery
St. Luke's University Health Network
Bethlehem, Pennsylvania

Amy L. Ladd, MD
Elsbach-Richards Professor of Surgery
Chief, Robert A. Chase Hand Center
Vice-chair Academic Affairs, Department of Orthopaedic
    Surgery
Assistant Dean for Student Advising
Stanford University Medical Center
Stanford, California

John Layne, PT, tDPT, MPT, MTC
Assistant Professor
University of St. Augustine for Health Sciences
St. Augustine, Florida

Adam Keith Lee, MD
Orthopaedic Trauma Surgeon
Division of Orthopaedic Surgery
Dignity Health Medical Group – St. Joseph's Hospital and
    Medical Center
Phoenix, Arizona

Kelly A. Lefaivre, BScH, MD, MSc, FRCSC
Associate Professor
Department of Orthopaedics
University of British Columbia
Vancouver, British Columbia, Canada

Rakesh P. Mashru, MD
Assistant Professor
Program Director, Orthopaedic Trauma Fellowship
Cooper University Healthcare
Camden, New Jersey

Ryan Martyn, MD
Fellow
Spine Institute of Arizona
Scottsdale, Arizona

**Elisabeth McGee, PhD, DPT, MOT, PT, OTR/L, MTC,
CHT, CHSE**
Director of Simulation Education and CICP Operations
University of St. Augustine for Health Sciences
St. Augustine, Florida

Sandra A. Miskiel, MD
Department of Orthopaedic Surgery
Cooper University Hospital
Camden, New Jersey

Maureen A. O'Shaughnessy, MD
Assistant Professor
Department of Orthopaedic Surgery
University of Kentucky
Lexington, Kentucky

Edward Perez, MD
Orthopaedic Trauma Surgeon
Broward Health Medical Center
Fort Lauderdale, Florida

Laura Phieffer, MD, FAOA, FAAOS
Professor - Clinical
Department of Orthopaedics
The Ohio State University Wexner Medical Center
Columbus, Ohio

Saqib Rehman, MD, MBA
Professor and Vice-Chair
Department of Orthopaedic Surgery and Sports Medicine
Director of Orthopaedic Trauma, Temple University
    Hospital
Lewis Katz School of Medicine at Temple University
Philadelphia, Pennsylvania

Andres Rodriguez-Buitrago, MD
Resident Physician
Department of Orthopaedics and Traumatology
Hospital Universitario Fundacion Sante Fe de Bogota
Bogota, Columbia

Carmen E. Quatman, MD, PhD
Associate Professor
Department of Orthopaedics
The Ohio State University Wexner Medical Center
Columbus, Ohio

Catherine Quatman-Yates, PT, DPT, PhD
Assistant Professor
Department of Physical Therapy
The Ohio State University Wexner Medical Center
Columbus, Ohio

Mark S. Rekant, MD
Associate Professor
Philadelphia Hand to Shoulder Center
Department of Orthopaedic Surgery
Thomas Jefferson University
Philadelphia, Pennsylvania

Daniela Furtado Barreto Rocha, MD
Orthopedic Trauma Research Fellow
Department of Orthopedics
Geisinger Medical Center
Danville, Pennsylvania

Julia M. Scaduto, APRN
Nurse Practioner, Foot and Ankle Surgery
Center for Bone and Joint Disease
Hudson, Florida

Adam P. Schumaier, MD
Resident Physician
Department of Orthopaedic Surgery
University of Cincinnati
Cincinnati, Ohio

Trevor J. Shelton, MD, MS
Orthopedic Sports Medicine Fellow
Department of Orthopaedic Surgery
Southern California Orthopedic Institute
Van Nuys, California

Bronwyn Spira, PT
Founder and CEO
Force Therapeutics
New York, New York

James P. Stannard, MD
Hansjörg Wyss Distinguished Professor and Chairman
Department of Orthopaedic Surgery
University of Missouri
Medical Director Missouri Orthopaedic Institute
Chief Medical Officer for Surgical and Procedural Services
University of Missouri Healthcare
Columbia, Missouri

Michael Suk, MD, JD, MPH, MBA
Professor and Chair, Department of Orthopaedic Surgery
Geisinger Commonwealth School of Medicine
Chair, Musculoskeletal Institute, Geisinger Health System
Chief Physician Officer, Geisinger System Services
Danville, Philadelphia

Diederik O. Verbeek, MD, PhD
Trauma Service, Department of Surgery
Maastricht University Medical Center
Maastricht, Netherlands

Sabrina Wang, PT, DPT, OTR/L, MOT
Orthopaedic Physical Therapy Residency Program Coordinator
Department of Rehabilitation Services
University of Florida – Jacksonville
Jacksonville, Florida

J. Tracy Watson, MD, FAAOS
Professor Orthopaedic Surgery,
Chief, Orthopaedic Trauma Service
Department of Orthopaedic Surgery
Saint Louis University School of Medicine
St. Louis, Missouri

Philip R. Wolinsky, MD
Professor, Department of Orthopaedic Surgery
University of California at Davis Medical Center
Sacramento, California

Geoffrey P. Wilkin, MD, FRCSC
Assistant Professor
Division of Orthopaedic Surgery
University of Ottawa
Ottawa, Ontario, Canada

Porter Young, MD
Resident Physician
Department of Orthopaedic Surgery & Rehabilitation
University of Florida – Jacksonville
Jacksonville, Florida

Terri Zachos, MD, PhD, DVM
Resident Physician, PGY-2
Department of Orthopaedic Surgery
University of California Davis Health System
Sacramento, California

Ryan Corbin Zitzke, MD
Orthopaedic Surgeon
Prisma Health Orthopedics
Sumter, South Carolina

Preface

I first met Dr. Stanley Hoppenfeld in the fall of 1997, when I was just beginning my residency at Montefiore Medical Center in Bronx, NY. I remember feeling like I was in the presence of orthopaedic royalty! Here he was, the surgeon who probably more than any other modern author, influenced our understanding and appreciation of the orthopaedic physical and neurological examination, and contemporary anatomic surgical approaches. It is without question, that his work influenced more than a generation of orthopaedic surgeons

In January 2000, Dr. Hoppenfeld and Vasantha L. Murthy, MD, coedited the first edition of the *Treatment and Rehabilitation of Fractures*. As a PGY-3 at the time, I recall Dr. Hoppenfeld coming into grand rounds with several boxes of the new publication and distributing them to the residents, each of whom respectfully asked him to sign their own personal copy. I still have my copy today.

Now a full two decades later, I am pleased to present the second edition the *Hoppenfeld's Treatment and Rehabilitation of Fractures*.

This book is intended for anyone interested in the aftercare treatment of fractures including all students of medicine, nursing, or physical or occupational therapy; postgraduate trainees in orthopaedic surgery, primary care sports medicine, or physical medicine and rehabilitation; and all physicians of all specialties.

In keeping with Dr. Hoppenfeld's original vision, the book is subdivided into anatomical sections with an emphasis on understanding the relationship between conservative or operative fracture care and the functional restoration of joint mobility to enhance patient outcomes. The book is inherently multidisciplinary and reflects a "total care" approach to fracture conditions.

I would be remiss if I did not formally acknowledge the many individuals who contributed to the development and production of this final work. First and foremost, a very special thank you to Dr. Hoppenfeld and his remarkable family for having the confidence and faith in our ability to complete this work. And to the faculty and residents of the Montefiore Medical Center Orthopaedic Residency Program, who were groundbreakers with the first edition and to whom Dr. Hoppenfeld devoted much of his storied academic career and to the faculty and residents at Geisinger Medical Center, where I now call home.

I am also thankful to the many chapter authors but especially grateful to my coeditor Daniel S. Horwitz, MD, who is not only an incredible partner in orthopaedic surgery, but also whose broad shoulders helped me carry this project over the finish line. And finally, kudos to the incredible team at Lippincott Publishing (Bob Hurley, David Murphy, Brian Brown, Stacey Sebring, and Oviya Balamurugan) who guided us through final production.

I hope that you will enjoy this book and will find it helpful for your future patient encounters!

MICHAEL SUK, MD, JD, MPH, MBA, FACS

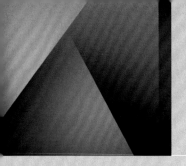

Contents

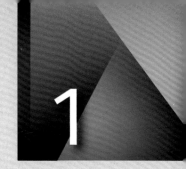

Introduction to Musculoskeletal Measures and Instruments

Diarmuid De Faoite
Beate Hanson

INTRODUCTION TO PATIENT-REPORTED OUTCOME MEASURES

As clinicians involved in fracture care, we have a vested interest in knowing how our patients fare postsurgical or nonsurgical treatment. However, defining "success" or "satisfaction" can be elusive and, in many respects, depends on our perspective.

In December 1895, Wilhelm Conrad Röentgen discovered x-rays by accident, the x in the name representing the unknown type of radiation he had discovered.[1] For the first time, physicians were able to view bony structures of the human skeleton, and the way we treat fractures forever changed. The x-ray became the first objective outcome measure for fracture care. Röentgen was awarded the Nobel Prize in Physics for this discovery in 1901. More than 120 years later, x-rays remain the gold standard in determining successful fracture alignment and accurate appropriate implant positioning.

Interpretation of x-rays requires the expertise of trained medical professionals and can provide helpful objective data such as alignment or bone cortical density. Interpretation of x-rays can lead to "clinician reported outcomes" and a determination of healing. While a clinical outcome, such as fracture healing, may be regarded as a "good" outcome by the treating physician, the same patient may continue to experience pain or impaired function and deem the same result as "poor." Recognizing these limitations of clinician-administered outcomes when researching patients' health-related quality of life led to the development of patient-reported outcomes (PROs).[2] These ensure that a good outcome in the eyes of the surgeon is also reflected in the experience of the patient.

PROs have established themselves in both clinical practice and clinical research. The Cochrane Collaboration defines PROs as "any reports coming directly from patients about how they function or feel in relation to a health condition and its therapy, without interpretation of the patient's responses by a clinician, or anyone else."[3]

TYPES OF PATIENT-REPORTED OUTCOME MEASURES

A patient-reported outcome measure (PROM) is a tool designed to elicit information from patients on their outcomes. There are two main types:

- Generic
- Disease-specific

Both are used to assess the healthcare provider's performance in improving a patient's condition.

Generic

As the name suggests, generic measures of outcome, such as the Short Form-36 (SF-36) Health Survey and the EQ-5D questionnaire, are applicable to a wide variety of patients.

Disease-Specific

Disease-specific (ie, validated for one or a few diseases) instruments are also commonly used. Some well-known examples include:

- KOOS: Knee Osteoarthritis Outcome Score
- OKS: Oxford Knee Score
- WOMAC: Western Ontario and McMaster Universities Osteoarthritis Index

The limitation of these disease-specific instruments is that they are not generalizable to other diseases of the lower extremity. Nor do they reveal how the disease impacts function. They measure neither patient satisfaction nor activity levels.

CHOOSING PROS

There are many considerations involved in selecting PROs. The suitability of PRO instruments may be an issue in certain populations or settings. As an example, PROMs are inappropriate for evaluating outcomes following acute injuries, such as fractures, because trauma patients may never return to their baseline (pretrauma) level of function. Because the injury was unexpected, information on a patient's preinjury condition is also generally not available.

Another of the difficulties in choosing an outcome measure is the wide variety of PROMs available, particularly when virtually all can be used to measure a specific PRO.[2] In addition, each outcome measure has a scoring system, which requires familiarity with the system in order for it to be understood and used effectively.

One book, published in 2009, which aimed to summarize all the major musculoskeletal outcome instruments in use ran to over 800 pages and highlighted more than 300 commonly used outcomes.[4] The number of PROs available today has only grown since the book's publication.

There are several methodological considerations associated with choosing an outcome measure. Of great importance is the validity of the instrument. Validity is the extent to which an instrument measures what it is supposed to measure.

The three main subtypes of validity are:

1. Content validity: refers to an instrument's comprehensiveness or how adequately the questions reflect its purpose.
2. Construct validity: a quantitative form of assessing validity. A construct is an item or concept such as pain or disability. It is evaluated by quantitatively comparing the relationship between a construct, for example, pain, and another variable, for example, use of pain medication.
3. Criterion validity: evaluates the instrument's correlation with a "gold standard" measure of the same topic—if one exists. For example, the Knee Society Score is regarded as the gold standard for total knee arthroplasty PROMs.[5]

The responsiveness (ability of the instrument to change as the status of the patient changes), internal consistency (the consistency of the questions in measuring the same outcome), and reproducibility (inter-observer agreement) of PROMs should also be considered when evaluating these instruments.

The authors of the PROM summary book demonstrated that not all of the instruments were validated or tested for inter- and intra-reliability.[4] Where a validation reference was provided, many of the PROMs were developed for one specific disease (eg, arthritis) and are not applicable for evaluating fracture healing after open reduction internal fixation.

In summary, surgeons wishing to use PROMs should thoroughly investigate their validation status prior to committing to their use.

CHALLENGES ASSOCIATED WITH PRACTICAL APPLICATION OF PROMS IN CLINICAL SETTINGS

Can the differences in perspectives on clinical progress between clinicians and patients be reconciled? This question was the focus of a study examining the ability of surgeons to assess patient expectations regarding orthopaedic trauma surgery outcomes. The authors investigated patients' and surgeons' postoperative perspectives on how well their preoperative expectations were met. Some 155 ankle fracture patients in three countries (the USA, Brazil, and Canada) were evaluated at 1 year postoperatively. The trauma expectation factor and trauma outcome measure questionnaires were administered both preoperatively and postoperatively.[6] The results revealed that surgeons have difficulty meeting or exceeding preoperative patient expectations of long-term outcomes after ankle fracture surgery. Brazilian and Canadian patients' expectations were more aligned (but never the same) as their surgeons. Patients in the US had markedly higher expectations. The study also indicated that culture and surgeon-patient communication have considerable influence on patient expectations.

CHALLENGES ASSOCIATED WITH PRACTICAL APPLICATION OF PROMS IN CLINICAL RESEARCH

While international multicenter studies are commonplace, using PROMs in clinical studies conducted with patients from different cultures can present difficulties. To ensure completeness of data collection, PROMs must be available in all local languages.

PROMs must be modified to ensure compatibility with the cultures in which they are used, particularly if developed in another country. For example, a team in the Netherlands translated the Patient-Reported Outcomes Measurement Information System (PROMIS) physical function item bank into Dutch.[7] The question for patients in the US, "Are you able to walk a block on flat ground?" was changed to "Are you able to walk 150 meters on flat ground?" for patients in the Netherlands.

THE FUTURE OF PROMS

Traditional questionnaires used to collect PROs are burdensome for both patients and healthcare staff. Due to the proliferation of different PROMs, results are difficult to compare across (or "among") settings. One systematic review of PROMs for total knee arthroplasty found that 38 articles reported using 47 different PROMS on over 85,000 patients.[5]

The PROMIS was designed to overcome these issues regarding lack of standardization.[8]

Developed with support from the National Institute for Health, it is a publicly available system of highly reliable, precise measures of patient-reported health status for physical, mental, and social well-being. Scores are referenced against US general population norms. The National Institutes of Health in the US funded the development of new PROs based on comprehensive literature reviews, focus groups, and cognitive interviews. The aims of these PROs were to provide efficient, precise, valid, and responsive measures of patient health and well-being. The end result was PROMIS. PROMIS researchers then introduced CAT (computerized adaptive testing), in which the next question in the PRO is based on the response to the previous question, to reduce the question burden to as few as four.[9]

The literature demonstrates clear agreement among researchers and across clinical studies on the utility, sensitivity, reliability, and validity of outcome measurement using PROMIS CATs.[10-12]

The use of PROMIS CATs could reduce the question burden on patients and clinicians. Using CAT, instead of traditional PROs with numerous questions, may increase compliance and minimize loss to follow-up in clinical trials.[13]

As patients become more comfortable with this technology, short PROMs, for example, PROMIS CATs, can be used with mobile technology (eg, smartphones).

In conclusion, orthopaedic surgeons continue to face challenges in objectively measuring success. Prior to surgery, meeting and/or exceeding patient expectations regarding short- and long-term outcomes continue to be elusive goals. This is all taking place against the trend in the modern world for greater connectivity. In medicine, we can see healthcare providers and organizations reaching out to the patient directly via easy-to-use and more patient-related daily activity levels and outcome.

Despite recent efforts to improve PROMs and related technology and instruments, culture, geography and surgeon-patient communication, comorbidities, and education exert considerable influence on patient expectations. These play critical roles in the utility of PROs.

REFERENCES

1. Roentgen WC. On a new kind of ray (first report) [German]. *Munch Med Wochenschr.* 1959;101:1237-1239. ·
2. Weldring T, Smith SMS. Patient-reported outcomes (PROs) and patient-reported outcome measures (PROMs). *Health Serv Insights.* 2013;6:61-68. doi:10.4137/HSI.S11093.
3. Patrick DL, Guyatt GH, Acquadro C. Chapter 17: Patient-reported outcomes. In: Higgins JPT, Green S, eds. *Cochrane Handbook for Systematic Reviews of Interventions Version 5.1.0.* [updated March 2011]. The Cochrane Collaboration; 2011. Available at http://handbook-5-1.cochrane.org. Accessed February 1 2018.
4. Suk M, Hanson BP, Norvell DC, Helfet DL. *Musculoskeletal Outcomes Measures and Instruments.* Vol. 2. 2nd ed. Stuttgart: Thieme; 2009:814.
5. Ramkumar PN, Harris JD, Noble PC. Patient-reported outcome measures after total knee arthroplasty: a systematic review. *Bone Joint Res.* 2015;4(7):120-127.
6. Suk M, Daigl M, Buckley RE, Lorich DG, Helfet DL, Hanson B. Outcomes after orthopedic trauma: are we meeting patient expectations? – a prospective, multicenter cohort study in 203 patients. *J Orthop Surg.* 2017;25(1):1-8.
7. Oude Voshaar MA, ten Klooster PM, Taal E, Krishnan E, van de Laar MA. Dutch translation and cross-cultural adaptation of the PROMIS® physical function item bank and cognitive pre-test in Dutch arthritis patients. *Arthritis Res Ther.* 2012;14:1-7.
8. Cella D, Yount S, Rothrock N, et al. The Patient-Reported Outcomes Measurement Information System (PROMIS): progress of an NIH roadmap cooperative group during its first two years. *Med Care.* 2007;45(5 suppl 1):S3-S11.
9. Patient-Reported Outcomes Information System. *PROMIS Scoring Guide: Version 1.0 Short Forms, Profile Short Forms, Computerized Adaptive Testing.* 2011. Available at https://assessmentcenter.net/documents/Assessment%20Center%20Glossary.pdf. Accessed November 5, 2020.
10. Schalet BD, Hays RD, Jensen SE, Beaumont JL, Fries JF, David Cella. Validity of PROMIS® physical function measures in diverse clinical samples. *J Clin Epidemiol.* 2016;73:112-118.
11. Schalet BD, Pilkonis PA, Lan Y, et al. Clinical validity of PROMIS® depression, anxiety, and anger across diverse clinical samples. *J Clin Epidemiol.* 2016;73:119-127.
12. Teresi JA, Ocepek-Welikson K, Kleinman M, Ramirez M. Giyeon Kim psychometric properties and performance of the patient reported outcomes measurement information system® (PROMIS®) depression short forms in ethnically diverse groups. *Psychol Test Assess Model.* 2016;58(1):141-181.
13. Burnham J, Meta F, Lizzio V, Makhni E, Bozic K. Technology assessment and cost-effectiveness in orthopedics: how to measure outcomes and deliver value in a constantly changing healthcare environment. *Curr Rev Musculoskelet Med.* 2017;10(2):233-239.

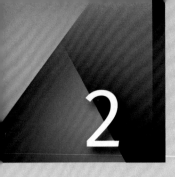

2

Trauma Basics

David J. Hak

BIOMECHANICS AND MECHANISMS OF INJURY

Fractures can occur as a result of a variety of injuries ranging from low energy (twisting injuries or ground-level falls) to high energy (motor vehicle accidents, pedestrians struck by vehicles, falls from heights, etc).

Bone is stronger in compression than in tension and is weakest in shear. The force of the injury is dissipated as the bone breaks. Lower energy injuries typically produce simple fracture patterns, while higher energy injuries result in variable degrees of comminution. The mechanisms of fracture (tension, compression, bending, or torsion) will produce different fracture patterns (**Figure 2.1**).

TENSION

The failure mechanism for bone loaded in tension is mainly debonding at the cement lines and pulling out of the osteons resulting in a transverse fracture. Tension fractures tend to occur in areas with a large proportion of cancellous bone.

COMPRESSION

The failure mechanism for bone loaded in compression is mainly oblique cracking of the osteons resulting in an oblique fracture at an angle of 30° due to the shear forces at this angle. These fractures tend to occur in the metaphyses of bones or in the vertebral bodies where there is more cancellous bone that is weaker than cortical bone.

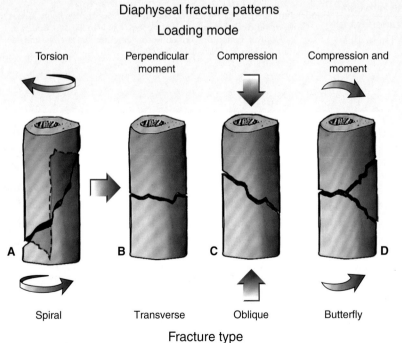

FIGURE 2.1 Characteristic fracture patterns based on the mechanism of injury. (Reprinted with permission from Weinstein SL, Flynn JM. *Lovell and Winter's Pediatric Orthopedics.* Philadelphia, PA: Wolters Kluwer; 2014.)

BENDING

Bone loaded in bending is subjected to compressive stresses on one side and tensile stresses on the opposite side. Bending causes transverse fractures as failure on the tension side progresses transversely across the bone. When bending is combined with compression, a separate triangular fragment, or "butterfly" fragment, may occur.

TORSION

When bone is twisted about its long axis, torque is produced within the structure.

Maximal tensile and compressive forces act on planes diagonal to the neutral axis resulting in a spiral shaped fracture.

SPECIAL FRACTURE PATTERNS IN CHILDREN

Children's bones are more plastic (deformable) and injury can result in incomplete fracture patterns. A **greenstick fracture** occurs due to mechanical failure on the tension side, but because the bone is not very brittle, it does not completely fracture, but rather exhibits bowing without complete disruption of the bone's cortex in the surface opposite the applied force. A **torus fracture** or **buckle fracture** is an incomplete fracture of a long bone shaft characterized by bulging of the cortex (**Figure 2.2**). This injury occurs from an axial loading force along the bone's long axis and normally occurs in the transition between metaphyseal and diaphyseal bone such as in the distal radius.

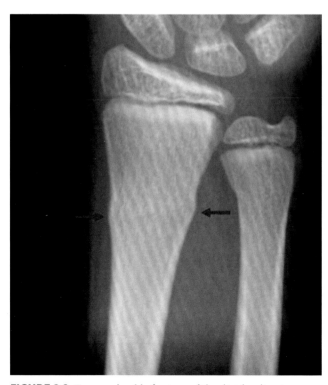

FIGURE 2.2 Torus or buckle fracture of the distal radius in a child.

COMMON CLASSIFICATIONS USED IN ORTHOPAEDIC TRAUMA

Numerous fracture classification systems have been developed to allow surgeons to differentiate different fracture patterns and organize them into clinically useful groups. A good classification system is valid, reliable, and reproducible. It should serve as a guideline for treatment, indicate risk and nature of potential complications, and provide information regarding anticipated prognosis. While the ideal classification system is difficult to achieve, it should provide a reliable method of communicating the pattern of injury and allow comparison of treatment results of similar fractures treated at different institutions or using different methods.

Fracture classification systems can be divided into three main types: nominal, ordinal, and scalar. Some classification systems may include a combination of nominal, ordinal, and scalar components. Nominal systems categorize fractures based on the accepted names and patterns of similar fracture lines. For instance, calcaneus fractures can be classified as either "tongue type" or "joint depression type" based on the location of the fracture. Ordinal systems classify fractures based on a numbered series. For example, fractures of the proximal humerus can be classified based on the number of separate displaced fracture fragments, such as 1-part, 2-part, 3-part, and 4-part. Scalar systems classify fractures based on specific measurements, such as displacement of <5 mm, 5 to 10 mm, and >10 mm.

TRADITIONAL FRACTURE CLASSIFICATION SYSTEMS

Most commonly used fracture classification systems were developed by individual surgeons to describe fractures limited to a specific anatomic area or a specific part of one bone. The developing surgeon's name is often attached to these classification systems, resulting in the frequency of classification eponyms. Common examples include:

- Pauwels classification of femoral neck fractures (**Figure 2.3**)
- Garden classification of femoral neck fractures
- Neer classification of proximal humerus fractures
- Schatzker classification of tibial plateau fractures
- Hawkins classification of talar neck fractures

While some of these classification systems may include the mechanism of injury, most are based on the radiographic appearance of the fracture. Assessments of these traditional classification systems have generally shown only poor to fair interobserver agreement and intraobserver reproducibility.

COMPREHENSIVE FRACTURE CLASSIFICATION SYSTEMS

Problems associated with traditional classification systems have led to the development of a comprehensive standardized classification system. The goal of these classification

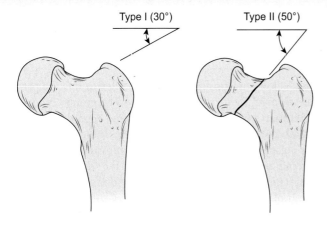

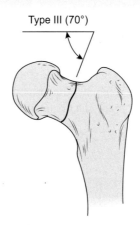

FIGURE 2.3 The Pauwels classification of femoral neck fractures. (Reprinted with permission from Koval KJ, Zuckerman JD. *Atlas of Orthopedic Surgery: A Multimedia Reference*. Philadelphia, PA: Lippincott Williams & Wilkins; 2004.)

systems is to facilitate communication in a consistent uniform fashion. While the primary role of many commonly used traditional classification systems is to aid surgeons in their day-to-day decision-making processes, the role of a comprehensive fracture classification is primarily in its usefulness for clinical research. By using a uniform comprehensive classification system, you can more accurately compare the results of different forms of treatment in a similar group of injuries.

Beginning in the 1970s, Maurice Müller began working with numerous colleagues on the AO Comprehensive Long Bone Classification System.[1] This alphanumeric system was designed to be internationally understandable and compatible with computerized databases. This classification system organizes fractures of long bones into hierarchical triads based on the severity of the bony injury. Each bone is given a specific numeric assignment (for example, humerus = 1, forearm = 2, femur = 3, tibia = 4). The location of the fracture in the bone is then specified as proximal, middle, or distal third. Fractures are then subdivided into three types, and each type is further subdivided into three groups. Types and groups are arranged in ascending order of severity. Groups are also further subdivided into subgroups using specific qualifications.

The Orthopaedic Trauma Association (OTA) has adopted and expanded the Müller long bone system, classifying fractures of other bones including the pelvis and spine, along with dislocation and pediatric fractures.[2,3] The initial version of the OTA Fracture and Dislocation was published in 1996, with the most recent update occurring in 2018.

SOFT-TISSUE INJURY CLASSIFICATION SYSTEMS

Open fractures are commonly classified using the Gustilo-Anderson classification system (**Table 2.1**).[4] The use of this classification system can help predict the rate of infection and fracture healing problems. The severity of soft-tissue injury in closed fractures can also be classified by the less frequently used Tscherne classification system (**Table 2.2**).[5]

VALIDATION OF FRACTURE CLASSIFICATION SYSTEMS

Validation of classification systems is important both for research and publication, since it is thought that the severity of the injury has an important impact on patient outcomes. Many current fracture classification systems have been stratified based on the presumed injury severity. However, fracture severity is not the only factor that impacts patient outcomes. Noninjury factors such as education level, overall health, and mental outlook may play an equally important role in patient outcomes.[6] The ability to apply a validated, reliable, and reproducible classification system will improve the ability to evaluate future clinical studies and published literature.

TABLE 2.1 Gustilo-Anderson Open Fracture Classification

Type	Description
I	Skin opening ≤1 cm; very clean; laceration most likely due to inside to outside mechanism; minimum muscle contusion; simple transverse or short oblique fractures
II	Laceration >1 cm; extensive soft-tissue damage, flaps, or avulsion; minimum to moderate crushing; simple transverse or short oblique fractures with minimum comminution
III	Extensive soft-tissue damage, including muscles, skin, and neurovascular structures; often a high-velocity injury with severe crushing component
IIIA	Extensive soft-tissue laceration with adequate bone coverage; segmental fractures, gunshot injuries
IIIB	Extensive soft-tissue injury with periosteal stripping and bone exposure; usually associated with massive contamination; requires soft-tissue coverage
IIIC	Vascular injury requiring repair

Adapted from Gustilo RB, Anderson JT. Prevention of infection in the treatment of one thousand and twenty-five open fractures of long bones: retrospective and prospective analyses. J Bone Joint Surg Am. *1976;58(4):453-458.*

TABLE 2.2	The Tscherne Classification of Soft-Tissue Injuries Associated With Closed Fractures
Type	Description
0	Minimum soft-tissue damage; indirect violence; simple fracture patterns *Example:* spiral fracture of the tibia in skiers
I	Superficial abrasion or contusion caused by pressure from within; mild to moderately severe fracture configuration *Example:* pronation fracture-dislocation of the ankle joint with soft-tissue lesion over the medial malleolus
II	Deep, contaminated abrasion associated with localized skin or muscle contusion; impending compartment syndrome; severe fracture configuration *Example:* segmental "bumper" fracture of the tibia
III	Extensive skin contusion or crush injury; may have severe underlying muscle damage; subcutaneous avulsion; compartment syndrome; associated major vascular injury; severe or comminuted fracture pattern

Reproduced with permission from Tscherne H, Gotzen L, eds. Fractures With Soft Tissue Injuries. *Berlin: Springer Verlag; 1984.*

REVIEW OF RADIOGRAPHIC LINES AND ANGLES

The language of orthopaedic trauma includes a number of named radiographic lines and angles. Those that have withstood the test of time provide a common language for communication between colleagues. In addition, many lines and angles have become a critical part of the systematic evaluation of orthopaedic conditions, defining the boundaries between normal and abnormal.[7]

Radiographic measurements often represent a continuum in which the normal and abnormal values overlap. The standard deviation of the measurements may be large. The accuracy and reproducibility of the measurements should be considered and may be influenced by many factors including the positioning of the patient and the x-ray beam. Variation in measurement is also seen based on patient age and sex. For extremity injuries, comparison with radiographs of the uninjured side may be helpful, especially in children. The *Atlas of Roentgenographic Measurement* by Keats and Sistrom provides an excellent reference for additional radiographic measurements.[8]

LINES AND ANGLES ABOUT THE WRIST

Distal radius fractures are common injuries that often occur as a result of a fall on an outstretched arm. The degree of angulation and thus indication for closed reduction or operative treatment are measured on wrist radiographs. On the

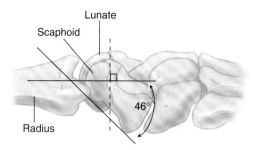

FIGURE 2.4 With the wrist in neutral position, the normal angle between the scaphoid and the lunate measures 46°. (Reprinted with permission from Wiesel SM. *Operative Techniques in Orthopedic Surgery.* Philadelphia: Wolters Kluwer; 2016.)

lateral view, the normal radial volar tilt should be 11° + 2°, and on the anteroposterior view, the normal radial inclination should be 24° + 2.5° (**Figure 2.4**). The acceptable degree of residual angulation will depend upon various patient factors including age, activity level, and hand dominance. Also measured on the lateral view is the scapholunate angle, which is normally 47° + 15°. Abnormalities in this angle can be seen with displaced scaphoid fractures and other conditions affecting the wrist joint.

LINES AND ANGLES ABOUT THE ELBOW

The measurement of various lines and angles about the elbow is primarily performed in relation to pediatric elbow fractures. On the lateral elbow radiograph, a line carried straight down from the anterior humeral cortex should pass through the middle third of the lateral condyle ossification center, but this relationship will often be distorted in the presence of an elbow fracture. The humeral-lateral condylar angle can also be measured on the lateral elbow radiograph and should normally be 40°. On the anteroposterior view of the arm, the carrying angle is an angle formed by the longitudinal axis of the humerus with the longitudinal axis of the forearm. This is normally around 15° of valgus. Malunited pediatric elbow fractures may lead to reduction in the normal carrying angle, a condition termed cubitus varus.

LINES AND ANGLES ABOUT THE HIP AND ACETABULUM

The neck shaft angle is formed by the intersection of a line drawn along the femoral shaft axis with a line drawn along the femoral neck (**Figure 2.5**). The normal neck shaft angle is 125° + 7°. Various congenital and development conditions may lead to an increased (coxa valgus) or decreased (coxa varus) neck shaft angle. Restoration of the normal femoral neck shaft angle is a common goal in the management of femoral neck and intertrochanteric hip fractures.

The iliopectineal line delineates the medial border of the anterior column of the acetabulum and will be disrupted in acetabular fractures involving the anterior column. The ilio-ischial line delineates the medial border of the posterior column of the acetabulum and will be disrupted in acetabular

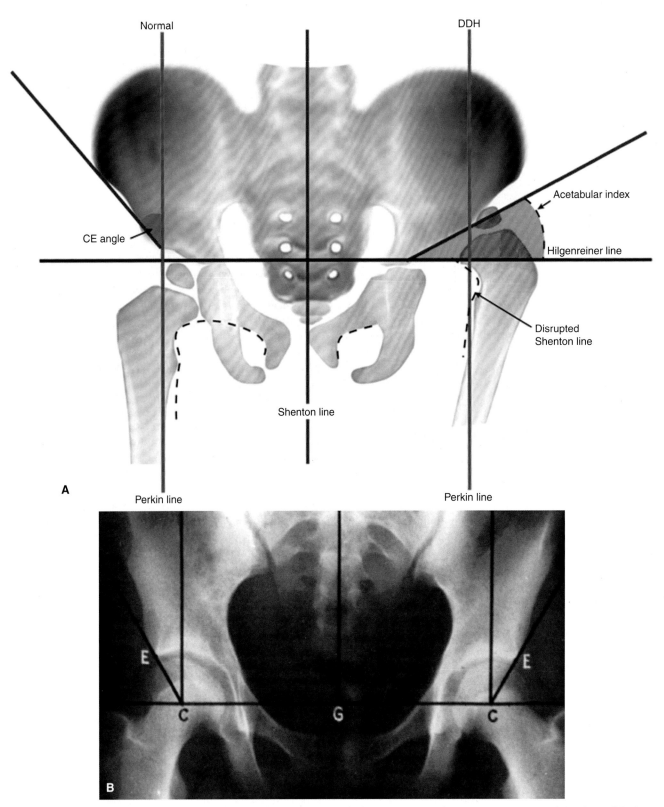

FIGURE 2.5 A and **B**, Common lines and angles around the hip and acetabulum. CE, center edge; DDH, developmental dysplasia of the hip. (Reprinted with permission from Weinstein SL, Flynn JM. *Lovell and Winter's Pediatric Orthopedics*. Philadelphia, PA: Wolters Kluwer; 2014.)

fractures involving the posterior column. On the anteroposterior view of the pelvis, the "tear drop" is seen just medial to the femoral head and represents the cortical border of the quadrilateral surface of the pelvis.

Pauwels developed a classification of femoral neck fractures based on the angle of the fracture relative to the horizontal plane (see **Figure 2.3**). In Type I fractures, this angle is <30°, Type II fractures are between 30° and 50°, while Type III fractures are >70°. With increasing verticality of the fracture line, there is increased shear stress on the fracture fixation. Outcomes of Type III fractures are generally poorer and may require a different fixation strategy to resist the shear forces to prevent loss of reduction.

LINES AND MEASUREMENTS ABOUT THE KNEE

Several lines and measurements are made on the lateral view of the knee. The Insall ratio compares the length of the patella with the length of the patella tendon. Normally this ratio is 1:1, but will be abnormal in the presence of patella ligament rupture, patella alta, or patella baja. The Blumensaat line is drawn along the superior aspect of the intercondylar notch and can also be used to assess normal patella position. This line is also used during retrograde femoral nailing to determine the correct position of the distal aspect of the intramedullary nail.

LINES AND MEASUREMENTS ABOUT THE ANKLE

Two angles are commonly measured in patients sustaining calcaneal fractures. The Böhler angle is formed by a line drawn from the superior aspect of the anterior calcaneal process to the superior aspect of the posterior articular surface with a line drawn from the superior aspect of the posterior articular surface to the superior aspect of the calcaneal tuberosity. The Gissane angle is the angle created by the strong thick cortical strut of bone along the superolateral aspect of the calcaneus that extends from the calcaneocuboid joint to the posterior margin of the posterior facet.

REFERENCES

1. Müller ME, Nazarian S, Koch P, Schatzker J. *The Comprehensive Classification of Fractures of Long Bones.* Berlin: Springer-Verlag; 1990.
2. Marsh JL, Slongo TF, Agel J, et al. Fracture and dislocation classification compendium – 2007: Orthopaedic Trauma Association classification, database and outcomes committee. *J Orthop Trauma.* 2007; 21(10 suppl):S1-133.
3. Slongo TF, Audigé L; AO Pediatric Classification Group. Fracture and dislocation classification compendium for children: the AO pediatric comprehensive classification of long bone fractures (PCCF). *J Orthop Trauma.* 2007;21(10 suppl):S135-S160.
4. Gustilo RB, Anderson JT. Prevention of infection in the treatment of one thousand and twenty-five open fractures of long bones: retrospective and prospective analyses. *J Bone Joint Surg Am.* 1976;58(4):453-458.
5. Tscherne H, Gotzen L, eds. *Fractures With Soft Tissue Injuries.* Berlin: Springer Verlag; 1984.
6. MacKenzie EJ, Burgess AR, McAndrew MP, et al. Patient-oriented functional outcome after unilateral lower extremity fracture. *J Orthop Trauma.* 1993;7(5):393-401.
7. Hak DJ, Gautsch TL. A review of radiographic lines and angles in orthopaedics. *Am J Orthop.* 1995;24(8):590-601.
8. Keats TE, Sistrom C. *Atlas of Roentgenographic Measurement.* 7th ed. St. Louis, MO: Mosby; 2001.

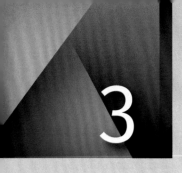

3

Bone Healing

James R. Lachman
Saqib Rehman

INTRODUCTION

The skeletal system, through coordinated biochemical and biomechanical processes, is capable of restoring mechanical and biological stability after injury. Compromise to the bone can be the result of direct injury, neoplasm, infectious microorganisms, and deprivation of essential nutrients when blood supply is disrupted.[1] The interaction of progenitor cells, inflammatory cytokines, growth factors, host biology, and mechanical environment provides a setting which enables bone to heal in an organized, predictable manner.[2]

When bone incurs a traumatic injury, a biochemical response is initiated secondary to direct cell damage. This sequence has classically been broken up into four phases: inflammation, soft callus formation, hard callus formation, and remodeling.[2,3] Injury occurs to the local bone and soft tissue, including the local vascular supply which causes the formation of a hematoma. Inside the hematoma are numerous mesenchymal stem cells (MSCs) which generate growth factors to aid in differentiation of osteoprogenitor cells. In the absence of surgical intervention, these cells, over a period of days, begin to form soft callus, which is composed primarily of cartilage. As this matrix becomes calcified, it becomes hard callus as osteoblasts and osteoclasts begin the balance of bony homeostasis. The final phase, called remodeling, involves restoration of a marrow cavity.[3]

In order for the phases of bone healing to carry out in the above path, a milieu conducive to healing must be present. The presence of appropriate nutrients and blood supply are basic requirements, and cells including osteoblasts, osteoclasts, chondrocytes, and endothelial cells must also be present. The extracellular matrix (ECM), which is produced by cells recruited to the fracture site, must provide a setting that promotes each successive phase of healing.[1-3]

CELL RESPONSIBLE FOR FRACTURE HEALING

MESENCHYMAL STEM CELLS

MSCs are stored in the bone marrow, adipose tissue, and the synovial lining. In the face of acute fracture, cytokines influence differentiation of MSCs to osteoprogenitor cells through interactions with specific cell surface antigens.[4,5] Mechanical environments also play a role in MSC differentiation favoring chondrocyte differentiation in mechanically less stable environments.

CHONDROCYTES, OSTEOBLASTS, AND OSTEOCLASTS

Chondrocytes and osteoblasts are key players in the mechanism of fracture healing. When a bone is injured, these cells differentiate from MSCs, which are brought to the fracture through vasculature and inherently present in the periosteum and endosteum surrounding the bone. Recent evidence suggests the periosteum as the main source of chondrocytes during the acute phase of fracture healing, while the periosteum and endosteum supply osteoblasts.[6] Depending on the signals present in the ECM, a pluripotent MSC will either differentiate into a chondrocyte or an osteoblast (**Table 3.1**).

Chondrocytes are the main producers of ECM proteins including proteoglycans and collagen.[7] When a fracture heals, the chondrocytes hypertrophy and undergo apoptosis. This allows for vascular invagination, and the cartilaginous matrix is then ossified through deposition of calcium by osteoblasts.[6,7]

Osteoblasts produce osteoid, which is the main component of bone made up of primarily type I collagen. They can be found on the surface of bone and are responsible for bone homeostasis by balancing bone formation with bone resorption done by osteoclasts.[2,6] Osteoblasts activity can be identified in vivo due to the presence of alkaline phosphatase, which is an enzyme that causes dephosphorylation.[8]

Osteoclasts are derived from the macrophage/monocyte cell line which originate from pluripotent MSCs. On bone surfaces, they reside in Howship lacunae, self-made pits where active bone resorption takes place. Their main function is to resorb bone in a remodeling process coordinated with osteoblasts. They resorb bone through a tartrate-resistant acid phosphatase, which is regulated by receptor activator of nuclear factor kappa beta ligand (RANKL) and a calcitonin receptor.[9]

TABLE 3.1 Cells Involved in Bone Healing

Chondrocytes	Chondrocytes develop from colony-forming unit fibroblast (CFU-F). These CFU-Fs become mesenchymal stem cells (MSCs) which are undifferentiated mesodermal cells capable of becoming multiple osteochondrogenic cells. Under specific conditions (BMP4 and FGF2 experimentally), MSCs differentiate into chondrocytes which are responsible for synthesizing extracellular matrix. In the bone, chondrocytes are present in lacunae. At the end of endochondral ossification, chondrocytes hypertrophy and apoptose.
Osteoblasts	Osteoblasts are terminally differentiated MSCs. They are single-nuclei cells which synthesize osteoid. This is highly cross-linked collagen with osteocalcin and osteopontin making up the organic matrix of the bone. In addition, they produce a calcium and phosphate based matrix. They, along with osteoclasts, are important in the regulation of acid-base balance through calcium and phosphate regulation.
Osteoclasts	Osteoclasts are large, multinucleated cells which develop from macrophages through the monocyte phagocytic system lineage. Differentiation into osteoclasts requires the presence of receptor activator of nuclear factor kappa beta ligand (RANKL) and macrophage colony-stimulating factor (M-CSF) produced by osteoblasts. This differentiation is inhibited by osteoprotegerin by preventing RANKL interaction with RANK. Osteoclasts live in cavities known as Howship lacunae which they form by digesting the underlying bone. They attach to the underlying bone through podosomes at the "sealing zone." They resorb bone at the "ruffled border" via the enzyme carbonic anhydrase. Lysosomes inside the osteoclast also help to break down the organic components of the bone through cathepsin and metalloprotease.

TYPES OF BONE HEALING

BACKGROUND

The type of healing that will occur depends on both the mechanical and biological environment present. The two types of bone healing are endochondral and intramembranous (**Figures 3.1** and **3.2**). These two modes are not independent of each other and often occur simultaneously in a coordinated fashion. Time to union, where the strength of the bone prior to fracture is restored, is the same in both types of bone healing.[3]

Endochondral ossification is the process whereby an existing cartilaginous matrix is replaced by the bone. Chondrocytes lay down mature cartilage and then slowly

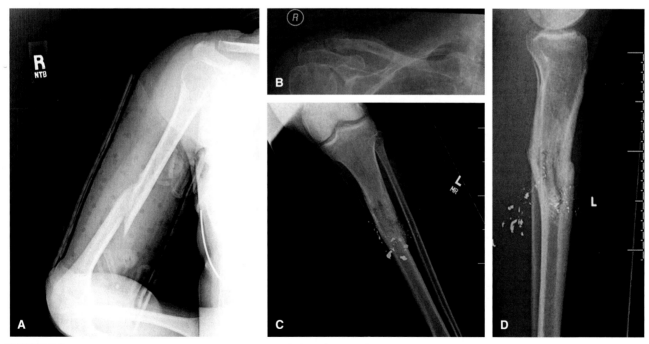

FIGURE 3.1 Nonoperative treatment resulting in endochondral ossification. **A**, An anteroposterior (AP) radiograph of a long oblique, mid-shaft humerus fracture in a 76-year-old female being treated nonoperatively in a Sarmiento brace. This brace allows significant motion at the facture site and so favors endochondral ossification. **B**, An AP radiograph 6 weeks after a distal 1/3 right clavicle fracture in a 45-year-old female treated in a sling. Note the callus formation indicative of motion at the fracture site and endochondral ossification. **C** and **D**, Eight-week follow-up AP and lateral radiographs of a gunshot wound tibia fracture in a 21-year-old male. The patient opted for nonoperative management in a cast, also an environment favoring endochondral ossification.

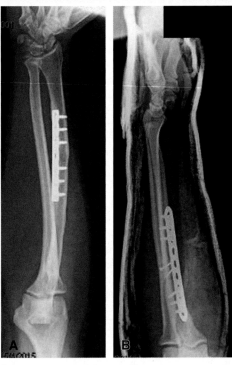
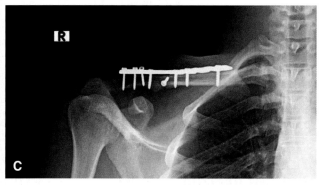

FIGURE 3.2 Constructs favoring intramembranous ossification. **A**, An anteroposterior (AP) radiograph of a forearm after open reduction and internal fixation of a radial shaft fracture using compression plating. This construct provides absolute stability and heals without callus with intramembranous ossification. **B**, A lateral radiograph of a forearm after an ORIF of an ulnar shaft fracture using interfragmentary compression with a lag screw and neutralization plating. This construct favors intramembranous ossification. **C**, An AP radiograph of a clavicle demonstrating interfragmentary compression and neutralization plating. This construct provides absolute stability.

hypertrophy and senesce. Vessels invade the cartilage, which allows osteoblasts to replace the chondrocytes in the scaffold, and begin laying down the bone. This process occurs both during normal human development and in fracture healing.[7] Historically, this type of bone healing was referred to as secondary bone healing, involved four stages (see below), and usually meant there was motion at the fracture site (**Figure 3.3**).

ENDOCHONDRAL OSSIFICATION (FIGURE 3.4)

Fracture Hematoma and Inflammatory Phase

In the first 24 hours after injury, a fracture hematoma forms. This is the result of local disruption of vasculature, periosteum and cortical bone, and the surrounding muscle.[10] Fracture hematoma is unlike hematoma or blood clot resulting from soft-tissue injury alone. Mizuno et al transplanted 4-day-old fracture hematoma to remote locations in a rat model, and it resulted in ectopic bone and cartilage formation.[11]

Macrophage, platelet, and neutrophil arrival at the fracture site mark the beginning of the inflammatory phase of bone healing. These cells release inflammatory cytokines including tumor necrosis factor alpha and beta (TNF-α, TNF-β) and interleukins 1, 6, 10, and 12 (IL-1, IL-6, IL-10, IL-12).[12,13] These inflammatory molecules play an integral role in enhancing the inflammatory response to recruit multiple cells from surrounding bone marrow and periosteum leading to growth factor production.

Fibroblast growth factor (FGF) and basic fibroblast growth factor (bFGF) are some of the earliest growth factors present at a fracture site hematoma. They help promote differentiation of MSCs to chondrocytes and osteoblasts during bone development and stimulate cartilage formation and increase the size of the fracture callus. Studies have demonstrated the promotive effects of FGF on angiogenesis and the presence of increased callus size and strength in the presence of FGF.[14]

Another of the growth factors detected early in the inflammation phase of bone healing is platelet-derived growth factor (PDGF). Nash et al demonstrated a stimulatory effect on fracture callus and early stability in a rabbit model when treated with PDGF. This study also showed advanced microscopic differentiation of the rabbit tibia treated with PDGF over the control.[15]

Bone morphogenetic proteins (BMPs) have been studied extensively and their stimulatory effects on bone healing are well known.[16-18] BMPs are capable of recruiting stem cells from distant sites and inducing osteoblast and chondrocyte differentiation, leading to ectopic bone formation. Clinically, recombinant BMPs (specifically rhBMP-2 and rhBMP-7) have been used in nonunion treatment and encouraging fusions.[18,19] Level 1 evidence suggests that rhBMP-2 improves the repair of open tibia fractures, while prospective case series have shown rhBMP-7 is effective in treating tibial and femoral nonunions.[20,21] A member of this superfamily, transforming growth factor-beta (TGF-β), is present at the fracture site during the first few days of the inflammatory phase and has a minor effect on callus size and strength.[22]

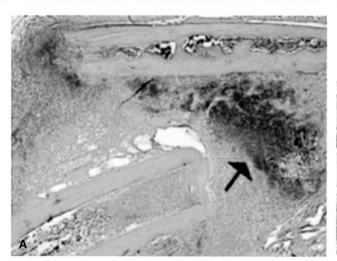 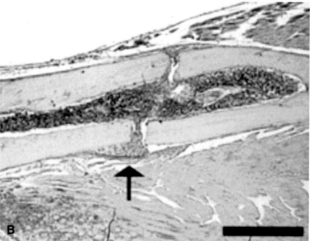

FIGURE 3.3 Effects of motion at the fracture site. Figures are cross sections of mice tibia. **A**, It demonstrates a fracture allowed to heal without stabilization. There is large callus formation evident (image taken 7 days after fracture) and cartilage can be seen forming around the fracture fragments (arrows). **B**, It demonstrates a stabilized fracture which heals with minimal fracture callus. No cartilage is present after 7 days but there are osteoprogenitor cells seen in the fracture site and the periosteal reaction can be appreciated (arrow). (Reprinted with permission from Thompson Z, Miclau T, Hu D, et al. A model for intramembranous ossification during fracture healing. *J Orthop Res.* 2002;20(5):1091-1098.)

Another early protein group present in the first few days of fracture healing include the **β-catenin/Wingless-type signaling proteins**. These are a family of extracellular cell-cell signaling proteins that are expressed by osteocytes. Some of these proteins include Wnt proteins, Fzd proteins, LRP5, LRP6, and β-catenin.[23] Through complex signaling pathways, the overall effect of these proteins is enhanced bone formation. The levels of these proteins increase over the first 3 to 5 days of bone healing and promote vascular ingrowth.[7,24]

The roles of other growth factors including insulin-like growth factor-1 (IGF-1) and growth hormone (GH) are less well understood. Some studies demonstrate stimulative effects of GH on fracture healing while others have not supported this finding.[7,25]

SOFT CALLUS PHASE

MSCs condensate around the fracture site and, as a response to the growth factors and cytokines present, differentiate into chondrocytes and osteoblasts. The stability of the fracture site determines the direction of differentiation (more instability at the fracture site lends to chondrocyte differentiation and enchondral ossification while stability at the fracture site promotes osteoblast differentiation and intramembraneous ossification).[26]

The production of cartilage stabilizes the fracture and forms the "soft callus" for which this phase of bone healing is named. Both enchondral and intramembranous ossifications occur simultaneously during this phase with the former being the primary mode. Stability at the fracture site promotes intramembranous ossification.

HARD CALLUS AND REMODELING PHASES

As the cartilaginous matrix is transformed through enchondral ossification, soft callus becomes hard callus. The final stage of this process involves chondrocyte maturation. The chondrocytes express collagen type X and begin to degrade the ECM. The cartilage becomes calcified and the chondrocytes undergo apoptosis. Through organized osteoclast and osteoblast activity, the newly formed bone remodels.[27,28]

INTRAMEMBRANOUS OSSIFICATION

Intramembranous ossification is the process of direct bone formation without cartilage precursors.[26] Direct deposition of bone through cells of mesenchymal origin leads to new bone formation without the creation of callus.[29] Again, this mode of bone formation occurs during skeletal development and during fracture repair where there is rigid fixation with minimal to no movement between fracture fragments. This has been historically referred to as "primary" bone healing, suggesting restoration of lamellar architecture of bone in a fracture which is stably fixed resulting in disappearance of the fracture lines on subsequent radiographs.[30] Bones heal directly through osteoclast-led cutting cones, which cut a linear path across the fracture site, and osteoblasts follow and lay down cortical bone.[30,31]

INFLUENCES ON BONE HEALING (FIGURE 3.5)

MECHANICAL ENVIRONMENT

It has long been understood that the mechanical environment surrounding a fracture influences healing.[31] For centuries, fractures have been stabilized by external means in order to improve patient comfort, prevent displacement, and encourage time to union. Over the past century, the understanding and techniques of surgical fracture stabilization have improved this process, and the effects of micro- and macromotion at the fracture site are better appreciated.

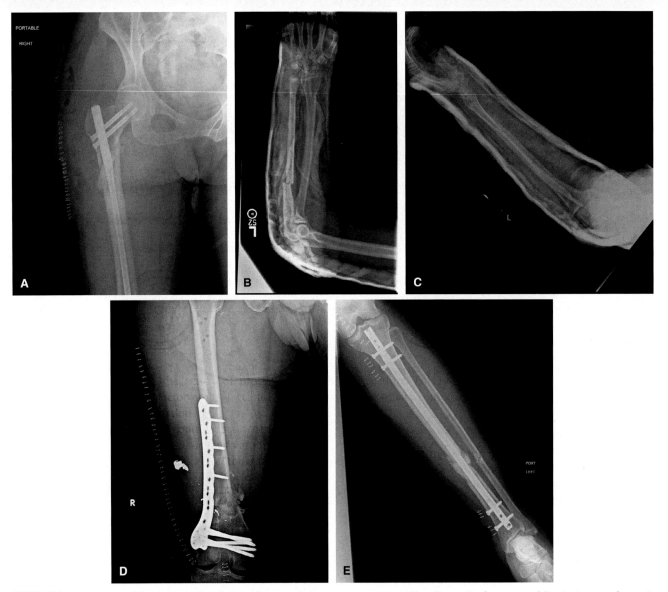

FIGURE 3.4 Constructs favoring endochondral ossification. **A**, An anteroposterior (AP) radiograph of a reverse obliquity intertrochanteric femur fracture treated with a cephalomedullary nail. **B** and **C**, AP and lateral radiographs of an ulnar shaft fracture initially splinted and subsequently lost to follow-up. **D**, An AP radiograph of the femur showing a gunshot wound supracondylar femur fracture treated with bridge plating. **E**, An AP radiograph showing a tibial shaft fracture (with associated fibular shaft fracture) treated with intramedullary nailing. All of these constructs allow micromotion if not motion at the fracture site and favor endochondral ossification.

Mechanical stability favors primary bone healing through intramembranous ossification. The concept of "absolute stability" in fracture fixation (fixing the fracture fragments with rigid internal fixation to prevent micromotion at the fracture site) optimized the mechanical environment for direct bone healing with "cutting cones" and no cartilage intermediate (**Figure 3.6**).[31,32] Mechanical instability favors endochondral ossification through the stages described above. Both primary and secondary bone healing rarely occur in isolation and often occur in a balanced and coordinate way. Strain theory, a principle first described by Perrin et al, states that intact bone has a normal strain tolerance of 2% before it fractures. Soft-tissue healing, also known as granulation tissue,

has a strain tolerance of 100%. Strain is the deformation of a material when a given force is applied to it. Hard callus will not bridge the fracture gap if the interfragmentary motion is too great.[33]

PHARMACOLOGIC ENVIRONMENT

Many pharmacologic agents, both prescription and recreational, contribute to nonunion or delayed union by modifying the biochemical environment present for healing bone. These agents can affect certain cellular pathways, local vascularity, or inhibit certain signaling molecules and hinder the inflammatory response.

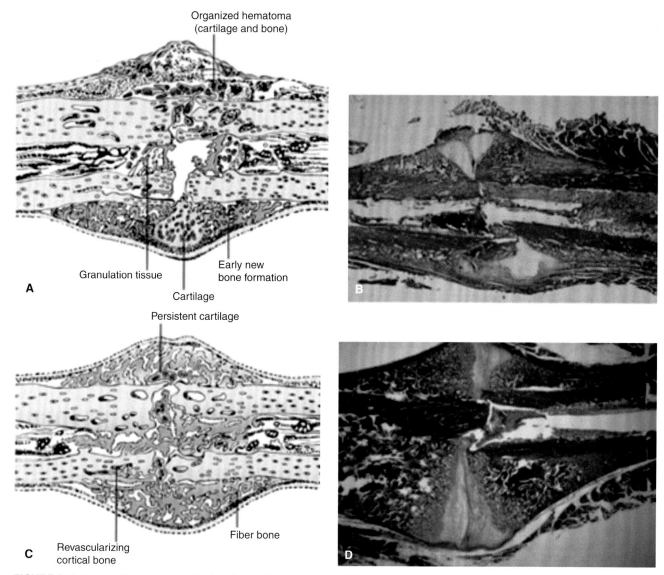

FIGURE 3.5 Stages of bone healing. **A**, This shows the early stages of fracture repair with fracture hematoma, early woven bone in subperiosteal regions, and cartilage formation. At this point, if the fracture is rigidly stabilized, there will be minimal fracture callus. **B**, A photomicrograph of a rat femur 9 days after injury showing. **C**, This shows progressive fracture callus formation bridging the fracture site with woven bone and uniting the gap between fragments. Cartilage remains in regions not yet reached by the ingrowing capillaries. **D**, The photomicrograph depicts a rat femur 21 days after injury demonstrating callus uniting the fracture fragments. (Reprinted with permission from Einhorn TA. The cell and molecular biology of fracture healing. *Clin Orthop Relat Res.* 1998;335:S7-S21.)

AGENTS WITH INHIBITING EFFECTS ON BONE HEALING

TOBACCO

Tobacco and nicotine and their effects on bone healing have been widely studied. Pure nicotine has been shown to increase fracture callus strength and bending stiffness in femur fractures in rats.[34] This process is not well understood.

Multiple studies implicate tobacco use with delayed healing in tibia fractures and in patients undergoing corrective osteotomies in the feet and spine.[35,36] Nicotine has been shown to inhibit tissue differentiation and angiogenesis in early fracture healing and can inhibit osteoblast function.[37,38] Cigarettes, the main source of tobacco in the above studies, contain hundreds of chemicals which could have independent and combined effects on fracture healing. A recent hypothesis suggested that TNF-α inhibition causes the deleterious effects on fracture healing seen in smokers.[38] More research is needed to better understand the details of the effect of tobacco, but avoiding its use during fracture healing appears to be the current recommendation.[35-38]

NONSTEROIDAL ANTI-INFLAMMATORY DRUGS

Nonsteroidal anti-inflammatory drugs (NSAIDs) are widely used agents to treat inflammation, pain, and swelling associated with acute injuries to the musculoskeletal system. NSAIDs work by inhibiting cyclooxygenases (COX-1 and COX-2). Nonselective NSAIDs inhibit both COX-1 and

Cutting cone | Reversal zone | Closing cone

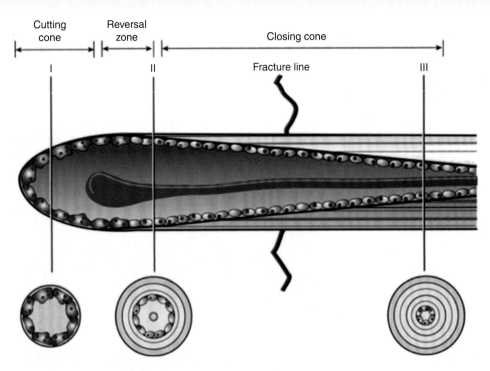

FIGURE 3.6 Cutting cones. Figure depicts an osteoclastic cutting cone (I) which crossed the fracture site in primary bone healing. The channel is then filled in by trailing osteoblasts (II, III). (Reprinted with permission from Court-Brown C, Heckman JD, McKee M, McQueen MM, Ricci W, Tornetta P. *Rockwood and Green's Fractures in Adults.* 8th ed. Philadelphia, PA: Wolters Kluwer Health; 2014.)

COX-2. COX-2, through the action of prostaglandin E_2, upregulates core-binding factor alpha-1 (Cbfa1), which is essential for osteoblast formation.[39]

The effects of NSAIDs are controversial when it comes to fracture healing. In a recent meta-analysis grouping together spinal fusion trials using NSAIDs, the authors fail to find any support for the hypothesis that NSAID use leads to increased rates of nonunion.[40]

CORTICOSTEROIDS

Corticosteroids are used in chronic inflammatory conditions, acute cases of swelling or pain and chronically in patients with obstructive lung disease. These agents, when present during bone healing, inhibit differentiation of MSCs into osteoblasts and chondrocytes.[41] They also have been shown to direct osteoblasts and osteocytes toward apoptosis. Once again, the exact effect of corticosteroids on in vivo fracture healing in humans is controversial.[41-43] Clinicians are advised to weight the potential risks and benefits prior to selecting to use these agents in the face of acute fracture.

PATIENT FACTORS WHICH AFFECT BONE HEALING

NUTRITIONAL STATUS

Deficiencies in nutrients essential for bone healing can be the result of insufficient intake, metabolic deficiencies, or endocrine abnormalities. The main nutrients found to be deficient are vitamin D and calcium.[44] Vitamin D deficiency is seen across the northern hemisphere during winter months and also in cultures where skin exposure is prohibited. Patients who are unable to metabolize calcium include gastric bypass patients who have undergone the Roux-en-Y

procedure. This procedure bypasses the duodenum which is the primary source for calcium uptake.[45]

AGE

Fragility fractures occur in the elderly population due to a decrease in bone quantity and quality. Rat models have shown that older rats have decreased expression of BMP-2 and were less capable of generating differentiation of osteoblasts when compared with younger patients.[17,46] Increased bone uptake combined with decreased bone deposition leads to net bone loss annually in elderly patients.

DIABETES MELLITUS

Diabetic patients with poor glycemic control have many known comorbidities including wound healing, peripheral vascular disease, and susceptibility to bacterial infection, but diabetes also negatively influences fracture healing. The exact mechanism is not well understood, but some hypothesize that the fracture callus is less cellular which causes fracture callus to have decreased strength.[47] Multiple studies have demonstrated increased time to union in long bone fracture as well as ankle fracture. These trends were not present in diabetics with adequate glycemic control.[48,49]

AGENTS FOR AFFECTING BONE HEALING

BACKGROUND

Many pharmacologic agents are available commercially which have stimulatory effects on healing bone. These agents have been and continue to be studied extensively in an effort to decrease time to union and improve quality of bone by modifying one of the four stages of fracture healing.

BISPHOSPHONATES

Bisphosphonates are a class of drug often referred to as "antiresorptives." They inhibit osteoclast function and limit bone turnover. Their structure is similar to pyrophosphate, and they are classified based on whether they contain nitrogen or not.[50]

The nonnitrogen containing bisphosphonates include etidronate, clodronate, and tiludronate. They are metabolized in the cell to compounds that replaced the terminal pyrophosphate of adenosine triphosphate (ATP) which forms a nonfunctional form of the compound. This inert ATP then competes for binding sites with unmodified ATP and initiates apoptosis in the osteoclast.[51] The net effect is a net decrease in bone breakdown.

Nitrogen containing bisphosphonates include pamidronate, neridronate, olpadronate, alendronate, ibandronate, risedronate, and zoledronate. They prevent the HMG-CoA reductase pathway by blocking the enzyme farnesyl diphosphate synthase.[51,52] The result is two metabolites which inhibit a process known as prenylation, which is essential for osteoclast contact between its ruffled border and bone (**Table 3.2**).[53]

Multiple studies have attempted to elucidate the effects of bisphosphonates on fracture healing.[54-56] A recent prospective trial aimed to compare healing rates of distal radius fractures in patients on bisphosphonates at the time of injury with those that were not. The authors found that

TABLE 3.2 Bisphosphonates

	Mechanism of Action
Nonnitrogenous	Absorbed and metabolized by osteoclasts. Due to their close structural similarity to inorganic pyrophosphate, they are incorporated into adenosine triphosphate (ATP) molecules. The enzyme aminoacyl-transfer RNA synthetase facilitates this. The accumulation of these nonfunctional ATP molecules leads to osteoclast apoptosis.
Etidronate	
Clodronate	
Tiludronate	
Nitrogenous	Nitrogen containing bisphosphonates bind to and inhibit farnesyl pyrophosphate synthase, part of the mevalonic acid pathway which creates cholesterol, sterols, and other lipids. This prevents the necessary modification of Rab, Rac, and Rho, proteins which are important in membrane formation and structure. This causes osteoclast apoptosis.
Pamidronate	
Neridronate	
Olpadronate	
Alendronate	
Ibandronate	
Risedronate	
Zoledronate	

current bisphosphonate use and surgical treatment led to healing times (measured radiographically) <1 week longer that those patients not on bisphosphonates, but concluded this small difference was not clinically significant.[54] In another study, researchers aimed to demonstrate the effects of risedronate on ulnar stress fractures in a rat model. The authors showed that high-dose bisphosphonate therapy did not adversely affect periosteal callus formation but impaired the radiographic healing of ulnar stress fractures by slowing down the remodeling phase.[55] Finally, a meta-analysis of randomized clinical trials examined the effects of early administration of bisphosphonates after fracture surgery. The author concludes that early administration of these drugs did not delay fracture healing time radiographically or clinically.[56]

Multiple adverse effects have been reported from long-term bisphosphonate using including osteonecrosis of the jaw, atrial fibrillation, chronic bone and muscle pain, and a very characteristic type of fracture.[57-60] Multiple studies demonstrated the "bisphosphonate fracture" described as a diaphyseal or subtrochanteric femur fracture (**Figure 3.7**). Bisphosphonates provide an overall reduction in hip fractures which far outweighs the small incidence of the "bisphosphonate fracture."[52,60]

STATINS

Statins have many effects on multiple body systems and were shown to also affect the HMG-CoA reductase pathway.[61] By inhibiting small GTP binding proteins such as Rho and Ras, statins inhibit osteoclast-directed bone catabolism in a similar way to bisphosphonates.[62]

Multiple studies have looked at statins use to promote fracture healing.[63-65] In a recent meta-analysis, statins were reported to cause a decreased rate of fracture and an increase in bone mineral density.[63] The effects of simvastatin on osteoporotic femur fractures in a rat model were examined in another study. The authors found a positive effect on bone density and histology in the group treated with standard dose statin.[64] Finally, a meta-analysis using the available observational studies demonstrating the positive effect statin use has on prevention of osteoporotic fractures examined the biases leading to those recommendations. The author concludes that unmeasured, confounding variables cannot explain the protective association between statins and fracture that have been observed in the literature.[61,65]

PARATHYROID HORMONE AND TERIPARATIDE

Parathyroid hormone (PTH) regulates calcium, vitamin D, and phosphate. PTH enhances the circulating levels of calcium by mobilizing it from stores in long bones through stimulation of osteoclasts. PTH does this by binding directly to osteoblasts, stimulating production of RANKL and inhibiting expression osteoprotegerin. The binding of RANKL to RANK stimulates osteoclasts.[66] The effects on PTH on

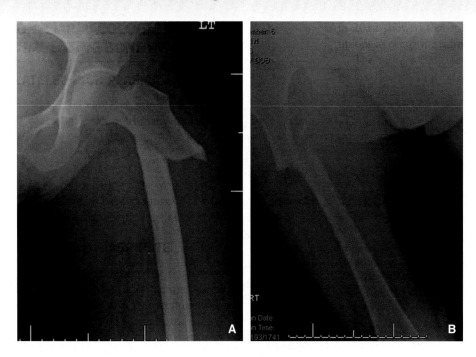

FIGURE 3.7 Bisphosphonate fractures. **A** and **B**, Anteroposterior hip radiographs illustrating the atypical subtrochanteric femur fractures attributed to long-term bisphosphonate use. Note the thickened cortex on either side of the fracture site.

fracture healing have been examined at the clinical level. In animal studies, PTH was able to partially reverse the effect of type 2 diabetes mellitus on bone mass, bone strength, and bone defect repair.[67]

Recombinant PTH, teriparatide, is thought to improve fracture healing by increasing the chondroprogenitor and osteoprogenitor cells in early fracture callus.[68] Multiple studies have demonstrated the positive effects of teriparatide on callus volume and load to failure in a rat femur fracture model as well as increasing proliferation rates and expression of prochondrocyte precursors and genes including pro-1α (II) collagen, pro-1α (X) collagen, and SOX-9 (**Figure 3.8**).[69,70]

GROWTH HORMONE

Human GH is made and released by the pituitary gland and causes systemic release of IGF-1, which is synthesized in the liver and can stimulate osteoblasts.[71] The action of IGF-1 is mediated through a tyrosine kinase receptor called insulin-like growth factor-1 receptor (IGF1R). This receptor is present on many cells and initiates intracellular signaling leading to cell growth and proliferation while inhibiting cell death.[72] Patients with "growth failure," which is caused by insulin-like growth factor deficiency (IGFD), have been successfully treated with IGF-1 and insulin-like growth factor binding protein-3 (IGFBP-3) and mecasermin, a synthetic analog of IGF-1 approved for the treatment of growth failure.[73]

Multiple studies have examined the effects of GH at the fracture site. In an animal model, mice with tibia fractures were injected with subcutaneous recombinant IGF-1 and MSCs. The authors noted increased fracture callus volume, toughness, and cellularity and recommended recombinant IGF-1 for use in patients with inadequate fracture repair.[74] Another animal model, looking at sheep tibia undergoing distraction osteogenesis, failed to demonstrate statistically significant differences between those tibiae treated with IGF-1 and the control group using packed autologous cancellous bone.[75] The results have been inconclusive, and further research is indicated.

BONE MORPHOGENETIC PROTEINS

Since the late 1980s, BMPs were studied for their impact on the induction of bone growth and synthesis. Historically, two recombinant BMPs were available for clinical use: rhBMP-2 and rhBMP-7 (also known as osteogenic protein-1 [OP-1]).[76]

Multiple prospective studies exist which have demonstrated the safety and efficacy of these two proteins.[20,77,78] rhBMP-7 was shown to be equally effective as autografted cancellous bone in promoting healing in a tibial nonunion model.[77] The BESTT (BMP-2 Evaluation in Surgery for Tibial Trauma) trial, a multinational, prospective, controlled, randomized study, looked at the effects of rhBMP-2 in open tibia fractures. The trial demonstrates a decreased rate of secondary interventions (returns to operating room), accelerated time to union, improved wound healing, and reduced infection rate when patients were treated with high-dose rhBMP-2.[19] The decrease in infection rates while using rhBMPs in reamed tibial nails, however, was not supported in a subsequent study.[78] In another prospective study, when OP-1 was used in the treatment of open tibia fractures, the authors noted significant decrease in rates of secondary interventions for delayed or nonunions and improvement in patient function at 12 months.[79]

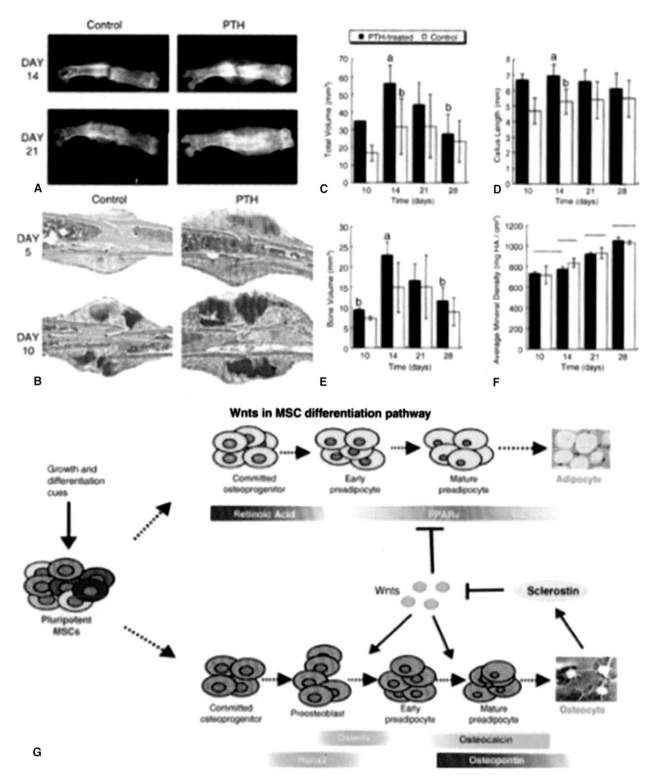

FIGURE 3.8 Parathyroid hormone (PTH) and fracture healing. Figure illustrates parathyroid hormones effect on fracture healing through the wnt pathway. Total callus formation and chondrogenesis induction were increased in fractures in rats which were treated with daily injections of PTH (1–34). **A**, Radiographs examining callus formation in the femurs of rats 2 and 3 weeks after injury. **B**, Safranin O staining of fracture slices 5 and 10 days after injury. Chondrogenic cells are stained red. **C-F**, Micro-CT analysis of callus and bone volume and mineral density. **G**, PTH exerts its effects through the wnt pathway, inducing the osteogenic and hypertrophic chondrogenic differentiation of progenitor cells, while inhibiting the adipogenic lineage. These effects are modulated by the wnt inhibitor, ssclerostin, which is secreted by osteocytes in a feedback loop. MSC, mesenchymal stem cell. (A-F, Reprinted with permission from Kakar S, Einhorn TA, Vora S, et al. Enhanced chondrogenesis and Wnt signaling in PTH-treated fractures. *J Bone Miner Res.* 2007;22(12):1903-1912 and G, From Wagner ER, Zhu G, Zhang BQ, et al. The therapeutic potential of the Wnt signaling pathway in bone disorders. *Curr Mol Pharmacol.* 2011;4(1):14-25.)

NONPHARMACOLOGIC MEASURES FOR STIMULATING BONE HEALING

PLATELET-RICH PLASMA

Platelet-rich plasma has long been thought to have positive effects on healing in many different body systems and bone healing is no different. After injury, activated platelets release growth factors (PDGF, TGF-β, VEGF, TGF-β1, BMP-2), which can stimulate vasculogenesis, MSC recruitment, and factors stimulating bone formation.[76,80]

Several studies have examined the effects on bone repair and fracture healing with less than consistent results.[81,82]

BONE MARROW ASPIRATE

Autografted bone has been used to aid in fusions, nonunion takedown and repairs, and fracture healing due to the inherent osteoinductive and osteoconductive growth factures it contains.[76] Harvesting allograft, and the associated morbidity, has forced clinicians to find other sources of these stimulatory effects. Bone marrow aspirate contains these promotive factors and can be harvested in a less invasive way.[83]

Many studies have demonstrated safety and stimulatory effects of using bone marrow aspirate (usually iliac crest bone marrow aspirate) on nonunions.[84-86] One theory on the effect of bone marrow aspirate is the direct delivery of MSCs to the fracture site, which have the potential to differentiate into osteoprogenitor cells.[85] No clinical study, however, that demonstrates this differentiation occurs exists. Another confounding factor in the bone marrow aspirate is the interhuman variability in cellularity and osteoblast progenitor cell prevalence.[86,87] Recently added systems allow for aspiration and concentration of MSC by use of centrifuge, but there is no known threshold concentration to ensure effectiveness.[88]

COMPLICATIONS OF FRACTURE HEALING

BACKGROUND

Complications in fracture healing can include those associated with the biological healing environment and those associated with the mechanical healing environment. These scenarios can lead to increased length of time to union, known as delayed union or failure of healing at all, known as nonunion. The three types of nonunion are atrophic, oligotrophic, and hypertrophic.

DELAYED UNION

Defined simply, delayed union is a failure of the fracture to unite in an expected amount of time for a specific anatomic location. Many studies cite 6 months as the differentiation point between delayed union and nonunion, and this number is determined on a case-by-case basis.[89] A survey of surgeons in 2004 of the Orthopaedic Trauma Association (OTA) defined a delayed union as, on average, 3.5 ± 1.4 months.[90] The repeat survey

in 2012 showed that most surgeons (70%) describe delayed unions as occurring during the first 12 weeks after fracture.[91]

The more recent survey of a similar group of OTA surgeons further illustrated the lack of standardized definitions but demonstrated some trends in modern-day clinical practice. Although 88% of surgeons agreed that determining fracture healing required both radiographic and clinical information, 37% of survey respondents believed long bone nonunion could be adequately assessed with a combination of radiographs and computed tomography scans.[91]

NONUNION

Nonunion is defined as failure to demonstrate expected radiographic and/or clinical signs of healing after the expected interval. They are classified based on appearance of fracture callus and vascularity. The surveyed surgeons in the OTA defined a nonunion, on average, as 6.3 ± 2.1 months in 2004.[90] It is both a clinical and radiographic diagnosis. Fracture healing was defined by Stojainovic et al as the ability of the patient to bear full weight on the affected limb (for a lower extremity nonunion), the absence of pain or tenderness at the fracture site with manual bending or compression, and reestablishment of cortical continuity on three of four cortices at the fracture site on radiographs and/or CT scans.[92]

ATROPHIC NONUNION

Atrophic nonunions are those where a fracture has failed to heal and demonstrates net bone resorption radiographically (**Figure 3.9**).[93] No fracture callus is visualized and the

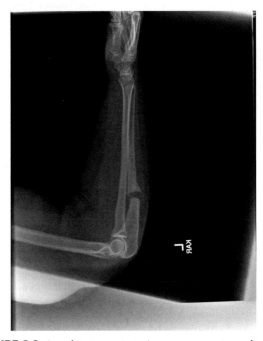

FIGURE 3.9 Atrophic nonunion. An anteroposterior radiograph of a forearm demonstrating net resorption and bone loss on either side of an ulnar shaft fracture. Due to the net bone loss, this would be classified an atrophic nonunion.

original fracture line is still present with loss of surrounding cortical bone. Multiple factors can contribute to the likelihood of developing an atrophic nonunion. Open fractures, infection, poor nutrition, tobacco use, corticosteroid use, and NSAID use have all been implicated in various studies as increasing the likelihood of nonunion (**Figure 3.10**).[91]

OLIGOTROPHIC NONUNION

Oligotrophic nonunion is defined as the failure of bony union with little callus formation but adequate blood supply (**Figure 3.11**). Some causes hypothesized to cause oligotrophic nonunion are malreduction with displacement or distraction of fracture fragments and also poor nutritional status.[94]

HYPERTROPHIC NONUNION

Hypertrophic nonunion develops from motion at the fracture site (**Figure 3.12**). Whether inadequate fixation or failure of fixation, macromotion at the healing fracture site causes hypertrophy developing callus. Blood supply is

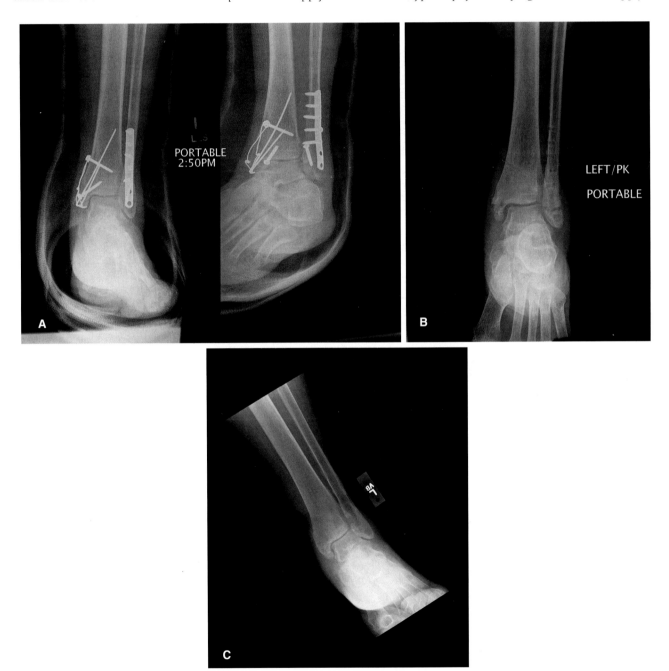

FIGURE 3.10 Infection as a cause for nonunion. **A**, An anteroposterior (AP) radiograph of a bimalleolar ankle fracture after ORIF. The patient returned to the clinic multiple times over the first six postoperative months with a draining wound and still visible fracture site. **B**, An AP radiograph of the same ankle after hardware removal in the operating room. **C**, An AP radiograph of the same ankle 3 months after hardware removal demonstration healing of the bimalleolar ankle fracture. Once the infection was eliminated, the fracture healed.

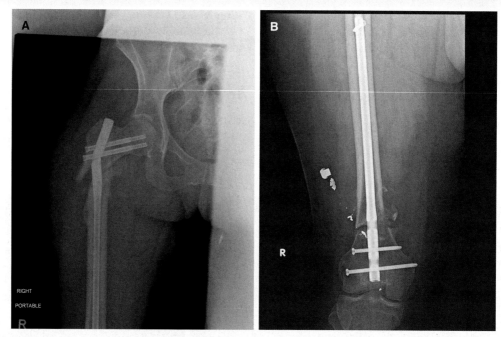

FIGURE 3.11 Oligotrophic nonunion. **A**, An anteroposterior (AP) hip radiograph demonstrating hardware failure 9 months after cephalomedullary nailing secondary to nonunion of a reverse obliquity intertrochanteric femur fracture. Note there is neither net resorption of bone nor excess fracture callus. **B**, An AP radiograph of a femur 7 months after retrograde intramedullary nailing. This is an oligotrophic nonunion.

adequate, but lack of mechanical stability prevents completion of fracture healing.[94] The fracture line is still present and is surrounded by a disorganized partially ossified cartilaginous matrix. Hypertrophic nonunions go on to union after adequate fixation and stabilization of the fracture.[95]

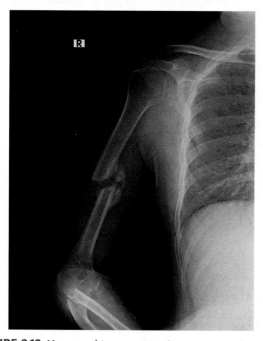

FIGURE 3.12 Hypertrophic nonunion. An anteroposterior radiograph of the humerus demonstrating excessive fracture callus with a still visible fracture line 7 months after injury. This is a classic location for hypertrophic nonunion.

REFERENCES

1. McKibbin B. The biology of fracture healing in long bones. *J Bone Joint Surg Br.* 1978;60-B(2):150-162.
2. Sathyendra V, Darowish M. Basic science of bone healing. *Hand Clin.* 2013;29:473-481.
3. Einhorn TA, O'Keefe RJ, Buckwalter JA, eds. *Orthopaedic Basic Science: Foundations of Clinical Practice.* 3rd ed. Rosemont, IL: American Academy of Orthopaedic Surgeons; 2007:331-348.
4. Dominici M, Le Blanc K, Mueller I, et al. Minimal criteria for defining multipotent mesenchymal stromal cells. The International Society for Cellular Therapy position statement. *Cytotherapy.* 2006;8(4):315-317.
5. Pittenger MF. Multilineage potential of adult human mesenchymal stem cells. *Science.* 1999;284(5411):143-147.
6. Bahney CS, Hu DP, Taylor AJ, et al. Stem cell-derived endochondral cartilage stimulates bone healing by tissue transformation. *J Bone Miner Res.* 2014;29(5):1269-1282.
7. Ferguson C, Alpern E, Miclau T, et al. Does adult fracture repair recapitulate embryonic skeletal formation? *Mech Dev.* 1999;87(1-2):57-66.
8. Eghbali-Fatourechi GZ, Lamsam J, Fraser D, et al. Circulating osteoblast-lineage cells in humans. *N Engl J Med.* 2005;352(19):1959-1966.
9. Drake FH, Dodds RA, James IE, et al. Cathepsin K, but not cathepsins B, L, or S, is abundantly expressed in human osteoclasts. *J Biol Chem.* 1996;271(21):12511 12516.
10. Epari DR, Schell H, Bail HJ, et al. Instability prolongs the chondral phase during bone healing in sheep. *Bone.* 2006;38(6):864-870.
11. Mizuno K, Mineo K, Tachibana T, et al. The osteogenetic potential of fracture haematoma. Subperiosteal and intramuscular transplantation of the haematoma. *J Bone Joint Surg Br.* 1990;72(5):822-829.
12. Barnes GL, Kosteniuk PJ, Gerstenfeld LC, Einhorn TA. Growth Factor regulation of fracture repair. *J Bone Miner Res.* 1999;14(11):1805-1815.
13. Rundle CH, Wang H, Yu H, et al. Microarray analysis of gene expression during the inflammation and endochonfral bone formation stages of rat femur fracture repair. *Bone.* 2006;38(4):521-529.
14. Bostrom MP, Saleh KJ, Einhorn TA. Osteoinductive growth factors in preclinical fracture and long bone defect models. *Orthop Clin North Am.* 1999;30(4):647-658.

15. Nash TJ, Howlett CR, Martin C, Steele J, Johnson KA, Hicklin DJ. Effect of platelet-derived growth factor on tibial osteotomies in rabbits. *Bone*. 1994;15(2):203-208.
16. Kwong FN, Harris MB. Recent developments in the biology of fracture repair. *J Am Acad Orthop Surg*. 2008;16(11):619-625.
17. Einhorn TA, Lee CA. Bone regeneration: new findings and potential clinical applications. *J Acad Orthop Surg*. 2001;9(3):157-165.
18. Gazit D, Turgeman G, Kelley P. Engineered pluripotent mesenchymal cells integrate and differentiate in regenerating bone: a novel cell-mediated gene therapy. *J Gene Med*. 1999;1(2):121-133.
19. Govender S, Csimma C, Genant HK, et al; BMP-2 Evaluation in Surgery for Tibial Trauma (BESTT) Study Group. Recombinant human bone morphogenetic protein-2 for the treatment of open tibial shaft fractures: a prospective, controlled, randomized study of four hundred and fifty patients. *J Bone Joint Surg Am*. 2002;84(12):2123-2134.
20. Kanakaris NK, Calori GM, Verdonk R. Application of BMP-7 to tibial non-unions: a 3 year multicenter study experience. *Injury*. 2008;39(suppl 2):S83-S90.
21. Lind M, Schumacker B, Soballe K. Transforming growth factor-beta enhances fracture healing in rabbit tibiae. *Acta Orthop Scand*. 1993;64(5):553-556.
22. Secreto FJ, Hoeppner LH, Westendorf JJ. Wnt signaling during fracture repair. *Curr Osteoporos Rep*. 2009;7(2):64-69.
23. Kim JB, Leucht P, Lam K, et al. Bone regeneration is regulated by Wnt signaling. *J Bone Miner Res*. 2007;22(12):1913-1923.
24. Chen Y, Whetstone HC, Lin AC, et al. Beta-catenin signaling plays a role in different phases of fracture repair: Implications for therapy to improve bone healing. *PLoS Med*. 2007;4(7):e249.
25. Trippel SB, Rosenfeld RG. Growth factor treatment of disorders of skeletal growth. *Instr Course Lect*. 1997;46:477-482.
26. Thompson Z, Miclau T, Hu D, Helms JA. A model for intramembranos ossification during fracture healing. *J Orthop Res*. 2002;20(5):1091-1098.
27. Colnot C, Thompson Z, Miclau T, Werb Z, Helms JA. Altered fracture repair in the absence of MMP9. *Development*. 2003;130(17):4123-4133.
28. Kronenberg HM. PTHrP and skeletal development. *Ann N Y Acad Sci*. 2006;1068:1-13.
29. Vu TH, Shipley JM, Bergers G, et al. MMP-9/gelatinase B is a key regulator of growth plate angiogenesis and apoptosis of hypertrophic chondrocytes. *Cell*. 1998;93(3):411-422.
30. Morshed S, Corrales L, Genant H, et al. Outcome assessment in clinical trials of fracture-healing. *J Bone Joint Surg Am*. 2008;90(suppl 1):62-67.
31. Le AX, Miclau T, Hu D, et al. Molecular aspects of healing in stabilized and non-stabilized fractures. *J Orthop Res*. 2001;19(1):78-84.
32. Repp F, Vetter A, Duda GN, Weinkamer R. The connection between cellular mechanoregulation and tissue patterns during bone healing. *Med Biol Eng Comput*. 2015;53:829-842.
33. Perren SM, Cordey J. The concept of interfragmentary strain. In: Uhthoff HK, Stahl E, eds. *Current Concepts of Internal Fixation of Fractures*. Heidelber, Berlin: Springer; 1980:63-77.
34. Hastrup SG, Chen X, Bechtold JE, et al. Effect of nicotine and tobacco administration method on the mechanical properties of healing bone following closed fracture. *J Orthop Res*. 2010;28(9):1235-1239.
35. Daftari TK, Whitsides TE, Heller JG, et al. Nicotine on revascularization of bone graft: An experimental study in rabbits. *Spine (Phila Pa 1976)*. 1994;19:904-911.
36. Castillo RC, Bosse MJ, MacKenzie EJ, et al. Impact of smoking on fracture healing and risk of complications in limb-threatening open tibia fractures. *J Orthop Trauma*. 2005;19(3):151-157.
37. Rothem DE, Rothem L, Soudry M, Dahan A, Eliakim R. Nicotine modulates bone metabolism-associated gene expression in osteoblast cells. *J Bone Miner Metab*. 2009;27(5):555-561.
38. Donigan JA, Fredericks DC, Nepola JV, et al. The effect of transdermal nicotine on fracture healing in a rabbit model. *J Orthop Trauma*. 2012;26(12):724-727.
39. Kurmis AP, Kurmis TP, O'Brien JX, Dalen T. The effect of nonsteroidal anti-inflammatory drug administration on acute phase or fracture-healing: a review. *J Bone Joint Surg Am*. 2012;94(9):815-823.
40. Dodwell ER, Latorre JG, Parisini E, et al. NSAID exposure and risk of nonunion: A meta-analysis of case-control and cohort studies. *Calcif Tissue Int*. 2010;87(3):193-202.
41. Pountos I, Georgouli T, Blokhuis TJ, Pape HC, Giannoudis PV. Pharmacological agents and impairment of fracture healing; what is the evidence? *Injury*. 2008;39(4):382-394.
42. Waters RV, Gamradt SC, Asnis P, et al. Systemic corticosteroids inhibit bone healing in a rabbit ulnar osteotomy model. *Acta Orthop Scand*. 2000;71(3):316-321.
43. Boguch ER, Ouellette G, Hastings DE. Intertrochanteric fractures of the femur in rheumatoid arthritis patients. *Clin Orthop Relat Res*. 1993;294:181-186.
44. Brinker MR, O'Connor DP, Monla YT, Earthman TP. Metabolic and endocrine abnormalities in patients with nonunions. *J Orthop Trauma*. 2007;21(8):557-570.
45. Wang A, Powell A. The effects of obesity surgery on bone metabolism: what orthopedic surgeons need to know. *Am J Orthop*. 2009;38(2):77-79.
46. Kanakaris NK, West RM, Giannoudis PV. Enhancement of hip fracture healing in the elderly: Evidence deriving from a pilot randomized trial. *Injury*. 2015;46(8):1425-1428.
47. Liuni FM, Rugiero C, Feola M, et al. Impaired healing of fracgility fractures in type 2 diabetes: clinical and radiographic assessments and serum cytokine levels. *Aging Clin Exp Res*. 2015;27:37-44.
48. Perlman MH, Thordarson DB. Ankle fusion in a high risk population: an assessment of nonunion risk factors. *Foot Ankle Int*. 1999;20(8):491-496.
49. Loder RT. The influence of diabetes mellitus on the healing of closed fractures. *Clin Orthop Relat Res*. 1988;232:210-216.
50. Eriksen EF, Díez-Pérez A, Boonen S. Update on long-term treatment with bisphosphonates for postmenopausal osteoporosis: a systematic review. *Bone*. 2014;58:126-135.
51. Compston J, Bowring C, Cooper A, et al. Diagnosis and management of osteoporosis in postmenopausal women and older men in the UK: National Osteoporosis Guideline Group (NOGG) update 2013. *Maturitas*. 2013;75(4):392-396.
52. Lenart BA, Lorich DG, Lane JM. Atypical fractures of the femoral diaphysis in postmenopausal women taking alendronate. *N Engl J Med*. 2008;358(12):1304-1306.
53. Serrano AJ, Begoña L, Anitua E, Cobos R, Orive G. Systematic review and meta-analysis of the efficacy and safety of alendronate and zoledronate for the treatment of postmenopausal osteoporosis. *Gynecol Endocrinol*. 2013;29(12):1005-1014.
54. Rozenthal TD, Vazquez MA, Chacko AT, Ayogu N, Bouxsein ML. Comparison of radiographic fracture healing in the distal radius for patients on and off bisphosphonate therapy. *J Hand Surg Am*. 2009;34(4):595-602.
55. Kidd LJ, Cowling NR, Wu AC, Kelly WL, Forwood MR. Bisphosphonate treatment delays stress fracture remodeling in the rat ulna. *J Orthop Res*. 2011;29(12):L1827-L1833.
56. Li YT, Cai HF, Zhang ZL. Timing of the initiation of bisphosphonates after surgery for fracture healing: a systematic review and meta-analysis of randomized controlled trials. *Osteoporos Int*. 2015;26(2):431-441.
57. Woo S, Hellstein J, Kalmar J. Narrative review: bisphosphonates and osteonecrosis of the jaws. *Ann Intern Med*. 2006;144(10):753-761.
58. Cummings SR, Schwartz AV, Black DM. Alendronate and atrial fibrillation. *N Engl J Med*. 2007;356(18):1895-1896.
59. Wysowski D, Chang J. Alendronate and risedronate: reports of severe bone, joint, and muscle pain. *Arch Intern Med*. 2005;165(3):346-347.
60. Shane E. Evolving data about subtrochanteric fractures and bisphosphonates. *N Engl J Med*. 2010;362(19):1825-1827.
61. Uzzan B, Cohen R, Nicolas P, Cucherat M, Perret G. Effects of statins on bone mineral density: a meta-analysis of clinical studies. *Bone*. 2007;40(6):1581-1587.
62. Laufs U, Liao JK. Direct vascular effects of HMG-CoA reductase inhibitors. *Trends Cardiovasc Med*. 2000;10(4):143-148.
63. Issa JP, Ingraci de Lucia C, Dos Santos KB, et al. The effect of simvastatin treatment on bone repair of femoral fracture in animal model. *Growth Factors*. 2015;33(2):139-148.
64. McCandless LC. Statin use and fracture risk: can we quantify the healthy-user effect? *Epidemiology*. 2013;24(5):743-752.
65. Ibrahim NI, Mohamed N, Shuid AN. Update on statins: hope for osteoporotic fracture healing treatment. *Curr Drug Targets*. 2013;14(13):1524-1532.
66. Poole K, Reeve J. Parathyroid hormone – a bone anabolic and catabolic agent. *Curr Opin Pharmacol*. 2005;5(6):612-617.
67. Hamann C, Picke AK, Campbell GM, et al. Effects of parathyroid hormone on bone mass, bone strength, and bone regeneration in mae rates with type 2 diabetes mellitus. *Endocrinology*. 2014;155(4):1197-1206.
68. Neer RM, Arnaud CD, Zanchetta JR, et al. Effect of parathyroid hormone (1-34) on fractures and bone mineral density in postmenopausal women with osteoporosis. *N Engl J Med*. 2001;344(19):1434-1441.

69. Nakajima A, Shimoji N, Shiomi K, et al. Mechanisms for the enhancement of fracture healing in rats treated with intermittent low-dose human parathyroid hormone (1-34). *J Bone Miner Res.* 2002;17(11):2038-2047.

70. Nakazawa T, Nakajima A, Shiomi K, et al. Effects of low-dose, intermittent treatment with recombinant human parathyroid hormone (1-34) on chondrogenesis in a model of experimental fracture healing. *Bone.* 2005;37(5):711-719.

71. Nauth A, Giannoudis PV, Einhorn TA, et al. Growth factors: beyond bone morphogenic proteins. *J Orthop Trauma.* 2010;24(9):543-546.

72. Locatelli V, Bianchi VE. Effect of GH/IGF-1 on bone metabolism and osteoporosis. *Int J Endocrinol.* 2014;2014:235060.

73. Rosenbloom AL. The role of recombinant insulin-like growth factor I in the treatment of the short child. *Curr Opin Pediatr.* 2007;19(4):458-464.

74. Myers TJ, Yan Y, Granero-Molto F, et al. Systemically delivered insulin-like growth factor-1 enhances mesechymal stem cell-dependent fracture healing. *Growth Factors.* 2012;30(4):230-241.

75. Bernstein A, Mayr HO, Hube R. Can bone healing in distraction osteogenesis be accelerated by local application of IGF-1 and TGF-beta1? *J Biomed Mater Res B Appl Biomater.* 2010;92(1):215-225.

76. De Long WG, Einhorn TA, Koval K, et al. Bone grafts and bone graft substitutes in orthopaedic trauma surgery. *J Bone Joint Surg Am.* 2007;89(3):649-658.

77. Friedlaender GE, Perry CR, Cole JD, et al. Osteogenic protein-1 (bone morphogenetic protein-7) in the treatment of tibial nonunions. *J Bone Joint Surg Am.* 2001;83(suppl 1 pt 2):S151-S158.

78. Aro HT, Govender S, Patel AD, et al. Recombinant Human Bone Morphogenetic Protein-2: a randomized trial in open tibial fractures treated with reamed nail fixation. *J Bone Joint Surg Am.* 2011;93(9):801-808.

79. McKee MD. Recombinant human bone morphogenic protein-7: applications for clinical trauma. *J Orthop Trauma.* 2005;19(10 suppl):S26-S28.

80. Slater M, Patava J, Kingham K, Mason RS. Involvement of platelets in stimulating osteogenic activity. *J Orthop Res.* 1995;13:655-663.

81. Bibbo C, Bono CM, Lin SS. Union rates using autologous platelet concentrate alone and with bone graft in high-risk foot and ankle surgery patients. *J Surg Orthop Adv.* 2005;14:17-22.

82. Guzel Y, Karalezli N, Bilge O, et al. The biomechanical and histological effects of platelet-rich plasma on fracture healing. *Knee Surg Sports Traumatol Arthrosc.* 2015;23(5):1378-1383.

83. Banwart JC, Asher MA, Hassanein RS. Iliac crest bone graft harvest donor site morbidity. A statistical evaluation. *Spine.* 1995;20:1055-1060.

84. Garg NK, Gaur S, Sharma S. Percutaneous autogenous bone marrow grafting in 20 cases of ununited fracture. *Acta Orthop Scand.* 1993;64:671-672.

85. Goel A, Sangwan SS, Siwach RC, Ali AM. Percutaneous bone marrow grafting for the treatment of tibial non-union. *Injury.* 2005;36:203-206.

86. Hernigou P, Poignard A, Beaujean F, Rouard H. Percutaneous autologous bone-marrow grafting for nonunions. Influence of the number and concentration of progenitor cells. *J Bone Joint Surg Am.* 2005;87:1430-1437.

87. Tiedeman JJ, Connolly JF, Strates BS, Lippiello L. Treatment of nonunion by percutaneous injection of bone marrow and demineralized bone matrix. An experimental study in dogs. *Clin Orthop Relat Res.* 1991;268:294-302.

88. Connolly J, Guse R, Lippiello L, Dehne R. Development of an osteogenic bone-marrow preparation. *J Bone Joint Surg Am.* 1989;71:684-691.

89. Marsh D. Concepts of fracture union, delayed union, and nonunion. *Clin Orthop Relat Res.* 1998;355:S22-S30.

90. Bhandari M, Guyatt GH, Swiontkowski MF, Tornetta P, Sprague S, Schemitsch EH. A lack of consensus in the assessment of fracture healing among orthopaedic surgeons. *J Orthop Trauma.* 2002;16(8):562-566.

91. Bhandari M, Fong K, Sprague S, Williams D, Petrisor B. Variability in the definition and perceived causes of delayed unions and nonunions: A cross-sectional, multinational survey of orthopaedic surgeons. *J Bone Joint Surg Am.* 2012;95(15):e109.

92. Stojadinovic A, Potter BK, Eberhardt J, et al. Development of a prognostic naïve Bayesian classifier for successful treatments of nonunions. *J Bone Joint Surg Am.* 2011;93(2):187-194.

93. Sathyendra V, Donahue HJ, Vrana KE, et al. Single nucleotide polumorphisms in ostegenic genes in atrophic delayed fracture-healing: A preliminary investigation. *J Bone Joint Surg Am.* 2014;96(15):1242-1248.

94. LaVelle DG. Delayed union and nonunion of fractures. In: Canale TS, eds. *Campbell's Operative Orthopaedics.* 9th ed. St. Louis, MO: Mosby; 1998:2579-2629.

95. Phieffer LS, Goulet JA. Delayed Unions of the Tibia. *J Bone Joint Surg Am.* 2006;88(1):205-216.

Wound Healing and Infection

Renee Genova
J. Tracy Watson
Bruce A. Kraemer

INTRODUCTION

Restoration of a patient's function, pain control, promotion of healing while minimizing potential complications such as infection and nonunion are fundamental goals in the management of the orthopaedic trauma patient. While some clinical pictures appear quite straightforward and evolve uneventfully, it is essential that the treating surgeon have a thorough understanding of the many factors involved in each step along the path to healing. He or she must be able to identify the modifiable risk factors in each individual case to optimize treatment so that outcomes may be maximized. It is also important to remember that fractures are as different as the individuals who present with them and taking a cookie cutter approach to all comers will likely leave the fracture, the patient, and the surgeon wanting.

WOUND HEALING

BASIC PATHOPHYSIOLOGY OF WOUND HEALING

Wound healing is an intricate process that can be summarized by dividing the cascade into four stages:

1. Hemostasis
2. Inflammation
3. Proliferation (granulation, vascularization, wound closure)
4. Remodeling

Each stage is affected by enzymes, growth factors, inflammatory cells, and signals both from the microenvironment in addition to our interventions.[1] Proper nutrition is required for our basic physiologic function, and these requirements are increased with the additional energy involved in wound healing. Oxygen is essential for normal physiology, and like nutrition, there are increased oxygen needs in the setting of wound healing.[1] In addition to the trauma itself, peripheral arterial disease, infection, diabetes, and tension on the tissues can all negatively affect oxygenation limiting wound healing potential.[1]

WOUND HEALING IN ORTHOPAEDIC TRAUMA

In addition to rudiments of basic wound healing, additional principles must be considered when addressing injuries and wounds in the orthopaedic trauma patient. These include, but are not limited to, open fractures, closed crush injuries, injuries to the distal lower extremity and associated fracture blisters, zone of injury, and internal fixation.

Fracture blisters are often present in the setting of pilon, tibial plateau, and calcaneus fractures and may continue to evolve along with swelling for days following the injury. Surgical incisions made through significant soft-tissue swelling or fracture blisters can lead to potentially preventable postoperative wound complications. Two types of fracture blisters are recognized: clear fluid–filled blisters and blood-filled blisters.[2,3] Both blister types are a result of the shearing forces experienced at the time of injury resulting in cleavage between layers of the dermal tissue. A clear fluid blister contains sterile scattered areas of retained epithelial cells, which can lead to faster reepithelialization and less morbidity than a hemorrhagic blister. A blood-filled blister (**Figure 4.1A and B**) may represent a more significant injury involving deeper layers of the dermis and is more likely to heal with scar formation rather than the uncomplicated reepithelialization seen with sterile fracture blisters.[4]

Severe contusion or blister formation is a direct factor contributing to the development of a wound complication.[5] Blisters are a hard sign indicating deep tissue involvement, and open surgical management is avoided until the blisters have resolved.[4] Varela et al[3] examined 51 patients with fracture blisters and found that the average time until the fracture blister was noted on clinical examination was 2.5 days after injury.

Blister care includes application of a nonadherent dressing with or without aspiration of the blister fluid and is followed by fracture reduction and application of a compressive dressing. Even when temporary spanning fixation has been utilized, a compressive dressing with multiple layers should be applied. This provides circumferential compression and

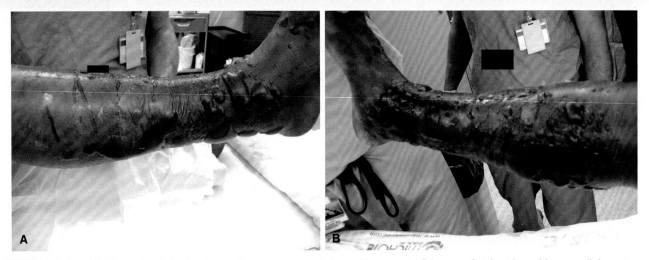

FIGURE 4.1 A and **B**, Hemorrhagic blisters indicating a more severe injury with necrosis of the superficial epidermal layers and deep tissue damage, as a result of internal degloving. Any invasive surgical approach should be delayed until soft-tissue recovery and reepithelization of the blisters have occurred.

minimizes the shearing effect on the injured tissue layers, which begins at the bone and progresses outward. The circumferential compression prevents delamination of the fascia from the muscle, the subcutaneous tissue from the fascia, and finally the epidermis from the dermis.

The wrinkle test is a reliable clinical sign used to determine skin integrity and suggests the resolution of soft-tissue edema. Presence of wrinkles and the ability to "pinch" up skin demonstrates that the interstitial third spacing of fluid is resolving and will allow the skin to be mobilized, enabling closure without undue tension. An additional adjunctive measure to help the soft tissues recover before surgery is the use of a pulsatile A/V foot pump compressive device placed in combination over a multilayered compressive dressing. The effectiveness of this technique is described in a consecutive series of 64 closed ankle fractures that were managed using an A/V foot pump system incorporated into the compressive dressing before surgery.[6] Use of this preoperative soft-tissue protocol was associated with the surgeon's ability to evaluate injury and expedite management. They found their soft-tissue complications and wound infections were also significantly reduced with the use of preoperative A/V compression foot pumps.

POSTOPERATIVE SOFT-TISSUE MANAGEMENT

Respecting the soft-tissue envelope is essential and should be considered a priority from the initial steps in management of a fracture until the patient is considered healed and appropriate for discharge. Management of the postoperative soft tissue starts preoperatively; it is critical that the appropriate surgical approach be utilized, with judicious incisions minimizing the undermining of skin flaps. Proper fixation with smaller implants that minimize fragment stripping and allow minimally invasive surgical techniques to be carried out is of primary importance during the fixation strategy. Meticulous soft-tissue handling is mandatory to minimize soft-tissue

complications. Gentle retraction with smooth retractors, avoidance of crushing the skin margins with forceps, use of shorter tourniquet times, and frequent irrigation of the tissues are all tenets of soft-tissue protection during surgery.[7] Minimizing operative time, specifically time the incisions are "open," has been found to be a primary predictor of post-op wound infection.[7] Open fractures, elevated postoperative glucose levels (≥125 mg/dL), and a surgery duration of more than 150 minutes with the wound "open" were associated with an increased risk for surgical site infection after open reduction and internal fixation of pilon fractures.[8] Thus, it is critical to perform thorough pre-op planning and develop a surgical tactic *before* incisions are made.

After all the planning and meticulous surgical technique, the closure should not be relegated to the most junior individual in the operating room. A tension-free closure is necessary to avoid wound compromise. If this cannot be obtained, the wound should be left open and later closed secondarily or closed with either a skin graft or a muscle flap. When treating pilon fractures, Leone advocates primary closure of the tibial incision, with delayed closure of the fibular incision or delayed split-thickness skin grafting of the fibular wounds to achieve coverage of the tibial component.[9]

Soft-tissue complications should be identified and treated early. McFerran et al[10] reported an overall local complication rate of 54%, with 40% of patients requiring an unplanned reoperation. Most of these complications occurred within 3 weeks of surgery; only two occurred more than 40 weeks after the index procedure. The authors concluded that the majority of complications were soft tissue initiated.[11]

WOUND MANAGEMENT

The management of a wound complication requires mature clinical judgment, and one should not live in denial and avoid immediate treatment. The best chance to avoid significant morbidity is to act aggressively as the situation requires. Superficial skin necrosis can be treated with local wound care, limb elevation, and close observation. If mild cellulitis with erythematous margins about the wound is present, the patient should be treated with oral antibiotics. If the cellulitis does not respond promptly or if a more significant cellulitis extending away from the margins of the wound is present, the patient should be admitted for intravenous antibiotics. Cultures taken from superficial skin drainage are historically unreliable and generally do not reflect the pathogenic infecting organism that may be deep to the incision.

At this time, negative-pressure wound therapy (NPWT) can be initiated and antibiotic therapy should be continued until all marginal erythema has resolved. However, if superficial skin loss results and the deep tissue or peritenon is intact, and deep tissue cultures are culture negative, these areas can be simply covered with a split-thickness skin graft once a healthy bed of granulation tissue has developed with the use of NPWT.

Full-thickness wound dehiscence generally results in immediate contamination of the underlying hardware and bone, is a very different situation from superficial wound necrosis, and requires aggressive debridement in the operating room followed by soft-tissue coverage as soon as feasible. This clinical scenario usually requires a rotational flap or free tissue transfer and should be performed before the onset of deep infection. During the initial debridements, deep tissue cultures should be obtained to rule out deep infection and guide specific antibiotic management. Additionally, the internal fixation should be visualized and its structural continuity and stability evaluated. If it is determined that the hardware provides stable fixation, it should be retained and soft-tissue coverage initiated. A 3- to 6-week course of intravenous antibiotics is recommended based on deep tissue culture results.

However, if at any time fixation demonstrates any instability, it should be removed and replaced with a stable fixation construct. Fracture reduction may be lost, and a late reconstructive procedure may be necessary once the soft tissues have healed. If deep cultures are positive, the situation is much more complex and a staged reconstruction for a potentially infected nonunion should be undertaken.

Negative-Pressure Wound Therapy

NPWT, frequently referred to as "vacuum-assisted closure" or "VAC," has recently demonstrated widespread use from management of decubitus ulcers to its use in postoperative wounds in many of the surgical subspecialty patient populations including orthopaedic trauma.

The NPWT system consists of three components: (1) porous dressing (sponge); (2) occlusive seal adhesive; (3) vacuum device with connector that together create the subatmospheric pressure environment that defines NPWT.

There exist a variety of sponge options, each with its own characteristics and unique contribution to the specifics of the NPWT environment. The most commonly used porous dressing (or sponge) in orthopaedic trauma surgery is the dry black sponge for its hydrophobic, reticulated large pore size foam, which provides for a more adherent application and significantly increased granulation and perfusion than a premoistened polyvinyl alcohol foam with smaller size pores.[12]

This therapy can be applied directly over high-risk surgical incisions that have been closed, referred to as an "incisional VAC." Placing such an incisional VAC on the surgical incision used for open reduction and internal fixation of a pilon fracture at the time of closure has been shown to reduce the risk of developing acute dehiscence and wound infection.[13] Another trial evaluated wound dehiscence and infection after high-risk lower extremity trauma. The relative risk of developing an infection was 1.9 times higher in standard dressing patients compared to patients treated with NPWT.[14,15]

Studies have demonstrated the stimulatory effects that NPWT has on local angiogenesis to increase local blood flow, and the ability to reduce the surface area of the wound as well as to increase the induction of cellular proliferation. The current data does not demonstrated its ability to reduce wound edema or the clearance of wound bacteria.[16]

Hyperbaric Oxygen Therapy

Healthy cells of nontraumatized tissues have a baseline oxygen requirement; naturally, cells of traumatized tissues have increased oxygen requirements compared to cells of nontraumatized tissues. Unfortunately, the same traumatized environment that increases the oxygen requirement of these cells is the very environment that decreases the oxygen available to them secondary to the traumatically induced edema.[17] In addition to limiting the oxygen available to the tissue, edema also diminishes the microcirculation that is integral in tissue healing and infection prevention and treatment in these traumatized tissues.[17] The downstream effect is growth of bacteria in an environment with limited exposure to circulating blood and antibiotics within it.

Specifically, fibroblast function is dependent on an oxygen tension of 30 mm Hg; therefore in the setting of decreased oxygen tension as can occur in the setting of a soft-tissue injury, these cells cannot mobilize and produce collagen matrix required for neovascularization and wound healing.[18]

Hyperbaric oxygen therapy (HBOT) has applications in diving medicine, carbon monoxide poisoning, gas gangrene, effects of radiation, and chronic wounds in the diabetic patient.[19] HBOT in conjunction with interdisciplinary wound care to decrease the risk of amputation in a patient with a diabetic foot ulcer is supported by a high level of evidence.[19] Animal models have demonstrated HBOT to minimize necrosis of muscle and reduce the edema in compartment syndrome,[20] and Radonic et al[21] suggested that HBOT decreased the rate of amputation in their military population sustaining combat injuries with prolonged ischemic periods. Others have also noted similar results in the setting of extensive bony and soft tissue injuries.[22]

Extracellular Matrix Materials

Extracellular matrix (ECM) materials such as urinary bladder matrix-extra cellular matrix (UBM-ECM) and dermal regeneration template (DRT) may facilitate definitive soft-tissue reconstruction by establishing a durable dermallike soft-tissue base acceptable for second-stage wound and skin coverage. Using these biomaterials, a new dermal layer can be established for second-stage wound and skin coverage options.[23] This approach may be suited in patients who are often poor surgical candidates for more advanced reconstructive procedures. Two materials are currently FDA approved. The first is an acellular, non–cross-linked, ECM scaffold derived from porcine bladder basement membrane. The material is applied in powder, single or multilayer sheets.[23] The ECM is typically applied in the operating room at the time of initial operative debridement. The UBM-ECM products have been found to facilitate healing despite the presence of exposed hardware and positive bacterial cultures, provided that all grossly devitalized bone has been removed (**Figure 4.2A**).[24] Once a bed of granulation tissue is achieved, the acellular dermal templates are applied directly over the clean wound (**Figure 4.2B**). Reapplication of the matrix may be required until a dermallike layer is established. Wounds can then heal secondarily or combined later with split-thickness skin grafting and NPWT (**Figure 4.2C**). Use of these extracellular porcine bladder matrices gives these patients additional options as they are combined with delayed skin grafting, local pedicle flaps, adjacent tissue rearrangements, and/or free tissue transfers.[25]

DRT Integra® Meshed Bilayer Wound Matrix (Integra Life Sciences Corporation), the second material available, is a porous matrix of cross-linked bovine tendon collagen and glycosaminoglycan and a semipermeable polysiloxane (silicone) layer. The meshed bilayer allows drainage of wound

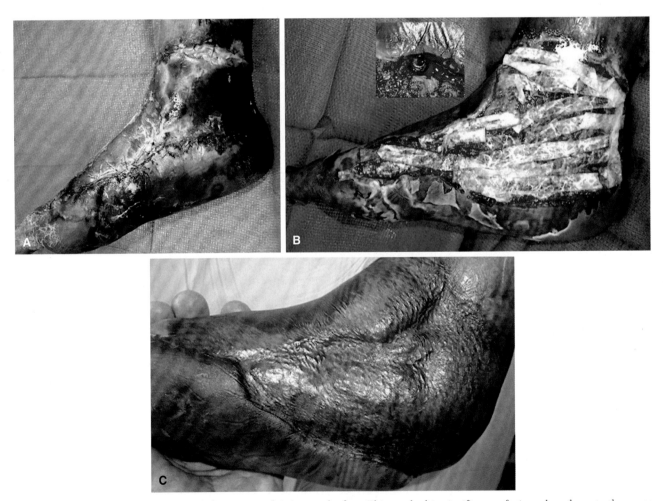

FIGURE 4.2 A, Soft-tissue necrosis secondary to a crush injury to the foot. This resulted in significant soft-tissue loss down to the superficial fascia of the foot. **B**, Following radical soft-tissue debridement, an acellular matrix has been placed directly over the deep tissues to develop a durable dermal layer that can eventually be skin grafted. Note, this matrix will facilitate granulation tissue formation even over exposed hardware (window). **C**, Split thickness skin grafting occurred over the reconstructed dermal layer, and this composite grafting technique provides durable soft-tissue covering with dermal and epidermal layers as opposed to skin grafting directly over muscle, bone, or fascia.

exudate and provides a flexible adherent covering for the wound surface. The collagen-glycosaminoglycan biodegradable matrix provides a scaffold for cellular invasion and capillary growth. Secondary procedures can be carried out once the basement tissue layer has been established.

Flap Coverage

The principle of aggressive wound debridement with early free flap wound coverage has dominated the management of wounds involving the distal third of the tibia and ankle. Free flap coverage is the workhorse coverage for those areas of significant soft-tissue loss secondary to massive wound necrosis. These are primarily used in cases of infected nonunion where eradication of infection requires radical debridement of involved bone and soft tissue. Unfortunately, the area most difficult to cover with muscle flaps is the lower third of the leg (**Figure 4.3**). The advent of fasciocutaneous flaps has stimulated great interest in the cutaneous circulation of the lower extremities and in alternatives to traditional, proximally based free flap procedures. Rather than sacrificing the whole vascular axis in the process of transferring a flap, flaps can be based on a single septocutaneous perforator of the tibial or peroneal vessels.[26]

Pedicled perforator flaps have several obvious advantages over free flaps. They can be performed expeditiously, and this is particularly beneficial in the management of soft-tissue defects in multiply injured patients, the elderly, and systemically compromised patients.[27] This reconstruction can replace like-with-like, by using tissues of similar texture, thickness, pliability, and color. This method avoids the complexity of multiple surgical sites, the need for special instrumentation, and the requirement for transfer of patients to specialty centers with the extra costs associated with free flaps and microsurgery.[27] Local flap surgery limits the scars and morbidity to one extremity. These are ideally suited to the smaller defects that result from wound dehiscence or wound breakdown resulting from the limited incisions currently used for pilon fixation.[28]

Pedicled perforator flaps have several potential disadvantages, particularly when used for major posttraumatic soft-tissue defects. The principal criticism is that the flap is raised within the zone of injury and its vascularity could be compromised. Appreciation of the vascular basis of such flaps and adequate assessment of degloving minimizes this risk. Incorrect raising of local skin flaps can interrupt superficial veins and cutaneous nerves, leading to edema and neuromata. Free flaps can be tailored to suit massive or irregular skin defects, whereas the design of a pedicled flap tends to be limited by the local anatomy and availability of skin and wound orientation. Local flaps can leave a significant cosmetic defect of the donor site, which may be difficult to camouflage.[28]

Failure of a local perforator flap leaves alternative methods including free flaps. As in free flaps, there is donor site morbidity. However, because the source artery and underlying muscle are preserved, morbidity is limited to only one region. For defects less than 6 cm wide, the donor site can be primarily closed.[29] In women, a problem can be the cosmetic deficit at the donor site. Another potential problem if the perforator is within the zone of injury is that the viability of the flap may be compromised. With few options, donor site defects may have to be accepted. Poor flap candidates may benefit from minimally invasive wound management such as NPWT and matrix materials.

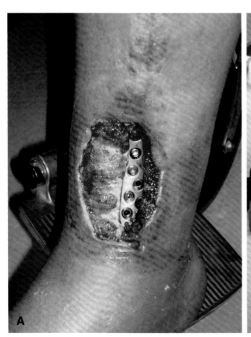
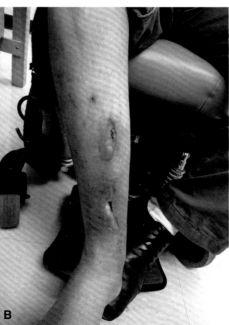

FIGURE 4.3 A and **B**, Wound breakdown over the distal third of the tibia following a medial "percutaneous" plating technique. Now exposed hardware is present. Even with limited incision techniques, this area is very sensitive to any additional surgical insult on top of the soft-tissue damage that occurs with distal third tibial fractures. This resulted in additional soft-tissue procedures to achieve competent wound closure with healthy soft tissues.

INFECTION

PATHOPHYSIOLOGY AND RISK FACTORS OF SURGICAL SITE INFECTION

It is believed that infection of surgical sites are acquired intraoperatively, making the sterile techniques in the operating room integral in the prevention of this potentially devastating complication.[30] It is therefore vital that the aseptic techniques such as hand washing, skin preparation, and sterilization procedures are strictly adhered as the first step to minimize the risk of a surgical site infection.[31]

Risk factors for infection can be either modifiable or not. Modification and optimization of many patient factors during the perioperative period may have a positive impact in preventing postoperative infections in orthopaedic trauma patients. These modifications include, but are not limited to, reversing malnutrition, nicotine cessation, tapering high-dose corticosteroid therapy, and maximizing oxygen delivery to the tissues.[30]

Often associated with malnutrition, a zinc deficiency in a patient makes them more likely to develop complications with wound healing. Supplementing a patient's zinc to reach serum levels above 95 µg/dL is associated with a significantly lower risk for postoperative wound complications.[32]

The detrimental effects nicotine has on our human physiology via a variety of mechanisms including many that negatively impact wound healing have been born out in the literature.[32] More important, however, is that smoking cessation decreases the risk of wound complications and fracture nonunion; the magnitude of the decrease in risk is commensurate with the duration of the smoking cessation.[32] It has been well established that hyperglycemia in a diabetic patient undergoing total joint replacement, spine surgery, and fracture surgery is associated with significantly increased rates of postoperative infections and other complications.[33-35] Recent data demonstrate that an increased perioperative blood glucose in nondiabetic patients undergoing operative fixation of a closed fracture was associated with an increased risk of surgical site infections.[36,37] The elevated blood glucose in these nondiabetic patients is attributed to the well-established phenomenon of stress-induced hyperglycemia. Identification of hyperglycemia in a nondiabetic trauma patient is therefore crucial as is the treatment of it with a goal perioperative blood glucose level less than 200 to 220 mg/dL (depending on the study) to statistically and predictably decrease the risk of a surgical site infection.

MANAGEMENT OF ORTHOPAEDIC INFECTION

Understanding the pathophysiology of infection in the setting of a fracture treated with open reduction and internal fixation is essential to appropriately treat the infection. Specifically, the formation of a biofilm establishes a sophisticated environment with multiple impediments to eradicating the infection including a hydrophobic structure that functions as a semi-impermeable barrier to the very antibiotic intended for the microbes of the biofilm.[38] For this and other reasons, simply administering even targeted intravenous antibiotics alone will not cure the musculoskeletal infection in the setting of retained hardware.

Therefore, to eradicate the infection, a methodical approach that addresses the pathogen, host factors, bony, and soft-tissue deficiencies is required including[38]:

1. Thorough and scrupulous debridement
2. Dead-space management
3. Soft-tissue and bone reconstruction using principles of the reconstruction ladder

Whether to remove the hardware can be a difficult decision, especially in the setting of a fracture that has not yet healed but has maintained stable fixation in the setting of an infection. Controversy exists as to if all hardware should be removed and the infection completely eradicated, or if merely suppressing the infection and maintaining stable fixation is more optimal to obtain fracture union.

Acute or Subacute Infection With Stable Hardware

When dealing with orthopaedic implant–related infections, the knee-jerk recommendation of nonsurgical consultants is often to remove all hardware, obtain deep cultures, and administer antibiotics. This is partially correct. Cultures are helpful, antibiotics are essential, but removal of stable, functioning hardware in the setting of the acutely infected fracture should be resisted resolutely. Although it is well known that the presence of inanimate material surfaces increases the risk of infection, lowers the inoculum necessary to cause infection, and reduces the chances of successful treatment, long-standing clinical experience teaches that skeletal stability reduces the infection rate.[4,39] This reduction is supported by the results of animal studies.[40,41] The mechanism by which instability promotes infection is not clear but may have to do with interference with revascularization of injured tissues, ongoing tissue damage, or increased micro–dead space. Although instability seems to interfere with the resolution of infection, the presence of infection does not necessarily prohibit bone healing. A logical strategy is to maintain stable internal fixation, which will facilitate union, and plan for hardware removal later if infection persists after the bone is healed.

For the treatment of acutely infected fractures, Berkes reported a 75% rate of fracture union and resolution of infection utilizing a standardized protocol of operative debridement, retention of *stable* fracture hardware, and culture-specific IV antibiotics (**Figure 4.4A-C**). Factors that were predictors of treatment failure included the injury being an open fracture (P = .03), the presence of an intramedullary nail (P = .01), a high association with smoking, and any infection with *Pseudomonas* species or other gram-negative organisms.[42]

Other authors have also identified factors that contribute to the successful salvage of acutely infected fractures. These include the maintenance of stable hardware, and that the time of surgery to infection diagnosis is less than 2 weeks.[43]

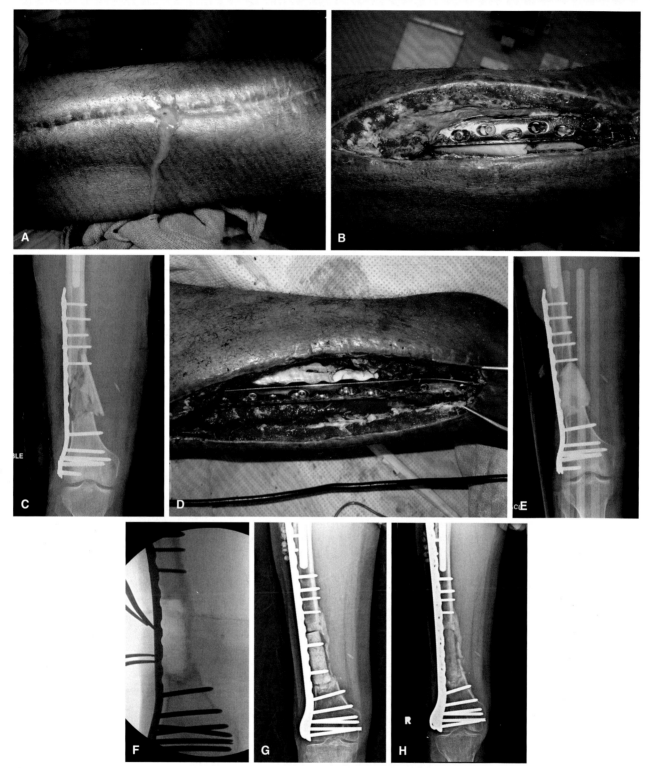

FIGURE 4.4 A, Eighteen days postoperative wound development of purulent drainage after open reduction and internal fixation of a periprosthetic midshaft femur fracture. **B**, At debridement, necrotic bone and soft tissue with gross purulence were discovered. **C**, Fracture construct appears to impart excellent stability. Hardware was retained following removal of necrotic bone and soft tissue. **D** and **E**, The defect was filled with antibiotic cement and competent lateralis flap rotated over the defect to achieve wound closure. **F**, A well-developed pseudoperiosteal membrane developed around the spacer and began bone incorporation medially along the membrane itself. **G** and **H**, At the time of grafting, the fixation was exchanged for a new longer plate. The spacer was carefully removed, preserving the membrane and developing bone. Reamer-irrigator-aspirator grafting was placed into the well-developed defect, and rapid consolidation occurred.

Another factor for successful salvage is the ability to achieve a thorough debridement of the fracture construct. If a collection of pus exists around an implant or under a flap or incision, it must be thoroughly drained. Incisions made for irrigation and debridement of infection should rarely be closed and should be placed carefully to avoid exposing hardware, bone, tendon, or neurovascular structures. If these are unavoidably exposed, consideration should be given to flap coverage of the wound. The ability to achieve competent wound closure is another predictor of successful salvage. The VAC (Kinetic Concepts, Inc.) dressing can be used while awaiting definitive coverage (**Figure 4.5A-C**).

As mentioned previously, culture-specific antibiotic treatment should be standard when treating these acutely infected stably fixed fractures. Furthermore, consideration to adding rifampin to culture-proven staphylococcal infections should be strongly considered. A randomized controlled trial to evaluate the utility in adding rifampin to conventional culture-proven staphylococcal infection associated with stable orthopaedic implants in patients with symptoms of infection that were acute or subacute in duration demonstrated a 100% cure rate in the group treated with ciprofloxacin-rifampin compared to the 58% cure rate in the group who received ciprofloxacin-placebo.[44]

In a study by Rightmire et al,[45] outcomes in patients with acute infections after fracture repair managed with retained hardware were reviewed. They evaluated the effectiveness of treating these patients with irrigation, debridement, and antibiotic suppression in the setting of retained hardware. A successful outcome was defined as a patient obtaining fracture union with original hardware in place.[45] There was a 68% success rate with an average of 120 days until fracture healing, and 36% of these patients went on to present with reinfection. The majority of the infected fractures that failed debridement and antibiotics with retained hardware failed within 3 months from the time of initial surgery. Patients who smoked were at a significantly higher risk of experiencing failure than nonsmokers. Smokers are estimated to have a risk of failure at least three to four times higher than nonsmokers in these studies.

It is important to consider all of the data at one's disposal when making the decision to remove hardware or not when treating these infections, including characteristics of the fracture, the type of fixation, virulence of the pathogen, physiology, and function of the patient.

Acute or Subacute Postoperative Infection With Unstable Hardware

Debridement

The presence of excessive motion, the displacement of hardware on radiographs, or the visualization of radiolucencies around screws, rods, or fixator pins denotes an unstable

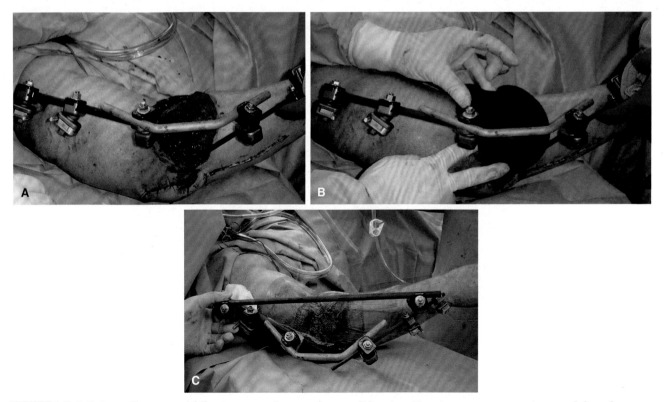

FIGURE 4.5 A-C, Open elbow wound following severe olecranon fracture dislocation. Negative pressure sponge is cut and shaped to cover the wound and wound margins. Sponge is then sealed over the wound and a negative pressure obtained following an occlusive overwrap dressing.

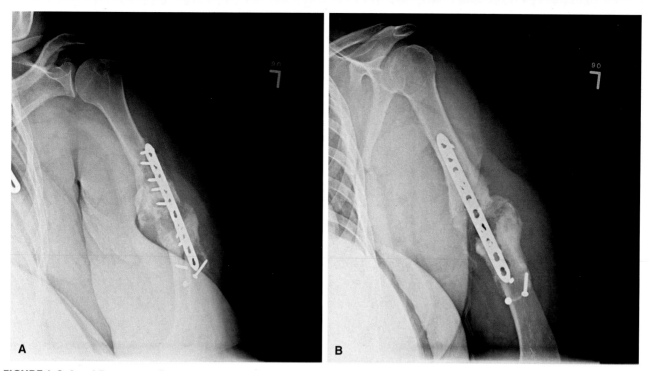

FIGURE 4.6 A and **B**, Humerus fracture nonunion with suspected infection presents 2 years post surgery. Hardware has failed and is providing no inherent stability, thus consideration for removal and staged reconstruction should be entertained.

situation (**Figure 4.6A and B**). This instability compromises the ability to overcome infection and to heal the fracture. In the face of unstable hardware or fracture malalignment, the hardware should be removed (**Figure 4.7**).

Animal studies with an infected fracture model document the detrimental effects of fracture-site instability.[40] The infection rates at 2 weeks postinfection were lower in internally fixed fractures with stable fixation compared to the infection rates that occurred in the unstable fractures with loose pins. Stability lowers the incidence of *Staphylococcus aureus* infection and other gram-positive organisms. However, gram-negative infections were worse in the internally fixed group and the infection could only be eradicated if the hardware was removed.[41]

Clearly, stability must be determined at the time of the initial debridement. Devascularized fragments of bone, missed at the original debridement or created during internal fixation, may be present in the fracture site. In most instances, this dead fragment cannot be extruded, and antibiotics will not penetrate it. The infection will never be eradicated unless the fragment is excised.[46]

Thin, scarred skin should be removed along with sinus tracts and avascular soft tissues. The dense fibrous sheath around infected hardware should be completely excised, with care taken not to strip periosteum from living bone with elevators or retractors. During debridement, the bone should be constantly visualized for evidence of punctate bleeding, which indicates adequate vascular inflow. This "paprika sign" is characteristic of living bone and is useful for establishing the limits of debridement.[46] The use of a

high-speed bur with the tourniquet down to remove cortical bone gently allows the surgeon to watch for this sign. The bur should be kept cool with irrigation.

Infection restricted to the medullary canal is debrided adequately by reaming. After removal of infected intramedullary nails, avascular material in the nail tract can be debrided by passing a flexible intramedullary reamer 1 to 2 mm larger in diameter than the nail down the tract. If this technique is used, the surgeon should avoid devitalizing cortical bone by stripping the periosteum and then reaming the endosteal vessels. This is commonly done when an unstable plate construct is converted to a nailing. There is substantial risk of creating a long sequestrum. Staging the procedures with a 6-week interval will reduce the risk.[43,46] To decrease the potential thermal effects of reaming, the tourniquet should not be inflated, progress should be slow, and irrigation should be used. A distal tibial medullary portal, or "blowhole," is useful to provide lavage throughout the canal to create a constant outflow.[43,47] The ability to achieve a culture-negative wound may require at least two sequential debridements.[48,49]

Defect Management

Removal of bone and hardware creates "dead" space, which will need to be filled with living tissue. Elimination of dead space and provision of durable soft-tissue coverage are both essential for the control of infection. In acute or subacute wound infections, closure is desirable; however, the wounds must frequently be left open. Coverage with free or rotational tissue transfer will be necessary. Bone defects may

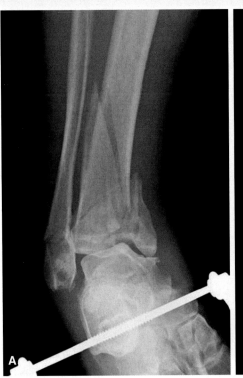
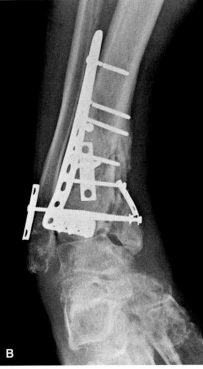

FIGURE 4.7 A and **B**, Preoperative pilon fracture radiographs and 6 months postoperative radiograph. Note fixation has failed and is providing no inherent stability at this time. This required hardware removal and initiation of a staged reconstruction for the infected nonunion.

be temporarily treated with local antibiotic delivery using antibiotic-impregnated beads or cement blocks (**Figure 4.8A-E**). The use of antibiotic beads has been shown to be effective in reducing the incidence of infection when used for dead space management during the initial stages of open fracture management. For type 2 open fractures, antibiotic bead pouches were shown to reduce infection rates from 15%-20% to 3%-4%. Likewise, when used for type 3 fractures, the infection rate was reduced from 20%-44% to 4%.[50,51]

The ability to utilize NPWT combined with antibiotic beads was thought to be an attractive combination therapy for dead space management in these injuries. Recent studies using a large complex musculoskeletal wound animal model compared the effectiveness of a bead pouch alone to the effectiveness of antibiotic beads combined with NPWT.[52] The antibiotic bead pouch group had sixfold less bacteria present in the wound compared to the NPWT plus antibiotic bead group. High levels of the antibiotic were consistently recovered from the augmented NPWT effluent, essentially demonstrating that the negative pressure device removed most of the eluded antibiotic away from the wound bead. The authors thought that although an attractive option for the management of dead space, NPWT reduces the overall effectiveness of local antibiotic beads and should not be combined.[52] Local antibiotic delivery systems are discussed in detail below.

External Fixation

After hardware removal, the bone is most commonly stabilized with external fixation. Once stability is achieved, the inflammatory phase of fracture healing and infection becomes markedly reduced, decreasing the complexity of the problem. The type of external fixator depends on wound location and fracture complexity. Less stable fractures require more complex frames to control motion at the bone ends. Because external fixators offer the ability to compress actively across fracture fragments, fracture gaps secondary to comminution and minimal bone loss can be closed directly by this maneuver. Fracture gaps secondary to malalignment can be corrected sequentially as bone union takes place. This can be accomplished with most circular and select monolateral fixators with three-dimensional adjustability.

Weight bearing should be allowed if possible because intermittent loading prevents additional bone loss from disuse atrophy. In the presence of periarticular infection, spanning external fixation provides satisfactory stability for the hard and soft tissues. This would allow for debridement and subsequent soft-tissue reconstruction because the pins are placed on either side of the joint out of the zone of soft-tissue reconstruction (**Figure 4.9A and B**).

Applying an Ilizarov circular fixator (Smith & Nephew, Memphis, TN) is advantageous for extra-articular locations because it allows weight bearing and correction of deformity or malalignment. Additionally, it can achieve compression or distraction at potential nonunion sites. The Ilizarov technique allows reconstruction of segmental skeletal defects and difficult infected fractures (**Figure 4.10A-D**).[53-55]

As external fixation devices and techniques have become more sophisticated, the ability to simultaneously correct a complex fracture deformity with a simplistic device has become more attractive. The Taylor Spatial Frame (TSF, Smith & Nephew, Memphis, TN) was designed to allow

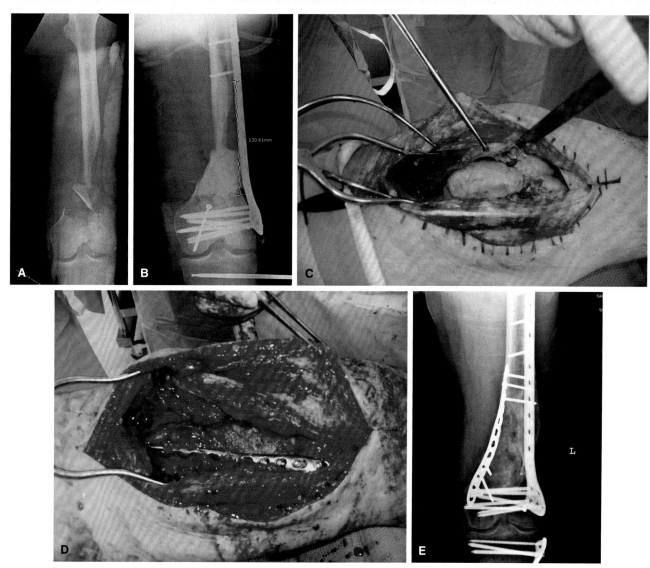

FIGURE 4.8 A, Fourteen-centimeter distal femoral defect as a result of an open fracture. **B**, Defect is filled with an antibiotic-laden cement spacer to develop a robust pseudoperiosteum (membrane) through which the spacer will be removed eventually and grafting carried out into the well-developed space. **C**, At surgery the membrane is identified and preserved, followed by removal of the spacer. **D**, Bone graft is placed in the well-circumscribed membrane-bound defect. **E**, Rapid consolidation occurs, bridging the defect by 3.5 months after grafting.

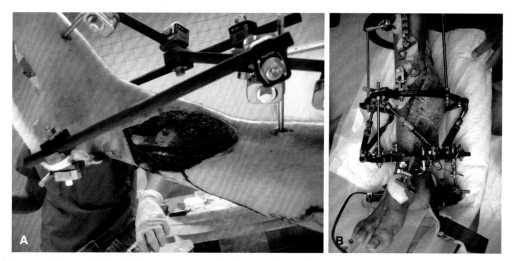

FIGURE 4.9 A, Large soft-tissue defect following an open pilon fracture. **B**, Defect management required a free flap followed by ring fixator for skeletal stability.

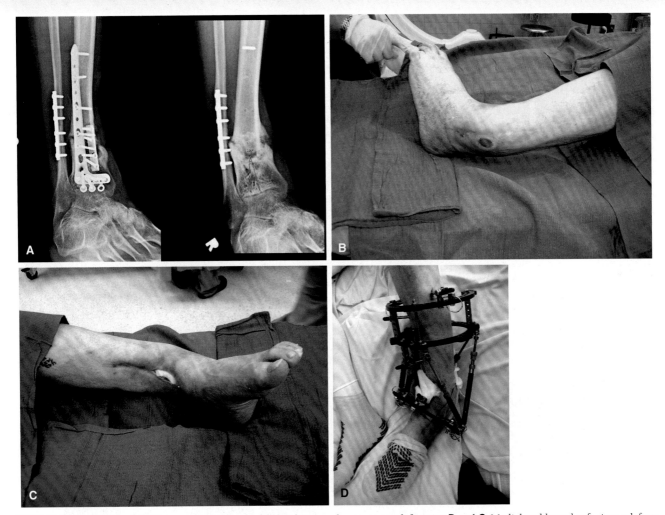

FIGURE 4.10 A, Infected tibial nonunion with unstable hardware and progressive deformity. **B** and **C**, Medial and lateral soft-tissue defects complicate this infected nonunion. **D**, Treatment with ring fixation to achieve deformity correction, bone reconstitution, and gradual soft-tissue closure, using distraction histogenesis techniques.

simultaneous correction in six axes (ie, coronal angulation, translation, sagittal angulation and translation, rotation and shortening). The hexapod-type frames allow the rings to be positioned in any orientation within their respective limb segment, ie, above the fracture site. The ability to apply a sophisticated ring fixator had been a very technically demanding technique that has been vastly simplified using this six-axis "hexapod" concept.

CHRONIC OSTEOMYELITIS

Debridement

Chronic infection after injury is largely a surgical disease and is rarely successfully treated by antibiotics alone. If infection persists after fracture union, hardware must be removed and avascular bone and soft tissue debrided. In general, previous incisions should be used, and all necrotic soft tissue should be removed. In the case of structures important to function and with questionable viability (tendons and ligaments), a staged approach can be taken. Care should be taken not to strip viable periosteum from bone.

Sclerotic or sequestered bone should be removed until all the remaining bone appears healthy and bleeds well. A high-speed bur, as described earlier, is a gentle way to accomplish bone removal.

Local Antibiotic Delivery

To prepare defects for grafting or coverage following debridement, antibiotic-impregnated polymethyl methacrylate (PMMA) beads, rods, or blocks are often placed to deliver a high concentration of antibiotics locally while avoiding systemic toxicity (**Figure 4.11A and B**). Antibiotic elutes from the PMMA by diffusion from the surface. Although most of the drug comes out in the first 24 hours, therapeutic levels of drugs have been detected in some cases for as long as 90 days. Tissue concentrations may be higher and persist longer than those seen in elution experiments. Local gentamicin concentrations around beads may be up to 200 times achievable tissue levels with systemic administration of the drug.[56] Serum and urine concentrations are at least 5 to 10 times less than tissue concentrations and are undetectable in many studies.

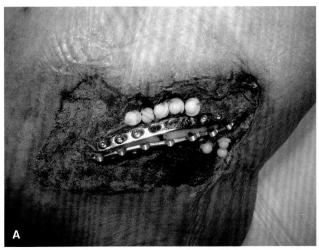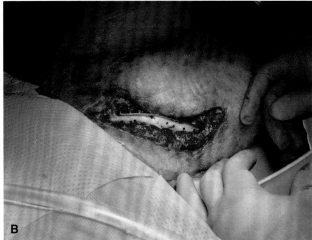

FIGURE 4.11 A and **B**, Antibiotic beads used to manage the dead space and provide high concentration of local antibiotics. Beads were used in the interim before removal of the infected clavicular plates.

Animal studies have suggested that treatment with antibiotic-impregnated PMMA beads for osteomyelitis is as good as or better than systemic antibiotic treatment.[57,58] The use of beads combined with systemic antibiotics significantly improved eradication of infection from rabbit wounds containing contaminated necrotic bone when compared with systemic antibiotics alone.[59] Necrotic bone gets no exposure to systemic antibiotics, whereas locally delivered antibiotics can achieve high concentrations.

In clinical studies of antibiotic bead treatment for chronic osteomyelitis, results have generally shown improved efficacy when the beads are used in conjunction with systemic antibiotics. Although many surgeons believe that antibiotic beads used to treat osteomyelitis should be removed, one retrospective study suggested that improved outcomes followed leaving the beads in situ.[60]

Many antibiotics have been used in beads. The antibiotic chosen must be water soluble, wide spectrum, well tolerated, heat stable, bactericidal in low concentrations, and available in powder form. Antibiotics can be mixed together. A common example in clinical use is tobramycin plus vancomycin. Palacos bone cement (Biomet Orthopedic, Inc., Warsaw, IN) is reported to elute antibiotics better than other cement types. We commonly use 2.4 g (two vials) of tobramycin powder added to a 40 g pouch of PMMA. More antibiotic can be added, but the volumetric ratio of 24 mL antibiotic to 120 mL Palacos cement is the limit for successful hardening. The mixture is made into beads in a commercially available mold or rolled by hand and strung on wire or suture. Beads can be stored in sterile containers at room temperature for long periods. When using antibiotic bead treatment, the wound should be closed, covered with a tissue flap, or covered with a semipermeable membrane (the antibiotic bead pouch technique).

After removal of an intramedullary rod, placement of antibiotic beads offers no mechanical support. Beads within the intramedullary canal must be removed within 10 to 14 days or subsequent removal may be extremely difficult.[50,61] Antibiotic cement rods can be custom-made at the time of surgery using varying chest tubes as molds.[61] Chest tubes are selected based on their inner diameter using the extracted nail as a template for the length and diameter of the fabricated rod (**Figure 4.12A and B**). A 3 mm guidewire is prebent and placed down the center of the chest tube mold to provide overall contour and dimensions of the fabricated rod. The liquid cement/antibiotic mixture is then poured into a cement gun and injected down the chest tube to surround the metal guide rod. Once the cement begins to cure, the chest tube is incised longitudinally and peeled off the intact cement rod. Following thorough medullary canal debridement, the antibiotic rod is inserted and does provide some mechanical stability. If additional debridements are necessary, the antibiotic rod is exchanged. At the time of definitive closure, the antibiotic rod is left intact in the canal, and the wound is closed directly over it. After a 6- to 8-week interval, bony reconstruction can be undertaken.

A variety of bioabsorbable carrier materials have been investigated to deliver antibiotics locally with an improved drug release and without a requirement for removal. These materials include demineralized bone matrix (DBM), bone graft,[62] lyophilized human fibrin, polyglycolic acid,[63] and polycaprolactone.[64] The material that has achieved the most clinical utility is calcium sulfate beads (**Figure 4.13**). The substance is osteoconductive and can also function as a bone graft substitute. Because the body absorbs it, calcium sulfate beads should release the entire load of antibiotic, whereas PMMA will only release ~20% of the impregnated drug. In a study of 25 patients with posttraumatic infected long bone defects, treatment with antibiotic-impregnated calcium sulfate beads eradicated the infection in 23 (92%) and healed 14 of 16 nonunions (nine required bone graft).[65] It has been noted that some patients have a sterile drainage that resolves when the pellets are absorbed.

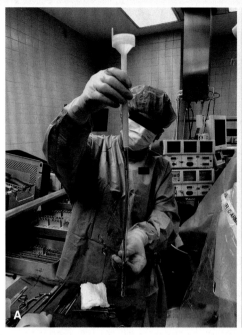

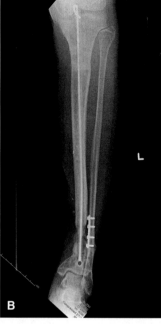

FIGURE 4.12 A, Antibiotic rod fashioned from a reaming guidewire, centered in a column of antibiotic cement. This was molded from a chest tube with the guidewire placed into the tube and then the tube injected with antibiotic-infused methyl methacrylate. **B**, The antibiotic rod is then inserted into the debrided medullary canal to manage the dead space, and provide stability and local antibiotic coverage.

Achieving Union: Reconstruction of Bone Defects After Debridement

Occasionally, the tissue remaining after adequate debridement has osteogenic potential, but union is prevented by excessive motion. Intervening fibrocartilaginous tissue has osteogenic potential, which can be exploited once torsional and axial instabilities are eliminated. The pluripotential cells that are present at the fracture site will selectively divide into the osteogenic precursor lineage in an environment of coupled stability and vascularity.[54] In this case, healing may be achieved by revision surgery with a variety of internal fixation devices. The stability afforded by nailing along with suppressive antibiotic therapy has been shown to produce excellent results. Select plating techniques often work well in metaphyseal infections once the soft tissues have been reconstructed and the wounds are under control.

Frequently, debridement will result in extensive gaps in the bone, which are beyond the healing capacity of the patient. If debridement includes significant portions of an articular surface, the reconstructive options are limited. Occasionally, resection of an infected joint can be treated with antibiotic-impregnated cement spacer, systemic antibiotics, and eventually prosthetic total joint arthroplasty. Often, however, it will require arthrodesis, resection arthroplasty, or amputation, particularly in compromised hosts or those infected with multiple or resistant organisms. When the resected bone involves mostly diaphysis or metaphysis, there are multiple reconstructive options to restore skeletal integrity.

Applied biologic stimuli for skeletal reconstruction are numerous; traditional techniques have included open autogenous bone grafting, intramedullary reaming, vascularized free-tissue transfers (muscle and bone), and distraction osteogenesis techniques. Other modalities that may provide a biologic "jump start" include electrical stimulation and ultrasound application. Recently, the injection or implantation of bone-growth factors and autogenous cellular grafts has been shown to augment healing in both animal and human nonunion studies. New composite bone grafting techniques[66] in conjunction with development of vascularized soft-tissue envelopes, the "Masquelet technique,"[67,68] as well as titanium segmental bone replacement[69] have all been shown to be successful approaches in reconstructing chronic segmental bone loss. Autogenous bone graft heals quickest and most reliably but is limited in quantity and involves donor site morbidity. Use of antibiotic-impregnated autogenous cancellous bone graft improves the eradication of infection and had no effect on the rate of graft maturation and incorporation.[70] Expanders can be added to autogenous bone graft to increase the volume available. Most function in osteoconduction, with variable and rather unpredictable

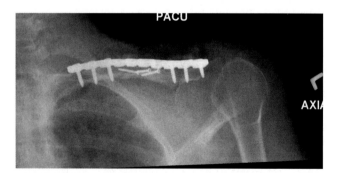

FIGURE 4.13 Calcium sulfate beads are still faintly visible above the clavicle plate, placed at the time of irrigation and debridement to manage the dead space and provide local antibiotic coverage. These beads rapidly degrade and disappear 10 to 12 weeks postimplantation.

degrees of osteoinduction. Examples include ceramics such as calcium phosphate, hydroxyapatite, tricalcium phosphates, or calcium sulfate. Bovine collagen composites with calcium phosphate (eg, collagraft) and demineralized bone matrix products function the same way. Alone, they are not able to stimulate sufficient bone to fill major gaps, but they may have a role when mixed with autograft. The exact indications and efficacy have not been clearly documented in the literature.

Allograft bone can be cancellous or cortical, or processed into components of bone such as demineralized bone matrix. Distraction osteogenesis is a technique for generating new bone by applying tension to healing mesenchymal tissues using external fixation techniques. In certain situations, other approaches such as primary shortening may be appropriate.

MASQUELET TECHNIQUE (MEMBRANE-DIRECTED BONE FORMATION)

The use of antibiotic spacers to develop a well-vascularized pseudomembrane has been developed as a precondition to bone grafting of critical sized defects. Masquelet first published his original clinical series in English in 2003.[68] He described a two-stage technique for the treatment of long bone defects that involved the formation of an induced membrane around a cement spacer. The spacer was removed at a second stage and replaced with autogenous iliac crest bone graft. He described a series of 35 patients treated with this technique for bone defects ranging from 5 to 25 cm.

Pelissier and other investigators have reported impressive results when performing this two-stage reconstructive procedure. Following the development of a healthy biologically competent wound, an antibiotic spacer is placed into the defect cavity and closed either by primary wound closure or by soft-tissue flap procedures. A tubular pseudomembrane is allowed to develop surrounding the spacer. Following complete wound healing, the antibiotic spacer is carefully removed preserving and maintaining the defect cavity and surrounding membrane. Traditional cancellous autografting was then placed directly into the tubularized membrane. Rapid reconstitution of the defect then occurred, with improved consolidation times and improved rates of union compared to historic rates of bone grafting large segmental defects (**Figure 4.4A-F**). Other authors have demonstrated similar improved union rates by placing composite grafts into these membranes, such as DBM plus bone morphogenic protein (BMP) adjuvants, vascularized free fibula grafts, and reamer-irrigator-aspirator–derived grafts. Many of these studies document the addition of culture-specific antibiotics to the cement spacer to facilitate the formation of infection-free membrane-directed bone formation. The improved graft performance is thought to be due to the induced membrane's ability to secrete various endogenous growth factors including VEGF, TGF-β1, and BMP-2.[67,71-73] These induced membranes have also been shown to favor the differentiation of human marrow stromal cells into an osteoblastic lineage.

DISTRACTION OSTEOGENESIS

There are two strategies for use of distraction osteogenesis in the face of bone deficits. The first involves acute shortening and compression at the fracture site after contouring the bone ends for stability, followed by corticotomy and lengthening at a separate metaphyseal location. Shortening acutely can be accomplished safely for defects up to 3 to 4 cm in the tibia and humerus.[74-76] More shortening can be tolerated acutely in a femoral defect up to 5 to 7 cm. In some situations, it is advantageous to decrease the transport distance and thus time in the frame. Shortening aids in soft-tissue coverage by decreasing tension and gaps in the open wound; this approach combined with negative-pressure dressings may allow wounds to be closed by delayed primary closure or healed by secondary intention or simple skin grafting.

Acute shortening more than 4 cm can cause the development of tortuous vasculature and actually produce a low flow state with detrimental consequences.[74,75] Open soft-tissue wounds when acutely compressed can become notably bunched and dysvascular with the development of significant edema and the possibility of additional tissue necrosis and infection. More than 4 cm may be safely accomplished in the femur; however, similar problems with wound edema and bunching may occur. A frame can be constructed to simultaneously compress at the fracture site and distract at a separate location. The second strategy involves putting on the frame with the limb at the correct length and alignment, and then using an internal lengthening of one or both segments to fill the gap. This is called bone transport, and the advantage is that the limb can be functional, even weight bearing, during the process.

Bone transport has a high rate of ultimate success, with many series reporting upward of 90% eventually healing with arrest of infection.[77,78] Unfortunately, most reports are small series, usually fewer than 20 patients, without comparison groups or controls. There is no donor site morbidity associated with transport because all the new bone comes from the injured leg. In addition, the leg can be functional and weight bearing during treatment. However, the treatment does require prolonged time in the external fixator, in some series up to 2 months per centimeter of gap filled. Substantial time is due to delayed healing of the docking site, which frequently requires bone grafting. Docking site healing problems occur in up to half the cases in some series. The prolonged time in the frame contributes to a high rate of complications, such as pin site infections, cellulitis, contracture, and edema.

CONCLUSIONS

Discussing and treating postoperative orthopaedic trauma complications is not the most glamorous part of our job. However, when carried out with a decisive evidence-based approach and communicating with the patient and entire treatment team, it can result in acceptable and successful outcomes.

What may be even more important is to consider these potential complications before they become a reality. Doing so early on allows for the identification of the modifiable patient-specific risk factors, the optimization of them, patient education, and avoidance of the detrimental denial that can exist when signs of infection or other complications present themselves. As mentioned earlier, the goals of our interventions include improving patient function and healing and do not include placating our own egos. It is imperative to maintain an objective eye in addition to relationships with our trauma surgeon, vascular surgeon, and plastic/reconstructive surgeon colleagues in order that we may work together to provide the appropriate treatment to all of our patients whether they are new patients, repeat patients, or long-standing patients.

REFERENCES

1. Sen CK, Roy S, Gordillo G. *13 - Wound Healing*. 4th ed. Philadelphia, PA: Elsevier Inc.; 2018. doi:10.1016/B978-0-323-35694-7.00013-8.
2. Giordano CP, Koval KJ, Zuckerman JD, Desai P. Fracture blisters. *Clin Orthop Relat Res*. 1994;(307):214-221. doi:10.1016/S0190-9622(09)80152-7.
3. Varela CD, Vaughan TK, Carr JB. Fracture blisters – clinical and pathological aspects. *J Orthop Trauma*. 1993;7(5):417-427.
4. Strauss EJ, Petrucelli G, Bong M, Koval KJ, Egol KA. Blisters associated with lower-extremity fracture: results of a prospective treatment protocol. *J Orthop Trauma*. 2006;20(9):618-622. doi:10.1097/01.bot.0000249420.30736.91.
5. Carr JB. Surgical techniques useful in the treatment of complex periarticular fractures of the lower extremity. *Orthop Clin North Am*. 1994;25(4):613-624. http://ovidsp.ovid.com/ovidweb.cgi?T=JS&PAGE=reference&D=med3&NEWS=N&AN=8090474.
6. Dodds MK, Daly A, Ryan K, D'Souza L. Effectiveness of "in-cast" pneumatic intermittent pedal compression for the pre-operative management of closed ankle fractures: a clinical audit. *Foot Ankle Surg*. 2014;20(1):40-43. doi:10.1016/j.fas.2013.09.004.
7. Thordarson DB. Complications after treatment of tibial pilon fractures: prevention and management strategies. *J Am Acad Orthop Surg*. 2000;8(4):253-265. doi:10.5435/00124635-200007000-00006.
8. Ren T, Ding L, Xue F, He Z, Xiao H. Risk factors for surgical site infection of pilon fractures. *Clinics*. 2015;70(6):419-422. doi:10.6061/clinics/2015(06)06.
9. Leone VJ, Ruland RT, Meinhard BP. The management of the soft tissues in pilon fractures. *Clin Orthop Relat Res*. 1993;(292):315-320. doi:10.1097/00003086-199307000-00041.
10. McFerran MA, Smith SW, Boulas HJ, Schwartz HS. Complications encountered in the treatment of pilon fractures. *J Orthop Trauma*. 1992;6(2):195-200. doi:10.1097/00005131-199206000-00011.
11. Watson J, Moed B, Karges D, Cramer K. Pilon fractures: treatment protocol based on severity of soft tissue injury. *Clin Orthop Relat Res*. 2000;(375):78-90. doi:10.1016/j.cpm.2012.01.001.
12. Gage MJ, Yoon RS, Egol KA, Liporace FA. Uses of negative pressure wound therapy in orthopedic trauma. *Orthop Clin North Am*. 2015;46(2):227-234. doi:10.1016/j.ocl.2014.11.002.
13. Brem MH, Bail HJ, Biber R. Value of incisional negative pressure wound therapy in orthopaedic surgery. *Int Wound J*. 2014;11(suppl 1):3-5. doi:10.1111/iwj.12252.
14. Stannard JP, Robinson JT, Anderson ER, Mcgwin G, Volgas DA, Alonso JE. Negative pressure wound therapy to treat hematomas and surgical incisions following high-energy trauma. *J Trauma*. 2006;60(6):1301-1306. doi:10.1097/01.ta.0000195996.73186.2e.
15. Stannard JP, Volgas DA, McGwin G, et al. Incisional negative pressure wound therapy after high-risk lower extremity fractures. *J Orthop Trauma*. 2012;26(1):37-42. doi:10.1097/BOT.0b013e318216b1e5.
16. Moués CM, Heule F, Hovius SER. A review of topical negative pressure therapy in wound healing: sufficient evidence? *Am J Surg*. 2011;201(4):544-556. doi:10.1016/j.amjsurg.2010.04.029.
17. Kawashima M, Tamura H, Nagayoshi I, Takao K, Yoshida K, Yamaguchi T. Hyperbaric oxygen therapy in orthopedic conditions. *Undersea Hyperb Med*. 2004;31(1):155-162. http://www.embase.com/search/results?subaction=viewrecord&from=export&id=L38958850%5Cnhttp://wx7cf7zp?h.search.serialssolutions.com?sid=EMBASE&issn=10662936&id=doi:&atitle=Hyperbaric+oxygen+therapy+in+orthopedic+conditions.&stitle=Undersea+Hyperb+Med&titl.
18. Hunt TK, Zederfeldt B, Goldstick TK. Oxygen and healing. *Am J Surg*. 1969;118(4):521-525. doi:10.1016/0002-9610(69)90174-3.
19. Goldman RJ. Hyperbaric oxygen therapy for wound healing and limb salvage: a systematic review. *PM R*. 2009;1(5):471-489. doi:10.1016/j.pmrj.2009.03.012.
20. Skyhar MJ, Hargens AR, Strauss MB, Gershuni DH, Hart GB, Akeson WH. Hyperbaric oxygen reduces edema and necrosis of skeletal muscle in compartment syndromes associated with hemorrhagic hypotension. *J Bone Joint Surg Am*. 1986;68(8):1218-1224. http://www.ncbi.nlm.nih.gov/pubmed/3021776.
21. Radonic V, Baric D, Petricevic A, Kovacevic H, Sapunar D, Glavina-Durdov M. War injuries of the crural arteries. *Br J Surg*. 1995;82(6):777-783. doi:10.1002/bjs.1800820620.
22. Dauwe PH, Pulikkottil BJ, Lavery L, Stuzin JM, Rohrich RJ. Does hyperbaric oxygen therapy work in facilitating acute wound healing: a systematic review. *Plast Reconstr Surg*. 2014;133(2):208e-215e. doi:10.1097/01.prs.0000436849.79161.a4.
23. Valerio IL, Campbell P, Sabino J, Dearth CL, Fleming M. The use of urinary bladder matrix in the treatment of trauma and combat casualty wound care. *Regen Med*. 2015;10(5):611-622. doi:10.2217/rme.15.34.
24. Kraemer BA, Geiger SE, Deigni OA, Watson JT. Management of open lower extremity wounds with concomitant fracture using a porcine urinary bladder matrix. *Wounds*. 2016;28(11):387-394. PMID: 27861131.
25. Fleming ME, O'Daniel A, Bharmal H, Valerio I. Application of the Orthoplastic reconstructive ladder to preserve lower extremity amputation length. *Ann Plast Surg*. 2014;73(2):183-189. doi:10.1097/SAP.0b013e3182a638d8.
26. Quaba A. Local flaps. In: Court-Brown CM, McQueen MM, Quaba AA, eds. *Management of Open Fractures*. London, England: Martin Dunitz Publishers; 1996:195-209.
27. Georgescu AV. Propeller perforator flaps in distal lower leg: evolution and clinical applications. *Arch Plast Surg*. 2012;39(2):94-105. doi:10.5999/aps.2012.39.2.94.
28. Quaba O, Quaba A. Pedicled perforator flaps for the lower limb. *Semin Plast Surg*. 2006;20(2):103-111. doi:10.1055/s-2006-941717.
29. Jakubietz RG, Jakubietz MG, Gruenert JG, Kloss DF. The 180-degree perforator-based propeller flap for soft tissue coverage of the distal, lower extremity: a new method to achieve reliable coverage of the distal lower extremity with a local, fasciocutaneous perforator flap. *Ann Plast Surg*. 2007;59(6):667-671. doi:10.1097/SAP.0b013e31803c9b66.
30. Uçkay I, Hoffmeyer P, Lew D, Pittet D. Prevention of surgical site infections in orthopaedic surgery and bone trauma: state-of-the-art update. *J Hosp Infect*. 2013;84(1):5-12. doi:10.1016/j.jhin.2012.12.014.
31. Beldi G, Bisch-Knaden S, Banz V, Mühlemann K, Candinas D. Impact of intraoperative behavior on surgical site infections. *Am J Surg*. 2009;198(2):157-162. doi:10.1016/j.amjsurg.2008.09.023.
32. Stephens B, Murphy A, Mihalko W. The effects of nutritional deficiencies, smoking and systemic disease on orthopaedic outcomes. *J Bone Joint Surg*. 2013;95(23):2153-2157. http://www.ejbjs.org/cgi/content/extract/81/12/1772.
33. Marchant MH, Viens NA, Cook C, Vail TP, Bolognesi MP. The impact of glycemic control and diabetes mellitus on perioperative outcomes after total joint arthroplasty. *J Bone Joint Surg Am*. 2009;91(7):1621-1629. doi:10.2106/JBJS.H.00116.
34. Liporace FA, Donley BG, Pinzur MS, Lin SS. Complications of ankle fracture in patients with diabetes. *J Am Acad Orthop Surg*. 2008;16(3):159-170.
35. Yang K, Yeo SJ, Lee BP, Lo NN. Total knee arthroplasty in diabetic patients: a study of 109 consecutive cases. *J Arthroplasty*. 2001;16(1):102-106. doi:10.1054/arth.2001.19159.
36. Karunakar MA, Staples KS. Does stress-induced hyperglycemia increase the risk of perioperative infectious complications in orthopaedic trauma patients? *J Orthop Trauma*. 2010;24(12):752-756. doi:10.1097/BOT.0b013e3181d7aba5.
37. Richards JE, Hutchinson J, Mukherjee K, et al. Stress hyperglycemia and surgical site infection in stable nondiabetic adults with orthopedic injuries. *J Trauma Acute Care Surg*. 2014;76(4):1070-1075. doi:10.1097/TA.0000000000000177.

38. Lowenberg D, Watson JT, Levin LS. Advances in the understanding and treatment of musculoskeletal infections. *Instr Course Lect*. 2015;64:37-49.

39. Mader J, Cripps M, Calhoun J. Adult posttraumatic osteomyelitis of the tibia. *Clin Orthop*. 1999;(360):14-21.

40. Friedrich B, Klaue P. Mechanical stability and post traumatic osteitis: an experimental evaluation of the relation between infection of bone and internal fixation. *Injury*. 1977;9(1):23-29. http://www.embase.com/search/results?subaction=viewrecord&from=export&id=L8149445%5Cnhttp://sfx.library.uu.nl/utrecht?sid=EMBASE&issn=00201383&id=doi:&atitle=Mechanical+stability+and+post+traumatic+osteitis%3A+An+experimental+evaluation+of+the+relation+be.

41. Merritt K, Dowd JD. Role of internal fixation in infection of open fractures: studies with Staphylococcus aureus and Proteus mirabilis. *J Orthop Res*. 1987;5(1):23-28. doi:10.1002/jor.1100050105.

42. Berkes M, Obremskey WT, Scannell B, Ellington JK, Hymes RA, Bosse M. Maintenance of hardware after early postoperative infection following fracture internal fixation. *J Bone Joint Surg Am*. 2010;92(4):823-828. doi:10.2106/JBJS.I.00470.

43. Ueng SW, Wei FC, Shih CH. Management of femoral diaphyseal infected nonunion with antibiotic beads local therapy, external skeletal fixation, and staged bone grafting. *J Trauma*. 1999;46(1):97-103. doi:10.1097/00005373-199901000-00016.

44. Zimmerli W, Widmer AF, Blatter M, Frei R, Ochsner PE. Role of rifampin for treatment of orthopedic implant – related staphylococcal infections a randomized controlled trial. *J Am Med Assoc*. 1998;279(19):1537-1541.

45. Rightmire E, Zurakowski D, Vrahas M. Acute infections after fracture repair: management with hardware in place. *Clin Orthop Relat Res*. 2008;466(2):466-472. doi:10.1007/s11999-007-0053-y.

46. Tetsworth K, Cierny G. Osteomyelitis debridement techniques. *Clin Orthop Relat Res*. 1999;(360):87-96.

47. Keating JF, Blachut PA, O'Brien PJ, Meek RN, Broekhuyse H. Reamed Nailing of open tibial fractures: does the antibiotic bead pouch reduce the deep infection rate? *J Orthop Trauma*. 1996;10(5):298-303. doi:10.1097/00005131-199607000-00002.

48. Cierny G, Mader JT, Penninck JJ. A clinical staging system for adult osteomyelitis. *Clin Orthop Relat Res*. 2003;414:7-24. doi:10.1097/01.blo.0000088564.81746.62.

49. Patzakis MJ, Greene N, Holtom P, Shepherd L, Bravos P, Sherman R. Culture results in open wound treatment with muscle transfer for tibial osteomyelitis. *Clin Orthop Relat Res*. 1999;(360):66-70.

50. Patzakis MJ, Zalavras CG. Chronic posttraumatic osteomyelitis and infected nonunion of the tibia: current management concepts. *J Am Acad Orthop Surg*. 2005;13(6):417-427.

51. Watson J, Gurley G. Transcutaneous oxygen tension monitoring in the preoperative evaluation of soft tissue injuries in closed fractures about the ankle. *Ortho Trans*. 1997;21:585-586.

52. Stinner DJ, Hsu JR, Wenke JC. Negative pressure wound therapy reduces the effectiveness of traditional local antibiotic depot in a large complex musculoskeletal wound animal model. *J Orthop Trauma*. 2012;26(9):512-518. doi:10.1097/BOT.0b013e318251291b.

53. Maiocchi A, Aronson J. *Operative Principles of Ilizarov: Fracture Treatment, Nonunion, Osteomyelitis, Lengthening, Deformity Correction*. Baltimore, MD: Williams & Wilkins; 1991.

54. Catagni MA, Guerreschi F, Holman JA, Cattaneo R. Distraction osteogenesis in the treatment of stiff hypertrophic nonunions using the Ilizarov apparatus. *Clin Orthop Relat Res*. 1994;(301):159-163. doi:10.1097/00003086-199404000-00025.

55. Tetsworth KD, Paley D. Accuracy of correction of complex lower-extremity deformities by the Ilizarov method. *Clin Orthop Relat Res*. 1994;(301):102-110. http://eutils.ncbi.nlm.nih.gov/eutils/elink.fcgi?dbfrom=pubmed&id=8156660&retmode=ref&cmd=prlinks%5Cnpapers2://publication/uuid/0DD12DAE-E5FD-4231-8DF9-ADBD8E9FCF8D.

56. Wahlig H, Dingeldein E, Bergmann R, Reuss K. The release of gentamicin from polymethylmethacrylate beads. An experimental and pharmacokinetic study. *J Bone Joint Surg Br*. 1978;60-B(2):270-275.

57. Evans RP, Nelson CL. Gentamicin-impregnated polymethylmethacrylate beads compared with systemic antibiotic therapy in the treatment of chronic osteomyelitis. *Clin Orthop Relat Res*. 1993;(295):37-42. http://www.ncbi.nlm.nih.gov/pubmed/8403668.

58. Seligson D, Mehta S, Voos K, Henry SL, Johnson JR. The use of antibiotic-impregnated polymethylmethacrylate beads to prevent the evolution of localized infection. *J Orthop Trauma*. 1992;6(4):401-406. doi:10.1097/00005131-199212000-00001. PMID: 1494090.

59. Chen NT, Hong HZ, Hooper DC, May JWJ. The effect of systemic antibiotic and antibiotic-impregnated polymethylmethacrylate beads on the bacterial clearance in wounds containing contaminated dead bone. *Plast Reconstr Surg*. 1993;92(7):1303-1305. http://ovidsp.ovid.com/ovidweb.cgi?T=JS&PAGE=reference&D=med3&NEWS=N&AN=8248406.

60. Henry SL, Hood G a, Seligson D. Long-term implantation of gentamicin-polymethylmethacrylate antibiotic beads. *Clin Orthop Relat Res*. 1993;(295):47-53. http://www.ncbi.nlm.nih.gov/pubmed/8403670.

61. Paley D, Herzenberg JE. Intramedullary infections treated with antibiotic cement rods: preliminary results in nine cases. *J Orthop Trauma*. 2002;16(10):723-729. doi:10.1097/00005131-200211000-00007.

62. Miclau T, Dahners LE, Lindsey RW. In vitro pharmacokinetics of antibiotic release from locally implantable materials. *J Orthop Res*. 1993;11(5):627-632. doi:10.1002/jor.1100110503.

63. Galandiuk S, Wrightson W, Young S, Myers S. Absorbable,delayed-release antibiotic beads reduce surgical wound infection. *Am Surg*. 1997;63:831-835.

64. Rutledge B, Huyette D, Day D, Anglen J. Treatment of osteomyelitis with local antibiotics delivered via bioabsorbable polymer. *Clin Orthop Relat Res*. 2003;(411):280-287. doi:10.1097/01.blo.0000065836.93465.ed.

65. McKee MD, Wild LM, Schemitsch EH, Waddell JP. The use of an antibiotic impregnated, osteoconductive, bioabsorbable bone substitute in the treatment of infected long bone defects: early results of a prospective trial. *J Orthop Trauma*. 2002;16(9):622-627. doi:10.1097/00005131-200210000-00002.

66. Lindsey R, Wood G, Ssadasivian K. Grafting long bone fractures with demineralized bone matrix putty enriched with bone marrow: pilot findings. *Orthopedics*. 2006;29(10):939-942.

67. Pelissier P, Martin D, Baudet J, Lepreux S, Masquelet AC. Behaviour of cancellous bone graft placed in induced membranes. *Br J Plast Surg*. 2002;55(7):596-598. doi:10.1054/bjps.2002.3936.

68. Masquelet AC. Muscle reconstruction in reconstructive surgery: soft tissue repair and long bone reconstruction. *Langenbecks Arch Surg*. 2003;388(5):344-346. doi:10.1007/s00423-003-0379-1.

69. Attias N, Lindsey RW. Management of large segmental tibial defects using a cylindrical mesh cage. *Clin Orthop Relat Res*. 2006;(450):259-266. doi:10.1097/01.blo.0000223982.29208.a4.

70. Chan YS, Ueng SWN, Wang CJ, Lee SS, Chen CY, Shin CH. Antibiotic-impregnated autogenic cancellous bone grafting is an effective and safe method for the management of small infected tibial defects: a comparison study. *J Trauma*. 2000;48(2):246-255. doi:10.1097/00005373-200002000-00009.

71. Pelissier P, Masquelet AC, Bareille R, Mathoulin Pelissier S, Amedee J. Induced membranes secrete growth factors including vascular and osteoinductive factors and could stimulate bone regeneration. *J Orthop Res*. 2004;22(1):73-79. doi:10.1016/S0736-0266(03)00165-7.

72. Viateau V, Guillemin G, Bousson V. Long-bone critical-size defects treated with tissue-engineered grafts: a study on sheep. *J Orthop Res*. 2007;25:741-749. doi:10.1002/jor.

73. Gruber HE, Riley FE, Hoelscher GL, et al. Osteogenic and chondrogenic potential of biomembrane cells from the PMMA-segmental defect rat model. *J Orthop Res*. 2012;30(8):1198-1212. doi:10.1002/jor.22047.

74. de Pablos J, Barrios C, Alfaro C, Canadell J. Large experimental segmental bone defects treated by bone transportation with monolateral external distractors. *Clin Orthop Relat Res*. 1994;(298):259-265. http://www.ncbi.nlm.nih.gov/entrez/query.fcgi?cmd=Retrieve&db=PubMed&dopt=Citation&list_uids=8118984.

75. Mekhail AO, Abraham E, Gruber B, Gonzalez M. Bone transport in the management of posttraumatic bone defects in the lower extremity. *J Trauma*. 2004;56(2):368-378. doi:10.1097/01.TA.0000057234.48501.30.

76. Mahaluxmivala J, Nadarajah R, Allen PW, Hill RA. Ilizarov external fixator: acute shortening and lengthening versus bone transport in the management of tibial non-unions. *Injury*. 2005;36(5):662-668. doi:10.1016/j.injury.2004.10.027.

77. Dendrinos GK, Kontos S, Lyritsis E. Use of the Ilizarov technique associated for treatment with of of the tibia infection. *Surgery*. 1995;77(6):835-846.

78. Marsh JL, Prokuski L, Biermann JS. Chronic infected tibial nonunions with bone loss. Conventional techniques versus bone transport. *Clin Orthop Relat Res*. 1994;(301):139-146. http://www.ncbi.nlm.nih.gov/pubmed/8156664.

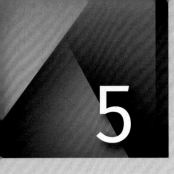

5

Biomechanics of Nonoperative and Operative Fracture Treatment

Amrut Borade

Harish Kempegowda

Terri Zachos

Daniel S. Horwitz

INTRODUCTION

Understanding and effective application of the biomechanical principles of fracture fixation are key to its success in achieving union and rehabilitation. The type of fixation chosen for each case is determined by multiple factors including soft-tissue status, fracture classification, age, and surgeon preference. Rehabilitation and return to activity are no doubt crucial determinants of the patient satisfaction after fracture treatment. The delicate balance between mobility and stability demands adequate stability to allow adequate mobility. In this chapter, we intend to explore the biomechanical principles of fracture fixation with special focus on their significance for rehabilitation and return to activity. A comprehensive review of fractures based on anatomical location is discussed; but it should be noted that pathological fractures, periprosthetic fractures, and pediatric fractures will not be addressed in this chapter.

GENERAL BIOMECHANICAL PRINCIPLES OF NONOPERATIVE TREATMENT OF FRACTURES

Nonoperative treatment options including functional braces, casts, and splints are helpful in providing temporary pain relief before definitive fixation is undertaken. They are stress sharing and promote secondary bone healing through callus formation, but they are rarely used nowadays for definitive treatment due to the requirements of immobilization. In addition, these options are quite cumbersome for the patients to use for a long-term duration. Casting works by immobilizing the joint above and below to prevent rotation

and translation of the fracture fragments. Functional fracture bracing works on the principle of hydraulic effect by containing the soft-tissue mass as a unit around the fracture between the joints. This hydraulic effect and loading of soft tissues during weight bearing enhances fracture healing while maintaining the fracture alignment. Splints are commonly used for upper extremities, especially hand injuries. Splints work as first-class lever systems with three pressure points acting on the extremities.[1] They support weak muscles and counteract the pull of stronger muscles. Static splints immobilize joints and maintain correct joint alignment. Dynamic splints provide a low magnitude force over a prolonged duration to facilitate remodeling of new tissue.[1]

GENERAL BIOMECHANICAL PRINCIPLES OF EXTERNAL FIXATION

External fixation is mainly used as a temporary method of fixation in cases of open fracture management in order to provide time for soft-tissue healing. Secondary bone healing with callus formation is initiated, but solid bone union is not the usual outcome. The factors determining the stability of the construct are the number of pins placed, the diameter of pins, the distance between the pins, the distance of the pins from the fracture, the diameter of rods, the number of rods, and the distance of the rods from the skin surface and from each other.[2] External fixator pins which traverse multiple soft-tissue planes may contribute to the loss of joint motion and stiffness. Small wire ring fixators, due to their unique design, are capable of allowing early mobilization and weight bearing.

GENERAL BIOMECHANICAL PRINCIPLES OF INTERNAL FRACTURE FIXATION

A thorough discussion of the biomechanical principles of fracture fixation requires explanation of some basic definitions. Strain of a body is defined as the change in length divided by initial length. Strain with reference to fracture is the relative change in fracture gap divided by the fracture gap (fracture gap strain ΔL/L).[3] Strain tolerance or elongation is the capacity to tolerate a certain amount of deformation before failure occurs.[4] Strength of the tissue is the ability to withstand force without failure. Lamellar bone undergoes failure at 2% elongation. Fibrous tissue-tendon-bone show decreasing tolerance for elongation in that order. The sequence represents conditioning of a fracture site for solid bony union. Solid bone union has the least tolerance for elongation.[4] Stability of fracture fixation is the degree of load-dependent displacement of fracture surfaces. Absolute stability designates a state of no relative motion at the location of the fracture under observation. It involves restricting mobility to the extent that little displacement occurs at the fracture site under functional load. It is classically achieved through compressive preload and friction. Relative stability designates a state of controlled motion at the fracture site. The influence of stability on the type of bone healing is well identified.[5] Amount of strain at the fracture site is a function of stability. Absolute stability maintains the strain at less than 2% and achieves primary bone healing (endosteal healing). Relative stability maintains strain between 2% and 10% and achieves secondary bone healing (healing with callus formation). Bone formation is impossible at strains greater than 10%.[3] Rigidity is the capacity to fight deformation and motion. Rigidity is the term mainly used with reference to tissues playing a role in healing. Fracture union is influenced by the interfragmentary movements occurring due to the interaction between the load at the fracture and the stability of fixation. Minimal interfragmentary movement with stiff fixation results in limited stimulation of callus formation.[4] Optimum interfragmentary movement with a relatively less stiff fixation stimulates callus formation and improves the healing process.[6] An unstable fixation results in nonunion.[6]

COMPRESSIVE PRELOAD AND FRICTION

Compressive preload (static compression which is more than traction forces acting at fracture site) creates close contact between the fracture fragments and contributes to absolute stability. Compressive preload does not tend to cause pressure necrosis. Friction is created by pressing fracture surfaces against each other. Friction along with the geometry of the fracture surfaces in contact (interdigitating) counteracts the tangentially acting shear forces produced by torque applied to the limb. This prevents sliding displacement.

LOAD BEARING AND LOAD SHARING IMPLANT

A load bearing implant bears the forces functioning at the fracture site. A load sharing implant adds to the frictional resistance between the fracture ends in providing the stability at the fracture site. In the load bearing situation, the implant assumes all the forces, and in the load sharing situation different levels of force distribution between the implant and the bone exist.[7,8]

FRACTURE CONFIGURATION AND STABILITY AFTER INTERNAL FIXATION

Fracture configuration plays a role in the choice of the implant utilized for fixation and the stability which can be achieved. Anatomic reduction can be easily achieved in simple transverse or oblique fractures. In complex fractures, absolute stability may or may not be achieved. For example, in fractures with butterfly fragments, interfragmentary screws can provide absolute stability. In comminuted fractures, relative stability is the desirable standard. Absolute and relative stability by themselves do not have prognostic significance for the outcome of fixation.

GENERAL BIOMECHANICAL PRINCIPLES OF INTRAMEDULLARY NAIL FIXATION

Internal fixation with intramedullary (IM) nailing is commonly utilized for treatment of diaphyseal fractures of long bones (**Figure 5.1**).[9,10] IM nails act as load sharing internal splints. The material properties, the cross-sectional shape, and the diameter are the chief factors playing roles in the structural stiffness of an IM nail. Load shared by the nail is dependent on factors including the nail size, the number of interlocking screws, and the distance of interlocking screws from fracture site. Torsion, compression, and tension are the physiologic loads acting on an IM nail.

Titanium alloy and 316L stainless steel are the most common materials used in IM nails. Titanium alloy has a modulus of elasticity approximately half of that of 316L stainless steel and approximately equal to that of the modulus of the cortical bone.[11] Clinical results with both titanium alloy and 316L stainless steel are found to be equivalent despite the reported laboratory differences. Torsional rigidity of the nail is influenced by its cross-sectional shape and contact with the endosteal bone within the medullary canal, but since most nails are similar in design, there is less than 15% difference in biomechanical stability between the available implants.[12] Bending rigidity is affected by the nail diameter. Bending rigidity for nails is proportional to the nail diameter to the third power and torsional rigidity is proportional to the fourth power.[11] Larger diameter creates the construct of a tight fit within IM canal which reduces the movement between the nail and bone. Surgeons usually determine the number of interlocking screws based on the fracture location,

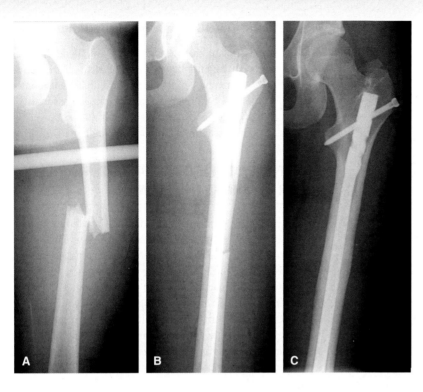

FIGURE 5.1 Anteroposterior radiographs of diaphyseal fracture of a femur (**A**) internally fixed with an intramedullary nail (**B**). Patient was allowed immediate weight bearing. Active and active-assisted range-of-motion exercises were started in immediate postoperative period. At 3 months, bony union was achieved. (**C**) Good range of motion of the hip (flexion 110°, extension 30°) and knee (0°-100°) with full weight bearing was achieved.

the severity of fracture comminution, and the fit of the nail within the canal. Midshaft fractures have the greatest fixation stability due to the isthmic cortical contact. Oblique and comminuted fractures rely on interlocking screws for stability similar to metaphyseal fractures. The closer the fracture is to the distal interlocking screws, the less cortical contact the nail has, which leads to increased stress on interlocking screws.[13] Interlocking screws restrict translation and rotation at the fracture site, yet minor movements occur between the nail and the screws permitting controlled motion and relative stability. Contemporary nails offer interlocking screws in multiple planes which offer additional stability. Multiple proximal and multiple distal interlocking screws and use of larger diameter IM nail can allow stable IM fixation of an unstable fracture pattern. Reaming of the medullary canal increases the contact area between the nail and the cortical bone, with an increase of 38% with every 1 mm of reaming. In addition, reaming makes the insertion of larger diameter nails possible which increases rigidity in bending and torsion.[14] Nails >9 mm in diameter have larger interlocking screws, and for all these reasons reamed nails generally provide better biomechanical fixation than unreamed nails.[15] Reaming has some disadvantages including diminishment of cortical wall thickness and generation of heat.

GENERAL BIOMECHANICAL PRINCIPLES OF INTERNAL FIXATION WITH PLATES

The extramedullary location of plates allows for application in diverse fracture patterns. A variety of plates are available including reconstruction plates, tubular plates, dynamic compression plates (DCPs), limited contact dynamic compression plates (LC-DCPs), locking compression plates (LCPs), and precontoured periarticular LCPs. With the introduction of newer designs of LCPs, reconstruction and tubular plates are less commonly used.

Plate length affects stiffness of the fixation construct. Increase in plate length increases the lever arm and decreases the pullout force acting on screws. The working length of a plate is the distance across a fracture site between the two nearest fixation points of the bone to the plate, and the addition of an extra screw nearest to the fracture site increases the axial stiffness to greatest extent. Working length of the plate influences the axial stiffness of the plate. DCPs have the ability to resist axial, torsional, and bending loads. When loaded axially in tension and compression, they convert the forces to shear stress at the plate-bone interface.[3] The axial forces are countered by frictional force between the plate and bone. The frictional force is measured by multiplying frictional coefficient between the plate and bone with force applied by screws in the plate. Screw torque when utilizing compression plating needs to be sufficient enough to prevent motion, but it should not exceed the shear resistance of the bone which can cause screw stripping and loss of fixation. DCPs may achieve primary bone healing through anatomic reduction and rigid fixation across a fracture sites, but this depends on the fracture pattern (**Figure 5.2**).

LCPs have uniquely designed screws with threaded heads which lock into the holes of the plate and provide the angular stability (**Figures 5.3** and **5.4**). LCPs do not rely on frictional force between the plate and bone to achieve compression and stability. Recently designed precontoured periarticular plates allow placement of multiple locking

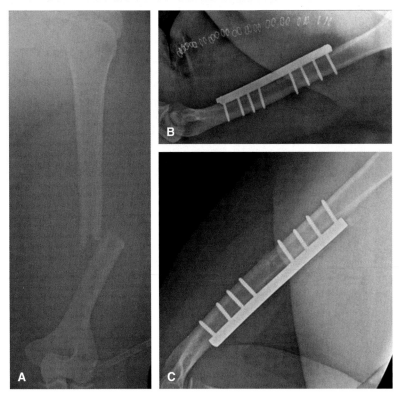

FIGURE 5.2 Anteroposterior radiographs of a humeral diaphyseal fracture (**A**) in a polytraumatized patient fixed with dynamic compression plate (**B**). Active and active-assisted exercises of the shoulder and elbow were started immediately. Patient was allowed partial weight bearing for utilizing crutch support. At 3 months, bony union was evident (**C**) with excellent range of motion of the shoulder (elevation 110°) and elbow (0°-120°).

screws in the periarticular zone creating angular stability and making early range of motion of the joint possible (**Figures 5.5** and **5.6**). While this is advantageous to maintain axial alignment and articular reduction, all the load at the fracture site is transmitted to the plate. LCPs carry more chances of implant failure as they act as load bearing implant. This predisposes to risk of loss of fixation and articular reduction on axial loading. For this reason, immediate weight bearing cannot be advised with LCPs. The recent instrumentation allows passing diaphyseal portion

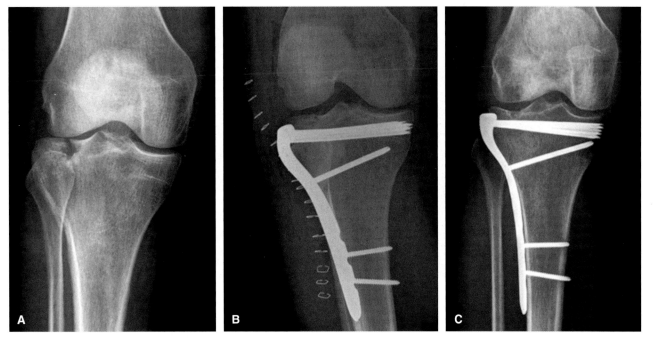

FIGURE 5.3 Anteroposterior radiographs of a lateral tibial plateau fracture (**A**) treated with anatomic reduction and rigid fixation with periarticular locking compression plate (**B**). Active and active-assisted exercises of the knee and ankle were started immediate postoperatively. Toe touch weight bearing was allowed preventing any axial loading. Partial weight bearing was initiated at 12 weeks progressing to full weight bearing. At 4 months, complete bony union (**C**) and good knee range of motion (0°-100°) was achieved.

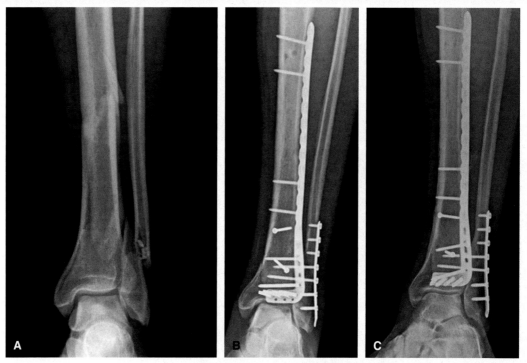

FIGURE 5.4 Anteroposterior radiographs of a pilon fracture (**A**) fixed with periarticular locking compression plate and interfragmentary screws (**B**). Active range-of-motion exercises of the ankle were initiated immediately postoperatively. Toe touch weight bearing was allowed initially to prevent any axial loading. Partial weight bearing was initiated at 12 weeks progressing to full weight bearing. At 4 months, bony union was achieved (**C**) with good range of motion of the ankle (dorsiflexion 40° and plantar flexion 20°).

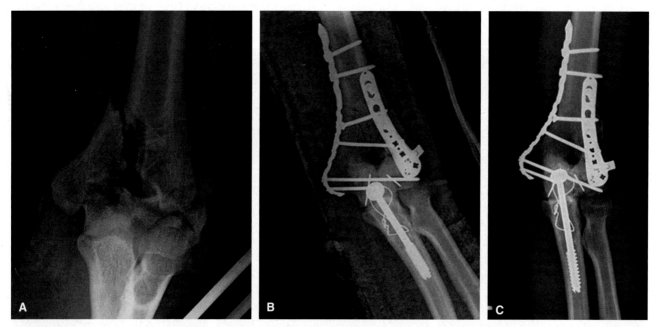

FIGURE 5.5 Anteroposterior radiographs of a distal humerus fracture (**A**) fixed with periarticular locking compression plates placed in perpendicular configuration (**B**). Active and active-assisted range-of-motion exercises were started with active flexion (to activate reflex arc of triceps) and passive extension (to prevent loading of triceps) taking into consideration the olecranon osteotomy. Patient was advised against any weight bearing or axial loading for initial 6 weeks. At 3 months, bony union was complete (**C**) with good range of motion of the elbow (10°-100°).

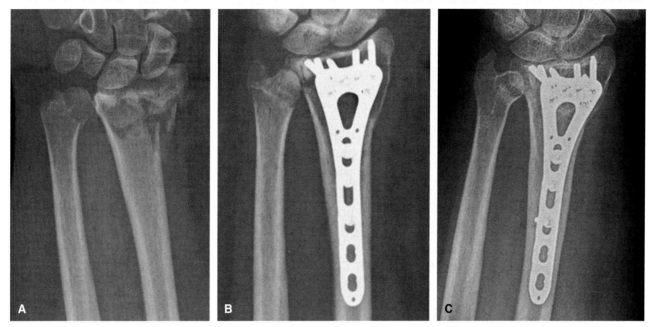

FIGURE 5.6 Anteroposterior radiographs of a distal radius fracture (**A**) fixed with periarticular locking compression plate (**B**). Immobilization was advised for initial 6 weeks taking into consideration the concomitant ulna fracture and osteoporosis. Active and active-assisted range-of-motion excercises were initiated at 6 weeks, but axial loading through the weight bearing was allowed only after bony union was achieved at 2 months (**C**). Good range of motion of the wrist was achieved at last follow-up (dorsiflexion 70°, palmar flexion 40°).

of LCP in percutaneous manner and minimizes the surgical soft-tissue injury. Unlike DCP, there is potential for motion between fracture fragments with LCP. The design of LCP can completely eliminate motion if desired. Depending upon the exact construct chosen, the number and the location of locking screws LCPs can provide either relative or absolute stability. LCPs facilitate secondary bone healing by optimizing the strain at the fracture site.[16] Combination holes in the LCP make blending of locked and compression plating possible.

DIFFERENT MODES OF PLATING

Compression Plate

A plate is used to achieve compression by bringing the two fracture fragments closer to each other and creating intimate opposition through different techniques (**Figure 5.7**).

Neutralization Plate

A lag screw is often used to counteract bending, shear, and rotational forces at a fracture site by direct compression. Since compression has already been achieved, the function of a plate is to maintain the reduction (**Figure 5.8**).

Bridge/Spanning Plate

This involves use of a plate as an *"extramedullary splint"* usually in cases of comminuted fractures. It is used to fix the two main fragments while the intermediate zone of comminution is bypassed and protected from devitalization (**Figure 5.9**).

Buttress Plate

A plate is contoured to match the contour of the underlying bone and is applied to a periarticular fracture. It creates direct compression in direction perpendicular to the long axis of bone and parallel to articular surface to maintain stability and to prevent collapse (**Figure 5.10**).

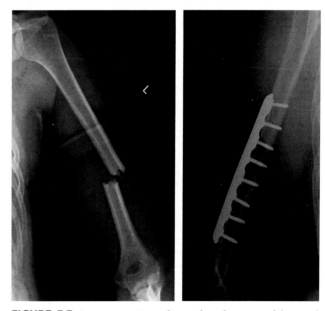

FIGURE 5.7 Anteroposterior radiographs of a case of humeral diaphyseal fracture treated with a dynamic compression plate applied as compression plate.

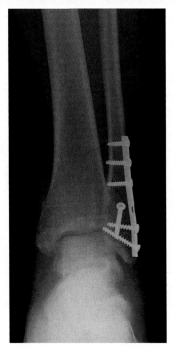

FIGURE 5.8 Anteroposterior radiograph of a case of oblique fracture of distal fibula fixed with a lag screw and a neutralization plate.

Antiglide Plate

A plate by virtue of its placement with respect to an oblique fracture acts to counteract the shear forces acting at the fracture site (**Figure 5.11**).

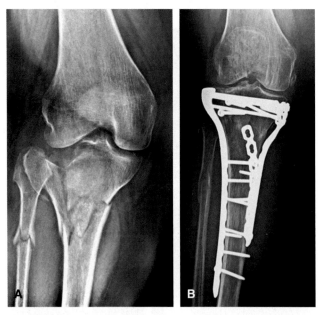

FIGURE 5.9 A and **B**, Anteroposterior radiographs of a case of bicondylar tibial plateau fracture fixed with posteromedial and lateral locking compression plates (LCPs). The posteromedial LCP is applied in buttress plate mode.

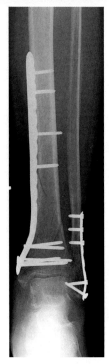

FIGURE 5.10 Anteroposterior radiograph of a case of comminuted distal tibia-fibula fracture treated with bridge plating.

BIOMECHANICAL PRINCIPLES OF SPECIAL CONSTRUCTS

A sliding hip screw, used for either a basicervical femoral neck fracture or an intertrochanteric femur fracture, works on the principle of controlled collapse (**Figure 5.12**). The screw plate angle closest to the combined force vector allows optimum sliding and impaction. Stability and the ability to resist medial displacement have been shown to be achieved with a sliding hip screw construct.[17] Cephalomedullary nails work on the same principle when used for these fractures.

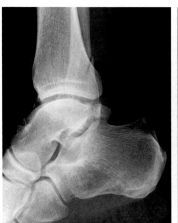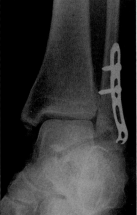

FIGURE 5.11 Radiographs of a case of oblique fracture of lateral malleolus treated with application of the antiglide plate.

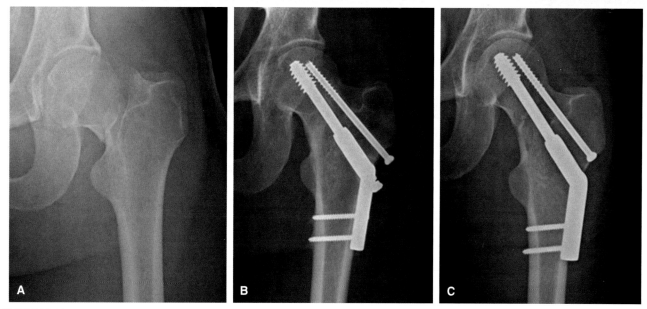

FIGURE 5.12 Anteroposterior radiographs of a basicervical femoral neck fracture (**A**) fixed with a sliding hip screw (**B**). Immediate weight bearing was allowed with the hip and knee range-of-motion exercises. **C**, At 2 months, union was achieved with collapse at fracture site as evident by protrusion of sliding hip screw. Full weight bearing with good range of motion of the hip (flexion 100°, extension 20°) and knee (10°-100°) was achieved.

CONCLUSION

Every fracture presents as a clinical problem with unique combination of variables. Appropriate application of the biomechanical principles of fracture fixation in each case enables implementation of effective rehabilitation protocol and helps achieve the best possible outcome.

REFERENCES

1. Duncan RM. Basic principles of splinting the hand. *Phys Ther.* 1989;69(12):1104-1116.
2. Moss DP, Tejwani NC. Biomechanics of external fixation: a review of the literature. *Bull NYU Hosp Jt Dis.* 2007;65(4):294-299.
3. Egol KA, Kubiak EN, Fulkerson E, Kummer FJ, Koval KJ. Biomechanics of locked plates and screws. *J Orthop Trauma.* 2004 Sep;18(8):488-493.
4. Perren SM. Physical and biological aspects of fracture healing with special reference to internal fixation. *Clin Orthop Relat Res.* 1979;138:175-196.
5. Perren SM. Evolution of the internal fixation of long bone fractures. The scientific basis of biological internal fixation: choosing a new balance between stability and biology. *J Bone Joint Surg Br.* 2002;84(8):1093-1110.
6. Kenwright J, Goodship AE. Controlled mechanical stimulation in the treatment of tibial fractures. *Clin Orthop Relat Res.* 1989:241:36-47.
7. https://www2.aofoundation.org.
8. Evans SL, Gregson PJ. Composite technology in load-bearing orthopaedic implants. *Biomaterials.* 1998;19(15):1329-1342.
9. Duan X, Li T, Mohammed AQ, Xiang Z. Reamed intramedullary nailing versus unreamed intramedullary nailing for shaft fracture of femur: a systematic literature review. *Arch Orthop Trauma Surg.* 2011;131(10):1445-1452.
10. Duan X, Al-Qwbani M, Zeng Y, Zhang W, Xiang Z. Intramedullary nailing for tibial shaft fractures in adults. *Cochrane Database Syst Rev.* 2012;1:CD008241.
11. Bong MR, Kummer FJ, Koval KJ, Egol KA. Intramedullary nailing of the lower extremity: biomechanics and biology. *J Am Acad Orthop Surg.* 2007;15(2):97-106.
12. Russell TA, Taylor JC, LaVelle DG, Beals NB, Brumfield DL, Durham AG. Mechanical characterization of femoral interlocking intramedullary nailing systems. *J Orthop Trauma.* 1991;5(3):332-340.
13. Lin J, Lin SJ, Chen PQ, Yang SH. Stress analysis of the distal locking screws for femoral interlocking nailing. *J Orthop Res.* 2001;19(1):57-63.
14. Wehner T, Penzkofer R, Augat P, Claes L, Simon U. Improvement of the shear fixation stability of intramedullary nailing. *Clin Biomech (Bristol, Avon).* 2011;26(2):147-151.
15. Fairbank AC, Thomas D, Cunningham B, Curtis M, Jinnah RH. Stability of reamed and unreamed intramedullary tibial nails: a biomechanical study. *Injury.* 1995;26(7):483-485.
16. Schütz M, Kääb MJ, Haas N. Stabilization of proximal tibial fractures with the LIS-System: early clinical experience in Berlin. *Injury.* 2003;34(suppl 1):A30-A35.
17. Bong MR, Patel V, Iesaka K, Egol KA, Kummer FJ, Koval KJ. Comparison of a sliding hip screw with a trochanteric lateral support plate to an intramedullary hip screw for fixation of unstable intertrochanteric hip fractures: a cadaver study. *J Trauma.* 2004;56(4):791-794.

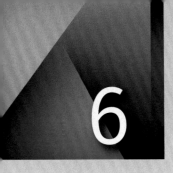

Assistive Modalities for Fracture Healing

Basem Attum
Andres Rodriguez-Buitrago
A. Alex Jahangir

INTRODUCTION

Annually, in the United States, there are approximately 6 million fractures per year, representing an annual economic loss estimated between US $3 to $6 billion.[1] Bone healing is a process that requires a precise interplay and coordination between multiple factors. Of the 6 million fractures, 5% to 10% will lead to nonunion or delayed union requiring additional procedures and increasing patient morbidity.[1-8] Modalities including *low-intensity pulse ultrasound* (LIPUS) and electrical stimulation for enhancing bone growth and fracture healing have been utilized to minimize the rate of nonunions and delayed unions and have the potential for enormous economic impact in fracture care.

LOW-INTENSITY PULSE ULTRASOUND

Low-intensity pulsed ultrasound (LIPUS) is considered a fracture enhancement technique accelerating fracture repair and promoting healing in stablished fracture defects.[1,3,4,6,8-11] Studies have reported a 30% to 38% reduction in time to union in acute fractures; in a majority of cases, a reduction in the incidence of delayed nonunions, and when present, it has shown to reduce the majority of nonunions (85% after 5.6 months and 86% after 5.5 months).[1,3-7,9-13]

HISTORY

The use of ultrasound for fracture healing dates back to the 1950s. Study results were contradicting, and in some cases, it was considered that its use was to be detrimental to bone health and healing.[4,5,8,14] Other studies, in which a lower intensity was used, reported that this technique could promote osteogenesis and decrease union times.[6,14] An animal study conducted by Duarte,[15] which exposed rabbits with fracture models to short bursts of low-intensity ultrasound for 15 minutes per day, was one of the first studies that concluded that ultrasound energy, with the appropriate parameters, can accelerate fracture healing.[15] Subsequent studies have proven its usefulness.[14]

MECHANISM OF ACTION

The use of LIPUS for accelerated healing of fresh fractures and established nonunions was approved by the Food and Drug Administration (FDA) in 1994 and 2000, respectively.[1,4,6-8,10] The literature has accepted the dose of LIPUS as a 20-minute daily therapy of 1 to 1.5 MHz sine waves repeating at 1 kHz, average intensity 30 mW/cm^2, pulse width 200 ms.[1-4,7,8,10,14] In vitro, low ultrsound wave intensities (<100 mW/cm^2) have shown to increase osteoblastic response.[4,9] In an intention to organize its effects over the cell, LIPUS can be thought to stimulate in two different and complementary ways.

1. **Mechanical stimulation.** Mechanical stimulation is transmitted via acoustic waves through soft tissue with the help of a water-based gel. Following Wolff's law, these waves provide forces that reach bone and travel across it as longitudinal and shear waves. These waves are thought to affect the integrin-cytoskeletal system and/or alter membrane spanning channel kinetics.[2,6,9,10]

   The importance of mechanical stimulation in bone healing is well understood with micromotion playing a key role. A study conducted by Greenleaf et al suggested that LIPUS might stimulate bone on a nanometer scale, because the displacement caused by it is almost 1000 times less when compared to micromotion values.[7,10] This mechanical stimulation will also cause a minimal, but sufficient, increase in temperature (near 1C°) altering enzymatic functions such as metalloproteinase 1 and collagenase 1.[1,2]

   Although it is only an observation, it has been theorized that this effect is proportional to bone's depth, being more effective in bone with less soft-tissue envelope such as the tibia.

2. **Response to pressure waves.** Alternate pressure waves cause stable cavitation and acoustic streaming, leading to shear forces and causing changes on membrane ion and molecule transport.[9,10,12] Although this cavitation-streaming mechanism has not been confirmed,[10] it is believed that pressure waves are transformed into mechanical forces substituting for physical forces normally applied to bone.[3,6] This mechanical force is then turned into biomechanical signals that affect all stages of the fracture healing.[2,3,10] This concept of streaming is based on an increase in flow among cells, increasing nutrient delivery to the cells.[6]

By these two overlapping and complementary mechanisms, LIPUS causes a myriad of changes inside the cell including gene expression, protein upregulation, and ion modifications that aim to promote inflammation and fracture repair. Although its effects have been well studied, there are still some gaps in the understanding of its mode of action and, the actual mechanism by which it promotes bone healing still is not well or fully understood.[3,5,6,9,10,13]

PHYSIOLOGIC CHANGES

Integrins

The mechanical stimulation, per se, will not cause a widespread response, and this stimulus has to be transduced into a biomechanical response. It has been proposed that integrin activation in osteoblasts plays an important role in a biomechanical response. Studies have shown an upregulation and activation of integrins after LIPUS treatment leading to focal adhesions.[7,10] In turn, this will cause an increase in the cell's capacity to attach to the surrounding matrix and initiate a cascade of intracellular responses (activation of FAK, PI3K, AkT, or ERK) enhancing the healing process.[7,10]

Cyclooxygenase-2 (COX-2)

Among the different changes in cells treated with LIPUS, COX-2 is the only one that has been linked to a transduction pathway[10]. The pathways by which LIPUS increases the production of COX-2 are variable, and the activation of PI2 kinase, AkT, ERK, and NF-KAPPA BETA has also been implicated.[10]

Warden et al[9] treated rodent osteosarcoma cells (UMR-106 cells) with a single dose of LIPUS and found that there was an upregulation of COX-2 genes after 20 minutes and secondary elevations not related to additional exposure. When compared to controls, there is a COX-2 mRNA upregulation, inducing production of prostaglandin E2 (PGE2), a key factor in fracture repair.[1,3,9,10] A persistent activation and stimulation of this pathway is consistent with accelerated fracture remodeling. Despite the fact that studies addressing COX-2 expression have consistently shown gene upregulation, its extent is not consistent and has shown to vary depending on the dose and duration of LIPUS.[7,10]

Vasculature

The existence of an adequate blood supply is crucial for bone healing. Histological results of different animal studies have led to the conclusion that LIPUS causes a significant increase in vascular endothelial growth factor (VEGF) production and vascularity around the fracture site, promoting endochondral ossification and mesenchymal cell migration.[1,3,6,7,10,11,16,17]

Ions

LIPUS has shown to increase potassium flow within cells. Calcium flow is greatly increased in chondrocytes, causing an activation and modulation in the second messenger system (eg, adenylate cyclase); additionally, there is an increase in the incorporation in cartilage and bone cells.[1,6,13] Ultimately, this leads to mineralization and increased bone mineral content (BMC).[7,10,12]

CELLULAR CHANGES (ENDOCHONDRAL OSSIFICATION)

The stimulus exerted by LIPUS on endochondral ossification appears to be a key determinant in the way fracture healing is stimulated. LIPUS causes positive effects in chondrogenesis, remodeling, and endochondral ossification periods; this is achieved not only by stimulating osteoblasts but all major cell types.[2,7,10,12] This effect has been demonstrated in different in vitro studies in which human osteogenic cells were stimulated with LIPUS.

When compared to controls, the use of LIPUS has shown statistically significant upregulation in countless osteogenic factors like aggrecan gene expression in chondrocytes which stimulate proteoglycan synthesis[1] and bone morphogenic proteins (BMP-2, BMP-4, BMP-6) which have shown consistent increases in their levels when compared to controls.[7] Although c-fos (proto-oncogene involved in osteoblast proliferation and differentiation) is upregulated, this elevation is only transitory when compared to COX-2 elevations.[9] Additionally, there is an upregulation of MMP-13 and mRNA levels for bone matrix proteins like alkaline phosphatase (ALP), bone sialoprotein (BSP), osteocalcin (OC), insulin growth factor (IGF-1), transforming growth factor B (TGF-B), and VEGF, among others.[3,6,7,9,10,12,13] These changes have not been consistent throughout the literature and some studies have not shown any difference in expression of BSP, IGF-1, or TGF-B expression.[7,9]

CALLUS AND BONE FORMATION

It is in this stage where all the preceding factors and changes stimulated by LIPUS work together, stimulating endochondral ossification, the key process by which LIPUS appears to exert its benefits and where many studies in the past decades have centered. As a direct consequence of the increased stimulation of COX-2, PGE2, ALP, and OC, LIPUS treatment causes a positive action on callus formation, enhancing its mechanical properties and increasing biomechanical strength and bone healing.[3,6,7,10,13]

Shimazaki et al[13] compared healing rates in rabbits previously treated with distraction osteogenesis, while Rutten et al[3] analyzed the histology of LIPUS treated fibulas; both studies concluded that LIPUS accelerates bone maturation in the initial phases, as well as osteoblast activity, endosteal bone formation, and increase in bone volume. These observations have also been noted by other in vivo studies in which it has been concluded that LIPUS accelerates endochondral ossification.[7,10] Azuma et al[16] performed an animal study in which they concluded that the use of LIPUS during different stages of bone healing increased bone stiffness. When dealing with complex factures, an RCT by Leung et al[12] found a decrease in tenderness, time to partial weight bearing, and removal for external fixator. These findings support the positive effect of LIPUS in bone healing of complex tibial fractures which are prone to potential complications.[8,12,14]

Different RCTs have shown LIPUS fracture enhancing properties, while others have not shown any difference when compared to controls regarding healing times.[8] Lubbert et al[14] evaluated the effect of LIPUS on 101 nonoperative treated clavicle shaft fractures and did not show any statistically significant difference in clinical healing (27.09 days in the placebo group vs 26.77 days in the treatment group), use of pain medications (32.88 tablets vs 37.21 tablets), visual analog scale score at 28 days of treatment (3.55 vs 3.51), or return to daily activities (household, work and sports). Additionally, Emami et al did not find any statistical difference in healing times of patients with tibial (closed or grade I open) fractures treated with LIPUS (155 days ± 22 days) versus **intramedullary** nail (125 days ± 11 days) (**Table 6.1**).[8]

CONCLUSION

Modern management of fractures is still limited to the traditional options. To date, studies involving LIPUS have focused on understanding its effects on cells and how it accelerates fracture healing. Still, we are lacking studies that also focus patient-reported outcomes. On the other hand, studies have not identified which patients will ultimately benefit from this technique, although recent literature has shown that patients who will most likely benefit from LIPUS use are those that are prone to have bad outcomes (smokers,

diabetics, concurrent use of steroids).[18] From an economic standpoint, the idea of promoting faster bone healing will lead a decrease in the economic burden of treating fractures, delayed unions, and nonunions even though there is an initial increase in costs.[11]

ELECTRICAL THERAPY

HISTORY

Electromagnetic fields for treatment have been explored since the 1800s.[18] In 1957, Fukada and Yasuda demonstrated a relationship between electricity and callus formation.[1] Four types of electrical fields have demonstrated potential cellular pathways, including growth factor synthesis, proteoglycan and collagen regulation, being affected.[19-23]

MECHANISM OF ACTION

Bone Tissue in Response to Electrical Stimulation

In order to understand the effect of electricity on bone healing, it is essential to understand the electrical activity that occurs in healthy and fractured bone. When bone is subjected to mechanical stress, osteocyte membranes are exposed to either electric potentials piezoelectrically generated or stream potentials that result from charged ionic flow in the bone canaliculi. In fractured bone, electrons migrate to the injured site and the distribution of electric potentials in the bone is altered.[24] Studies have shown that electrical fields affect the migration and proliferation of cells involved in bone remodeling, alkaline phosphatase activity, and gene regulation of connective tissue cells for structural extracellular matrix proteins resulting in the increase of cartilage and bone production.[25,26] This has been observed through in vitro systems including limb rudiments, osteoblasts, chondrocytes, and osteoprogenitor cells and has been seen with direct current, capacitive coupling, inductive coupling, and combined magnetic fields.

Direct Coupling

Direct coupling is used to produce a localized electric current between electrodes that are inserted at the fracture site. Originally the anode was placed on the skin with a battery pack worn at the waist. Implantable batteries acting as anodes were later developed to deliver a consistent 20 µA current. Advantages to this method are that patients are uniformly compliant and there is a constant current of approximately 20 µA and 1.0 V delivered to the fracture site.

Direct current acts by stimulating proteoglycan and collagen synthesis while creating an optimal environment for bone formation by lowering pO_2 and raising PH in the vicinity of the cathode.[1,27] Overall success rates have been documented to be between 62.5% and 78%.[27,28] In 1979, the FDA approved the use of DC for the use of nonunions and spinal fusions.[1]

TABLE 6.1 Potential Benefits of LIPUS

- Treatment of skin wounds and ulcers
- Noninvasive procedure
- Shorter healing time
- No side effects
- Outpatient basis
- Reduced costs

LIPUS, low-intensity pulse ultrasound.

Inductive Coupling

Pulsed electromagnetic field (PEMF) was developed to induce electrical fields in bone similar in magnitude and time course to endogenous electrical fields produced in response to strain.[1] External coils on the device produce a complex quasirectangular signal of pulse bursts with a repetition rate of 15 Hz and a peak amplitude of approximately 20 G producing a current of 20 mV and 10 μA/cm^2 in tissue.[27]

A broad range of frequencies are used, but the majority of the energy lies at the lower end of the spectrum.[29]

This method is thought to encourage mineralization and angiogenesis, increase DNA synthesis, and alter cellular calcium content on osteoblasts.[30] In an endochondral ossification model using demineralized bone matrix–induced osteogenesis, PEMF treatment caused an increase in chondrogenesis concomitant with and upregulation of TGF-B thereby enhancing fracture repair[16]. A several fold increase in BMP-2 and BMP-4 mRNA occurred in chick calvarial osteoblasts in vivo after 15 days of stimulation with this same signal.[31]

PHYSIOLOGIC CHANGES

Stages of Maturation and PEMF

PEMF is thought to affect osteoblasts differently depending on the stage of maturation. During the active proliferation stage, accelerated cellular proliferation, enhanced cellular differentiation, and increased bone tissue–like formation have been seen. During the differentiation stage, osteoblasts have enhanced cellular differentiation and increased bone tissue–like formation. This is in contrast to the mineralization stage where decreased bone formation occurs.[32]

Enchondral Ossification and PEMF

Animal and cell culture models suggest that enchondral ossification is also stimulated by increasing cartilage mass and production of TGF-B1. PEMF has been shown to have an effect on TGF-B1. Querkov et al found that a 130% increase in TGF-B1 was seen after 4 days of stimulation.[20] A time-dependent increase in TGF-B1 was shown in a conditioned media of hypertrophic nonunion cells by day 2 and atrophic nonunions in day 4.[19] Evidence also suggests that PEMF increases chondrogenesis and subsequent enchondral ossification. This cartilage mass increase due to enhanced chondrogenesis provides greater surface area to serve as a larger scaffold for bone formation. As cartilage forms quicker, enchondral bone formation is accelerated.[20]

Calcium/Calmodulin Pathway and PEMF

It is believed that PEMF stimulation leads to an increase in activity of the calcium/calmodulin pathway through various mechanisms. Transmembrane channels cause stimulation with PEMF through increasing cytosolic calcium concentrations while signal transduction is mediated by the release of intracellular calcium leading to increases in cytosolic calcium and activated calmodulin. Studies on osteoblast-osteoclast cocultures have shown that indirect coupling fields disrupt the interaction between calcitonin and its receptor systems causing osteoclast insensitivity to calcitonin.[33]

PEMF and BMPs

PEMF exposure has been postulated to increase mRNA expression of several BMPs. In a calvarial model of chick embryos exposed to PEMF, BMP-2 mRNA levels were increased by exposure 2.7-fold on day 15 and 1.6-fold on day 17 of incubation suggesting that upregulation of mRNA in BMP-2 and BMP-4 is related to and possibly mediates the bone inductive effect on PEMF.[31] Exposure to PEMF reproducibly and markedly increased the levels of mRNA for BMP-4, -5, and -7 in a time-dependent manner with a maximum increase after 24 hours of exposure.[34] MG63 (osteoblast-like cells) responds to PEMF with a reduction in cell proliferation and an increase in ALP-specific activity, collagen synthesis, and osteocalcin levels. Terminally differentiated MLO-4 (a seven transmembrane protein in osteocyte-like cells) did not show an effect on PEMF on cell number or osteocalcin levels, but TGF-B1 and PGE2 levels were increased and nitrogen dioxide was altered.

Three randomized control trials **(RCT)** have been published on PEMF. Sharrard et al found a significant difference when PEMF was used between those who healed or progressing to heal compared to those who went on to nonunion.[35] Scott and King demonstrated a healing rate of 60% in the protocol group (PEMF group) but none in the control group in a study of patients with long bone nonunions.[36] Griffin et al had 89% of nonunions in long bone fractures unite in the PEMF group compared to 50% in the control group.[29]

Indications for PEMF treatment include treatment for nonunions, failed fusion, and congenital pseudoarthrosis.[1]

Capacitive coupling

Capacitive coupling (CC) was developed by Brighton and Pollack.[37] This method uses disk electrodes coupled to the skin via conductive gel to produce a broad uniform electric field in the fracture site. This induced field is driven by an oscillating electric current.[1] When the device is used for 24 hours, a 60 kHz sine wave is generated, in turn, this produces a 5 V peak to peak current.[27] When applying CC, cast immobilization is applied and two small windows are cut out for the application of the electrodes. These electrodes are moistened before application, and when they dry, the monitor detects the loss of contact and sets off an alarm indicating that the pads need to be remoistened. The pads are worn 24 hours a day and changed weekly. The device uses a 9-V battery that needs to be changed every day.[1] Brighton et al found that field strength was the dominant factor affecting bone cell proliferative response to a capacity coupled field.[38]

CC electric fields induce the proliferation of osteoblastic cells (MC3T3-E1) and increase levels of TGF-B1 mRNA by a mechanism involving the calcium/calmodulin pathway.[39] Bone cells produce two types of TGF-B, active and latent forms. Activation of the latent form of TGF-B is one of the major control mechanisms of TGF-B activity. Zhuang et al found that mRNA levels of TGF-B1 increased significantly upon 2 hours or longer of stimulation and that increased TGF-B1 activity is probably a result of increased TGF-B1 mRNA.[39] A CC osteoblast culture model found that CC decreased the cAMP response to parathyroid hormone (PTH) and desensitizes osteoblasts to PTH.[40] Other studies with human fibroblasts have shown an increase in calcium translocation and the number of insulin receptors in response to an electric field.[41] These electric fields trigger the opening of voltage-gated sensitive calcium channels as the primary event followed by an increased level of intracellular calcium.

Current indications for CC are nonunion of the long bone and the scaphoid and as an adjunctive treatment in spinal fusions.

Combined Magnetic Field

Combined magnetic field uses an external pair of coils that produce to parallel low energy, magnetic fields. This alternating magnetic field is a sinusoidal wave of 76.6 Hz with an amplitude of 400 mG peak to peak and the static field set at 200 mg.[27] Growth factor synthesis in response to electric and electromagnetic fields showed an increase in IGF-2 mRNA and protein, which suggests that IGF-2 may mediate the proliferation of osteoblast-like cells.[42]

CONCLUSION

There are different mechanisms by which it is thought that electrical therapy assists in the fracture healing process. More clinical studies are needed to show that this method of treatment is effective. The current literature is mainly focused on animal models, and until more clinically studies are performed, skepticism of the efficacy of treatment will continue to limit this method of treatment.

REFERENCES

1. Nelson FRT, Brighton CT, Ryaby J, et al. Use of physical forces in bone healing. *J Am Acad Orthop Surg*. 2003;11(5):344-354. doi:10.5435/00124635-200309000-00007.
2. Claes L, Willie B. The enhancement of bone regeneration by ultrasound. *Prog Biophys Mol Biol*. 2007;93(1-3):384-398. doi:10.1016/j.pbiomolbio.2006.07.021.
3. Rutten S, Nolte PA, Korstjens CM, Van Duin MA, Klein-Nulend J. Low-intensity pulsed ultrasound increases bone volume, osteoid thickness and mineral apposition rate in the area of fracture healing in patients with a delayed union of the osteotomized fibula. *Bone*. 2008;43(2):348-354. doi:10.1016/j.bone.2008.04.010.
4. Romano CL, Romano D, Logoluso N. Low-intensity pulsed ultrasound for the treatment of bone delayed union or nonunion: a review. *Ultrasound Med Biol*. 2009;35(4):529-536. doi:10.1016/j.ultrasmedbio.2008.09.029.
5. Busse JW, Bhandari M, Kulkarni AV, Tunks E. The effect of low-intensity pulsed ultrasound therapy on time to fracture healing: a meta-analysis. see comment. *CMAJ*. 2002;166(4):437-441.
6. Malizos KN, Hantes ME, Protopappas V, Papachristos A. Low-intensity pulsed ultrasound for bone healing: An overview. *Injury*. 2006;37(1):56-62. doi:10.1016/j.injury.2006.02.037.
7. Harrison A, Lin S, Pounder N, Mikuni-Takagaki Y. Mode & mechanism of low intensity pulsed ultrasound (LIPUS) in fracture repair. *Ultrasonics*. 2016;70:45-52. doi:10.1016/j.ultras.2016.03.016.
8. Watanabe Y, Matsushita T, Bhandari M, Zdero R, Schemitsch EH. Ultrasound for fracture healing: current evidence. *J Orthop Trauma*. 2010;24(suppl 1):S56-S61. doi:10.1097/BOT.0b013e3181d2efaf.
9. Warden SJ, Favaloro JM, Bennell KL, et al. Low-intensity pulsed ultrasound stimulates a bone-forming response in UMR-106 cells. *Biochem Biophys Res Commun*. 2001;286(3):443-450. doi:10.1006/bbrc.2001.5412.
10. Pounder NM, Harrison AJ. Low intensity pulsed ultrasound for fracture healing: A review of the clinical evidence and the associated biological mechanism of action. *Ultrasonics*. 2008;48(4):330-338. doi:10.1016/j.ultras.2008.02.005.
11. Hannemann PFW, Essers BAB, Schots JPM, Dullaert K, Poeze M, Brink PRG. Functional outcome and cost-effectiveness of pulsed electromagnetic fields in the treatment of acute scaphoid fractures: A cost-utility analysis Orthopedics and biomechanics. *BMC Musculoskelet Disord*. 2015;16(1):1-10. doi:10.1186/s12891-015-0541-2.
12. Leung K-S, Lee W-S, Tsui H-F, Liu PP-L, Cheung W-H. Complex tibial fracture outcomes following treatment with low-intensity pulsed ultrasound. *Ultrasound Med Biol*. 2004;30(3):389-395. doi:10.1016/j.ultrasmedbio.2003.11.008.
13. Shimazaki A, Inui K, Azuma Y, Nishimura N, Yamano Y. Low-intensity pulsed ultrasound accelerates bone maturation in distraction osteogenesis in rabbits. *J Bone Joint Surg Br*. 2000;82:1077-1082.
14. Lubbert PHW, van der Rijt RHH, Hoorntje LE, van der Werken C. Low-intensity pulsed ultrasound (LIPUS) in fresh clavicle fractures: A multi-centre double blind randomised controlled trial. *Injury*. 2008;39(12):1444-1452. doi:10.1016/j.injury.2008.04.004.
15. Duarte LR. The stimulation of bone growth by ultrasound. *Arch Orthop Trauma Surg*. 1983;101(3):153-159. doi:10.1007/BF00436764.
16. Azuma Y, Ito M, Harada Y, Takagi H, Ohta T, Jingushi S. Low-intensity pulsed ultrasound accelerates rat femoral fracture healing by acting on the various cellular reactions in the fracture callus. *J Bone Miner Res*. 2001;16(4):671-680. doi:10.1359/jbmr.2001.16.4.671.
17. Siska PA, Gruen GS, Pape HC. External adjuncts to enhance fracture healing: What is the role of ultrasound? *Injury*. 2008;39(10):1095-1105. doi:10.1016/j.injury.2008.01.015.
18. Mollon B, da Silva V, Busse JW, Einhorn TA, Bhandari M. Electrical stimulation for long-bone fracture-healing: a meta-analysis of randomized controlled trials. *J Bone Joint Surg Am*. 2008;90(11):2322-2330. doi:10.2106/JBJS.H.00111.
19. Aaron RK, Boyan BD, Ciombor DM, Schwartz Z, Simon BJ. Stimulation of growth factor synthesis by electric and electromagnetic fields. *Clin Orthop Relat Res*. 2004;(419):30-37. doi:10.1097/01.blo.0000118698.46535.83.
20. Guerkov HH, Lohmann CH, Liu Y, et al. Pulsed electromagnetic fields increase growth factor release by nonunion cells. *Clin Orthop Relat Res*. 2001;(384):265-279. http://www.ncbi.nlm.nih.gov/pubmed/11249175.
21. Lohmann CH, Schwartz Z, Liu Y, et al. Pulsed electromagnetic fields affect phenotype and connexin 43 protein expression in MLO-Y4 osteocyte-like cells and ROS 17/2.8 osteoblast-like cells. *J Orthop Res*. 2003;21(2):326-334.
22. Ciombor DM, Aaron RK. The role of electrical stimulation in bone repair. *Foot Ankle Clin*. 2005;10(4):579-593.
23. Heermeier K, Spanner M, Träger J, et al. Effects of extremely low frequency electromagnetic field (EMF) on collagen type I mRNA expression and extracellular matrix synthesis of human osteoblastic cells. *Bioelectromagnetics*. 1998;19(4):222-231.
24. Huang CP, Chen XM, Chen ZQ. Osteocyte: the impresario in the electrical stimulation for bone fracture healing. *Med Hypotheses*. 2008;70(2):287-290.
25. Qiu Q, Sayer M, Kawaja M, Shen X, Davies JE. Attachment, morphology, and protein expression of rat marrow stromal cells cultured on charged substrate surfaces. *J Biomed Mater Res*. 1998;42(1):117-127.
26. Wiesmann H-P, Hartig M, Stratmann U, Meyer U, Joos U. Electrical stimulation influences mineral formation of osteoblast-like cells in vitro. *Biochim Biophys Acta Mol Cell Res*. 2001;1538(1):28-37. doi:10.1016/S0167-4889(00)00135-X.
27. Ryaby JT. Clinical effects of electromagnetic and electric fields on fracture healing. *Clin Orthop Relat Res*. 1998;(355 suppl):S205-S215. http://www.ncbi.nlm.nih.gov/pubmed/9917640.

28. Brighton CT, Friedenberg ZB, Mitchell EI, Booth RE. Treatment of non-union with constant direct current. *Clin Orthop* 124: 106-123,1977.

29. Griffin XL, Warner F, Costa M. The role of electromagnetic stimulation in the management of established non-union of long bone fractures: what is the evidence? *Injury*. 2008;39(4):419-429.

30. Bassett CA. Fundamental and practical aspects of therapeutic uses of pulsed electromagnetic fields (PEMFs). *Crit Rev Biomed Eng*. 1989;17(5):451-529.

31. Nagai M, Ota M. Pulsating electromagnetic field stimulates mRNA expression of bone morphogenetic protein-2 and -4. *J Dent Res*. 1994;73(10):1601-1605.

32. Diniz P, Shomura K, Soejima K, Ito G. Effects of pulsed electromagnetic field (PEMF) stimulation on bone tissue like formation are dependent on the maturation stages of the osteoblasts. *Bioelectromagnetics*. 2002;23(5):398-405.

33. Shankar VS, Simon BJ, Bax CMR, et al. Effects of electromagnetic stimulation on the functional responsiveness of isolated rat osteoclasts. *J Cell Physiol*. 1998;176(3):537-544.

34. Yajima A, Ochi M, Yukito H, Sakaguchi K, Wang P-L. Effect of pulsing electromagnetic fields on gene expression of bone morphogenetic proteins in cultured human osteoblastic cell line. *J Hard Tissue Biol*. 2000;9(2):63-66.

35. Sharrard WJW. A double-blind trial of pulsed electromagnetic fields for delayed union of tibial fractures. *J Bone Joint Surg Br*. 1990;72(3):347-355. http://www.ncbi.nlm.nih.gov/pubmed/2187877.

36. Gareth S, King JB. A prospective, double-blind trial of electrical capacitive coupling in the treatment of non-union of long bones. *J Bone Joint Surg Am*. 1994;76(6):820-826.

37. Brighton CT, Pollack SR. Treatment of recalcitrant non-union with a capacitively coupled electrical field. A preliminary report. *J Bone Joint Surg Am*. 1985;67(4):577-585. http://www.ncbi.nlm.nih.gov/pubmed/3872300.

38. Brighton CT, Friedenberg ZB, Mitchell EI, Booth RE. Treatment of nonunion with constant direct current. *Clin Orthop Relat Res*. 1977(124):106-123.

39. Zhuang H, Wang W, Seldes RM, Tahernia AD, Fan H, Brighton CT. Electrical stimulation induces the level of tgf-β1 mrna in osteoblastic cells by a mechanism involving calcium/calmodulin pathway. *Biochem Biophys Res Commun*. 1997;237(2):225-229. http://www.sciencedirect.com/science/article/pii/S0006291X97971187%5Cnhttp://linkinghub.elsevier.com/retrieve/pii/S0006291X97971187.

40. Brighton CT, McCluskey WP. Response of cultured bone cells to a capacitively coupled electric field: inhibition of cAMP response to parathyroid hormone. *J Orthop Res*. 1988;6:567-571.

41. Bourguignon GJ, Bourguignon LY. Electric stimulation of protein and DNA synthesis in human fibroblasts. *FASEB J*. 1987;1(5):398-402.

42. Ryaby JT, Fitzsimmons RJ, Khin NA, et al. The role of insulin-like growth factor II in magnetic field regulation of bone formation. *Bioelectrochemistry Bioenerg*. 1994;35:87-91.

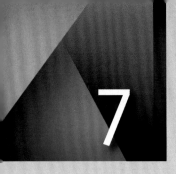

7

Nutritional Supplementation of Fracture Healing

Robert M. Corey
Lisa K. Cannada

INTRODUCTION

Fracture healing is a complex set of events that involves the coordination of different processes. These processes have been described in earlier chapters and include initial inflammatory response, soft and hard callus formation, initial bony union, and bony remodeling. This well-coordinated series of events follows a specific sequence that can be affected by a number of biological factors, such as patient age, medical comorbidities, and bone quality. Advanced age is one factor that can inhibit fracture repair, while another factor that affects bone metabolism is nutrition. Bone density, fracture risk, and fracture healing are all influenced by nutritional status.[1,2]

In order to properly evaluate the nutritional status of a patient, we first must define our terms. The terms "malnutrition" and "nutrient deficiency" are frequently used interchangeably in orthopaedic literature.[2-4] According to the World Health Organization, malnutrition encompasses both deficiencies and excess of nutrients.[5] A thin person is not always the representative example of nutritional deficiencies. Nutrient deficiencies may be prevalent in persons with obesity and play a contributing factor to the development of diabetes mellitus (DM) in this patient population.[6] For the purposes of this chapter, we define malnutrition as any disorder of nutrition, including excess of nutrients (ie, obesity) or deficiency of nutrients.

DEFINITION OF MALNUTRITION

As discussed by Cross et al,[2] malnutrition has been defined using a variety of different methods in the orthopaedic literature. These include serologic laboratory values,[3,7,8] anthropometric measurements,[9-12] and standardized nutrition scoring systems[13-15] (**Tables 7.1** and **7.2**). In relation to surgical site infection (SSI) or impaired wound healing, the most common definitions of malnutrition are a serum lymphocyte count <1500 cells/mm^3 and a serum albumin concentration of <3.5 g/dL.[2,3,7,14,16] The total lymphocyte count is calculated by multiplying the serum white blood cell count by the percentage of lymphocytes in the differential. Low serum prealbumin[8,9,15,17] serum transferrin levels <200 mg/dL[2,3,16,18] are also considered signs of malnutrition. Although not a universally established assessment of nutrition, a low zinc level (95 µg/dL) has also been associated with impaired wound healing following orthopaedic surgery.[16]

Albumin, prealbumin, and transferrin are visceral proteins that are sensitive indicators of marginal nutritional deficiency, and they can be used to detect acute nutritional changes because of their shorter half-lives.[7,12] However, prealbumin has not been used extensively in order to assess perioperative nutrition. This parameter is thought to be too sensitive to accurately reflect protein-caloric nutrition,[9] and as such, no established definition of malnutrition using prealbumin exists in the orthopaedic literature. The normal range of prealbumin is approximately 16 to 35 mg/dL.[19] Similarly, controversy exists regarding the validity of the total lymphocyte count as a marker for nutrition.[20] Despite this, total lymphocyte count is still frequently used in the literature as a marker for nutrition.[3,7,9,18] Albumin level is one of the most recognized and simplest markers of nutritional status.

"Under nutrition" has also been defined in the orthopaedic literature by way of anthropometric measurements, such as calf circumference,[9,21] arm muscle circumference,[9,11,12,21] and triceps skinfold.[10] Undernutrition in adults has been defined as calf circumference <31 cm or an arm muscle circumference <22 cm.[21] Arm muscle circumference of 60% to 90% of the standard for one's sex is a marker of moderate malnutrition, while circumference <60% is a marker for severe malnutrition.[11] Although the triceps skinfold test is a poorly described tool for assessing nutrition, it continues to be used in the literature.[10]

Anthropometric measurements function as an indirect gauge of under nutrition by providing insight into body composition.[9] Body fat and skeletal muscle are not depleted

TABLE 7.1

Measure	Normal	Low
Serum lymphocyte count		
Serum albumin concentration		
Serum prealbumin concentration		
Serum transferrin		
Serum zinc		

until late in the course of malnourishment; thus, anthropometric tools cannot be used to detect acute changes in nutritional status.[7] Despite this, these tools are good indicators of chronic changes in nutritional status.[10] The advantages of anthropometric measurements are that these tests are inexpensive and can be easily performed.

Standardized malnutrition screening tools and malnutrition assessment tools are used to define malnutrition. The Rainey-MacDonald nutritional index (RMNI) has been used in several studies.[9,13,14] It is calculated from serum albumin and serum transferrin:

$$RMNI = (1.2 * serum\ albumin) +$$
$$(0.013 * serum\ transferrin) - 6.43.$$

A zero or negative score indicates nutritional depletion. The RMNI has not been validated.[9,22]

The multiquestion Mini Nutritional Assessment (MNA) has been shown to be reliable in assessing malnutrition in the geriatric population (**Figure 7.1**).[9,21,23] The MNA includes questions of a variety of topics, such as anthropometric measures and dietary habits, which allows for complex measurement of malnourishment, taking into account multiple variables that affect nutritional status.

A difference exists between screening nutrition tools and assessment tools. However, Ozkalkanli et al[15] demonstrated that the odds ratio of the association between malnutrition (ie, assessment tools) or the risk of malnutrition (ie, screening tools) and morbidity in orthopaedic surgery were 3.5 and 4.1, respectively. Thus, both tools can be used to predict increased morbidity following orthopaedic surgery.

The World Health Organization classified obesity as Class 1-Body Mass Index (BMI) 30.0 to 34.9 kg/m^2, Class 2-BMI 35.0 to 39.9 kg/m^2, and Class 3-BMI >40.0 kg/m^2 (**Table 7.3**).[5] The American Diabetes Association lists four diagnostic criteria for DM: (1) hemoglobin A1C > 6.5%, (2) fasting plasma glucose (>8 hours) levels >125 mg/dL (or 7 mmol/L), (3) two-hour plasma glucose >200 mg/dL (11.1 mmol/L) during an oral glucose tolerance test, and (4) classic symptoms of hyperglycemia (ie, polydipsia, polyuria) or hyperglycemic crisis and random plasma glucose >200 mg/dL (11.1 mmol/L) (**Table 7.4**).[19]

MECHANISMS BY WHICH MALNUTRITION MAY INCREASE INFECTION RISK

Both superficial and deep SSI after orthopaedic spinal surgery have been linked to several markers of malnutrition, including serologic laboratory values, DM, hyperglycemia, and obesity.[24-29] Because the risk of deep infections has been shown to be higher in patients with neuromuscular conditions, most research in spine surgery has been performed in order to identify risk factors that may increase the risk of infection. The relationship between blood glucose impairment and DM and deep infections has also been well studied,[30-35] as multiple studies have shown DM to be a risk factor for deep infection.[30-32,36] Jamsen et al reported that preoperative hyperglycemia (blood glucose levels >110 mg/dL) was associated with a higher risk of prosthetic joint infection,[34]

TABLE 7.2 Methods of Evaluating Malnutrition

Method	Advantages	Parameters
Standardized Scoring System	• Standardized • Easy to interrupt • Allows for different consideration for variables	• Rainey-MacDonald nutritional index • Mini Nutritional Assessment
Serologic Lab Values	• Sensitive indicator • Most commonly used method	• Total lymphocyte <1500 cells/mm • Serum albumin level <3.5 g/dL • Serum transferrin <200 mg/dL
Anthropometric Measurements	• Indirect indicator • Cheap • Easy to perform • Sensitive for long-term changes	• Calf muscle circumference <31 cm • Arm muscle circumference <22 mm • Triceps skinfold measurement

Mini Nutritional Assessment
MNA®

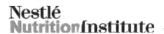

Last name:		First name:	
Sex:	Age:	Weight, kg:	Height, cm:	Date:

Complete the screen by filling in the boxes with the appropriate numbers. Total the numbers for the final screening score.

Screening

A Has food intake declined over the past 3 months due to loss of appetite, digestive problems, chewing or swallowing difficulties?
0 = severe decrease in food intake
1 = moderate decrease in food intake
2 = no decrease in food intake ☐

B Weight loss during the last 3 months
0 = weight loss greater than 3 kg (6.6 lbs)
1 = does not know
2 = weight loss between 1 and 3 kg (2.2 and 6.6 lbs)
3 = no weight loss ☐

C Mobility
0 = bed or chair bound
1 = able to get out of bed / chair but does not go out
2 = goes out ☐

D Has suffered psychological stress or acute disease in the past 3 months?
0 = yes   2 = no ☐

E Neuropsychological problems
0 = severe dementia or depression
1 = mild dementia
2 = no psychological problems ☐

F1 Body Mass Index (BMI) (weight in kg) / (height in m)^2
0 = BMI less than 19
1 = BMI 19 to less than 21
2 = BMI 21 to less than 23
3 = BMI 23 or greater ☐

IF BMI IS NOT AVAILABLE, REPLACE QUESTION F1 WITH QUESTION F2.
DO NOT ANSWER QUESTION F2 IF QUESTION F1 IS ALREADY COMPLETED.

F2 Calf circumference (CC) in cm
0 = CC less than 31
3 = CC 31 or greater ☐

Screening score (max. 14 points)

12 - 14 points: Normal nutritional status
8 - 11 points: At risk of malnutrition
0 - 7 points: Malnourished ☐☐

References
1. Vellas B, Villars H, Abellan G, et al. Overview of the MNA® - Its History and Challenges. J Nutr Health Aging. 2006;**10**:456-465.
2. Rubenstein LZ, Harker JO, Salva A, Guigoz Y, Vellas B. Screening for Undernutrition in Geriatric Practice: Developing the Short-Form Mini Nutritional Assessment (MNA-SF). J. Geront. 2001; **56A**: M366-377
3. Guigoz Y. The Mini-Nutritional Assessment (MNA®) Review of the Literature - What does it tell us? J Nutr Health Aging. 2006; **10**:466-487.
4. Kaiser MJ, Bauer JM, Ramsch C, et al. Validation of the Mini Nutritional Assessment Short-Form (MNA®-SF): A practical tool for identification of nutritional status. J Nutr Health Aging. 2009; **13**:782-788.
® Société des Produits Nestlé SA, Trademark Owners.
© Société des Produits Nestlé SA 1994, Revision 2009.
For more information: www.mna-elderly.com

FIGURE 7.1 Mini Nutritional Assessment form.

while another Jamsen study demonstrated an increased risk of infections in orthopaedic patients with hemoglobin A1C >6.5%.[37]

Malnutrition is thought to predispose patients to SSI[3,30,38] by impairing wound healing[9,13,18] and prolonging inflammation via several mechanisms, including impaired fibroblast proliferation and collagen synthesis.[39] Decreased lymphocyte count is thought to impair the ability of the immune system to eradicate or prevent infection. Obesity contributes to SSI through multiple mechanisms. First, obesity makes it difficult to achieve adequate wound closure. Additionally, wound healing is impaired through fat

TABLE 7.3 Classification of Obesity (World Health Organization)

- Class 1-Body Mass Index (BMI) 30.0 to 34.9 kg/m²
- Class 2-BMI 35.0-39.9 kg/m²
- Class 3-BMI >40.0 kg/m²

necrosis. Both mechanisms can lead to problems with local wound healing.[39] Obesity is associated with increased surgical time, which further increases the risk of infection.[31] DM predisposes patients to SSI by preventing the adequate utilization of glucose for energy and adequate oxygenation delivery secondary to glycosylation of hemoglobin and microvascular and macrovascular disease, which results in ischemic tissue that is more susceptible to infection.[39] Obesity may also contribute to increased infection rates by increasing operative time. In obese patients, the exposure and implant placement may take more time due to the patient's body habitus.[31,39]

VITAMINS, NUTRITIONAL FACTORS, AND BONE QUALITY

Aging is often accompanied by malnutrition. Deficiency of nutritional factors appears to be strongly implicated in fractures in the osteoporotic elderly.[1] Nutritional personalized programs could prevent bone loss and thus fragility fractures in aged people. Many compounds in food and plants act on bone metabolism, stimulate osteoblastogenesis, inhibit osteoclastogenesis, and reduce inflammatory condition.[40,41]

Oxidative stress plays a vital role in pathophysiology of aging. Oxidative stress is an imbalance between free radicals and antioxidant mechanism, and it damages macromolecules and cellular functions. Following bone fracture, damaged tissue increases free radicals. Free radicals are also produced in response to inflammatory stimuli, and TNF-α increases intracellular oxidative stress.[42] Oxidative stress is associated with osteoporosis and may be reduced by dietary antioxidants. Polyphenols have a positive role in the prevention of cardiovascular diseases, cancer, and osteoporosis.

TABLE 7.4 Diagnostic Criteria for Diabetes Mellitus (American Diabetes Association)

- Hemoglobin A1C >6.5%
- Fasting plasma glucose (>8 h) levels >125 mg/dL (or 7 mmol/L)
- Two-hour plasma glucose >200 mg/dL (11.1 mmol/L) during an oral glucose tolerance test
- Classic symptoms of hyperglycemia (ie, polydipsia, polyuria) or hyperglycemic crisis and random plasma glucose >200 mg/dL (11.1 mmol/L)

They act by increasing trabecular bone volume and bone mass, enhancing bone formation, and inhibiting bone resorption.[43-47]

Among dietary antioxidants, lycopene reduces the levels of bone turnover markers and the risk of osteoporosis. Carotenoids are important in bone remodeling. They function by reducing fracture risk by decreasing bone resorption and increasing bone formation. Vitamin C inhibits the differentiation of precursor cells in mature osteoclasts and reduces the bone resorption.[48,49] It has been shown to be essential for the maintenance of differentiated functions of osteoblasts, including those in fracture repair.[50] Vitamin C supplementation has also been shown to accelerate fracture healing in an animal model.[51]

While vitamin A is necessary for bone development, it has been shown to have negative effects in the event of high intake. Excess vitamin A leads to an increased incidence of hip fractures, and it is associated with poor bone quality.[52] Proper balance between carotenoids and vitamin A is important for a proper bone development.

Vitamin deficiency in elderly patients is common, particularly in osteoporotic patients. Improvement of their vitamin intake may help treat and prevent osteoporosis. Increasing the administration of dietetic antioxidants could protect bone from osteoporosis and could lead to reduction in fractures with personal and social benefits. Additionally, antioxidants could help in the acceleration of fracture healing.[49]

Fatty acids have beneficial effects in several diseases, including osteoporosis.[53-56] Their mechanism of action occurs through anti-inflammatory effects by decreasing the production of proinflammatory cytokines, such as TNF-α, IL-1β, and IL-6.[57] In vivo and in vitro studies have shown that the dietary fatty acids may play an important role in enhancing bone formation and suppressing the production of bone absorption.[58,59] Isoflavones, including genistein, have been demonstrated to have an anabolic effect on bone metabolism, potentially delaying osteoporosis. They function in protein synthesis and gene expression to bone formation and bone resorption.[60] The anabolic effect may be correlated to the binding of estrogens receptor β in osteoblastic cells.[61] The potential role of isoflavones is to prevent bone loss in aging. Oral administration of soybean extract, which contains isoflavone, has been demonstrated to increase bone components in rats, confirming an anabolic effect on bone metabolism.[62] The activity of alkaline phosphatase, a marker enzyme in differentiation of osteoblastic cells, increases in the presence of genistein.

Zinc, an essential trace element, is involved in the differentiation of osteoblastic and osteoclastic cells and is required for growth, development, and maintenance of bone health.[63] Zinc may increase the concentration of OPG in osteoblastic cells. The presence of zinc during fracture repair increases alkaline phosphatase activity and stimulates osteocalcin production; therefore, zinc supplementation may promote fracture healing.[64] Zinc levels in osteoporotic subjects are much lower than those in controls. The combination of zinc and genistein has a synergistic effect on osteoblastic cells; it enhances bone mineralization and increases bone mass.[65]

Calcium (Ca) is an essential structural component of bone; its levels are correlated to bone mineral density and to the risk of osteoporosis and fragility fractures. An active lifestyle and daily consumption of dairy products maintains bone health and reduces osteoporosis. Dairy products may represent the best dietary sources of Ca due to their high calcium and nutrients content. Please see Chapter 3 for a detailed discussion on the effects of calcium and bone health.

VITAMIN D

Vitamin D is integral in the control of blood calcium levels, and vitamin D insufficiency is common among the elderly population[66,67] leading to bone loss and increased risk of fragility fractures. The National Osteoporosis Guideline Group recommends a daily intake of at least 1000 mg of calcium, 800 IU of vitamin D, and 1 g/kg body weight of protein as a general measure for osteoporosis prevention. These nutritional factors, as discussed earlier, play an important role in osteoporosis and fracture healing process by enhancing bone formation and reducing bone absorption.

The term vitamin D typically refers to cholecalciferol (ie, vitamin D_3). Calcifediol (ie, 25-hydroxyvitamin D_3) and calcitriol (ie, 1,25-dihydroxyvitamin D_3) are hydroxylase forms of vitamin D_3.[68] Ergocalciferol (ie, vitamin D_2) is a less potent, plant-derived form of vitamin D that is frequently found in commercially available oral vitamins.[68] These terms are often used interchangeably in the literature.[68] Additionally, literature and clinical laboratories inconsistently report vitamin D levels in either ng/mL or nmol/L (1 ng/mL = 2.5 nmol/L).[69]

Vitamin D is obtained through dietary sources, oral supplements, and exposure to sunlight. A small number of foods contain naturally occurring vitamin D, but fortified foods such as milk and breakfast cereals are the major dietary source of the vitamin. In vivo conversion of 7-dehydrocholesterol to vitamin D_3 by ultraviolet B radiation in the skin is the primary source of vitamin D.[68]

Vitamin D_3, synthesized in the skin or obtained from dietary sources, is inactive and must be converted through hydroxylation in the liver into 25-hydroxyvitamin D. 25-Hydroxyl-vitamin D is then converted in the kidney into 1,25-dihydroxyvitamin D, the active form of vitamin D (**Figure 7.2**). Activated vitamin D is thought to act through a single, common vitamin D receptor that binds to specific DNA sequences known as vitamin D response elements, currently found on more than 200 genes in a wide distribution of tissues.[69,70]

The production of 1,25-dihydroxyvitamin D is tightly regulated by a homeostatic interaction among parathyroid hormone (PTH), calcium, and phosphate in the kidneys. Increased PTH, in response to low serum calcium levels, stimulates production of 1,25-dihydroxyvitamin D. Low serum phosphate also stimulates production of 1,25-dihydroxyvitamin D. This process is inhibited by fibroblast growth factor, which is produced by osteocytes. High levels of 1,25-dihydroxyvitamin D stimulate the enzymatic production of 24,25-dihydroxyvitamin D, the inactive form of vitamin D, thereby self-regulating the action of 1,25-dihydroxyvitamin D.[68]

The principal function of vitamin D is to maintain serum calcium homeostasis. Vitamin D stimulates active intestinal absorption of calcium and phosphate. In the kidney, vitamin D (with PTH) increases distal renal tubule reabsorption of calcium. Vitamin D also stimulates mobilization of calcium from bone via receptor activator of nuclear factor-dB ligand-induced osteoclast genesis. In the absence of vitamin D, calcium and phosphate intestinal absorption is reduced by as much as 50%, and PTH is maximally produced in order to maintain the normal calcium-to-phosphate ratio essential for collagen matrix mineralization.[71] This can result in secondary hyperparathyroidism and increased osteoclastic bone resorption.

Vitamin D deficiency is estimated to affect about 1 billion people worldwide and is linked to multiple medical maladies including cancer, diabetes, cardiovascular disease, and musculoskeletal health.[72] Vitamin D deficiency has been associated with fragility fractures and tibial nonunions.[73,74] Approximately 40% of elective sports-related orthopaedic surgery patients have low vitamin D levels.[75] However, the direct consequence of having a low serum 25-OH vitamin D level and orthopaedic injury, such as fracture nonunion or infection, is unknown.

Robertson et al recently examined the effectiveness of vitamin D treatment in managing low serum vitamin D levels in orthopaedic trauma patients. Their retrospective review consisted of 201 patients at a Level 1 trauma center. The authors concluded that although vitamin D therapy improved the majority of the patients' vitamin D-25-OH level, most patients with vitamin D-25-OH level did not normalize. The authors also demonstrated that most patients with an initial deficiency had the largest improvement.[76]

An association between nonunion and undiagnosed metabolic and endocrine abnormalities has also been demonstrated. Brinker et al showed that 84% of patients who met the authors' screening criteria (1, an unexplained nonunion that occurred despite adequate reduction and stabilization, 2, a history of multiple low-energy fractures with at least one progressing to a nonunion, and 3, a nonunion of a nondisplaced pubic rami or sacral ala fracture) had one or more new diagnoses of metabolic or endocrine abnormalities. The most common newly diagnosed abnormality was vitamin D deficiency, followed by calcium imbalances, central hypogonadism, thyroid disorders, and PTH disorders. Although the study did not prove a causal link between metabolic and endocrine abnormalities and either the development or healing of nonunions, 84% of the patients who met the authors' screening criteria were found to have metabolic or endocrine abnormalities, and eight patients achieved bony union following medical treatment alone. The authors recommended that all patients with nonunion who meet their

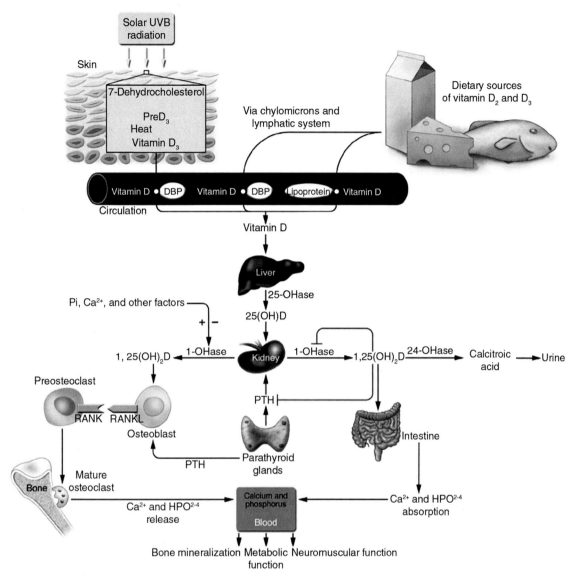

FIGURE 7.2 Pathway for vitamin D synthesis. (Reproduced with permission from Holick MF. Resurrection of vitamin D deficiency and rickets. *J Clin Invest.* 2006;116(8):2062-2072.)

screening criteria should be referred to an endocrinologist for evaluation because they are likely to have undiagnosed metabolic or endocrine abnormalities that may be interfering with bone healing.[77]

The diagnosis and management of hypovitaminosis D and other endocrine and metabolic abnormalities is no longer the sole responsibility of primary care physicians. Initiatives such as Own the Bone by the American Orthopaedic Association have attempted to improve patient education and physician communication regarding osteoporosis and treatment, including vitamin D and calcium supplementation.[78] Orthopaedic trauma, spine, and arthroplasty patients >50 years old, patients with a fragility fracture, those being treated for osteoporosis, and patients with a nonunion should be screened for vitamin D insufficiency. Laboratory evaluation should include 25-hydroxyvitamin D and serum calcium levels as well as a PTH level to evaluate

for secondary hyperparathyroidism.[68] Hydroxyvitamin D has a 2- to 3-week half-life and is the preferred clinical measure of vitamin D status. If appropriate, a referral to a metabolic bone specialist may be helpful in identifying other underlying metabolic abnormalities.

There is no universal protocol for oral vitamin D supplementation in the setting of decreased levels. Most observational and randomized studies have used doses of vitamin D ranging from 400 to 1000 IU per day. Daily supplementation in lower doses is thought to be more efficacious in comparison to large annual doses. Vitamin D3 has also been shown to be more effective than vitamin D2 in maintaining levels over time.[79] Vitamin D toxicity is rare and limited to a few case reports in the literature. It presents primarily as hypercalcemia.[80] The Institute of Medicine recommended daily allowance of vitamin D is up to 4000 IU per day.[81]

Given the uncertainty of the optimal therapeutic dose as well as the rarity of vitamin D toxicity, multiple differing vitamin D recommendations have been made in the literature. Although the Institute of Medicine affirmed the role of vitamin D in bone health, conflicting evidence in the literature led to their more conservative recommendation of 20 ng/mL. We agree with Patton et al[68] and recommend a target 25-hydroxyvitamin D level of between 30 and 40 ng/mL. The threshold for treatment, however, is based on the PTH response to vitamin D levels <30 ng/mL, similar to recent recommendations from Osteoporosis Canada and the International Osteoporosis Foundation. This threshold also accounts for temporal variations in individual levels of vitamin D.[82,83]

For patients with insufficient vitamin D levels of between 25 and 30 ng/mL, a daily oral dose of 2000 to 4000 IU of vitamin D_3 is often effective. For patients with levels <25 ng/mL, 50,000 IU of vitamin D_2 administered weekly for 8 to 12 weeks is preferred. In addition, we recommend 1000 mg of daily calcium supplementation for adults aged ≤50 years and 1200 mg of daily calcium for adults aged >50 years. Vitamin D levels are rechecked at 3-month intervals after initiation of treatment.[68]

CARTILAGE HEALING

Articular cartilage consists of extracellular matrix (ECM) and chondrocytes. The ECM is formed by water (65%-80%), collagen (95% type II), and proteoglycans (chondroitin sulfate and keratin sulfate). Collagen in the ECM provides form and tensile strength. Proteoglycans and water give the cartilage stiffness, resilience, and endurance.

Chondrocytes are sparse in the adult cartilage, which is not a vascularized tissue. Their nutrition comes from the synovial fluid, and adequate circulation of the fluid through the sponge-like cartilage matrix is crucial. The low baseline metabolic rate and small cell-to-matrix ratio of chondrocytes also diminish the reparative capacity of articular cartilage. Motion of the joint is responsible for most of the circulation. Rigid internal fixation of articular fractures and early weight bearing of immobilized joints allow cyclical compression of the cartilage and circulation of the synovial fluid. If the defect in the cartilage does not go through the calcified plate, the body attempts repair with hyaline cartilage. This may be seen at superficial articular cartilage lesions. If the calcified plate is violated, as in osteochondral lesions, the subchondral capillaries bring an inflammatory reaction, which fills the defect with granulation tissue and, eventually, fibrocartilage. The quality of this fibrocartilage can be improved by passive or active motion of the joint. Basic and clinical research has shown the potential of artificial matrices, growth factors, perichondrium, periosteum, transplanted chondrocytes, and mesenchymal stem cells to stimulate the formation of cartilage in articular defects.[84-86]

Glucosamine sulfate and chondroitin are the most common supplements marketed to those with osteoarthritis (OA).[87] They both have been used to treat OA since the 1980s. Literature with regard to fracture healing is limited.

Glucosamine is an amino saccharide that is a substrate for the biosynthesis of chondroitin sulfate, hyaluronic acid, and other cartilage molecules. It is prepared commercially from crustacean shells. In addition to providing structural support, it may also have anti-inflammatory activity. Oral glucosamine is well tolerated and does not elevate serum glucose levels in humans. There have been case reports of an increased INR in patients taking warfarin who ingest glucosamine. It is recommended to allow 4 to 6 months for an adequate therapeutic trial.[88] Chondroitin is a glycosaminoglycan normally present in the cartilage matrix that helps maintain articular fluid viscosity, inhibit enzymes that break down cartilage, and stimulate cartilage repair. Chondroitin is a constituent of the ECM, increasing the load-bearing properties of cartilage by increasing its water content. These supplements have been heavily marketed to arthritis pain sufferers.

Several early studies have shown a benefit of using either glucosamine or chondroitin, although these studies were small.[89] A large, 6-month randomized controlled trial sponsored by the National Institutes of Health, the glucosamine/chondroitin Arthritis Intervention Trial (GAIT), compared the use of glucosamine, chondroitin, or a combination of the two to celecoxib and placebo in the treatment of knee OA. The trial failed to show significant benefit with respect to pain or joint space width using supplement either alone or in combination. However, a subgroup of patients with moderate to severe pain taking the combination of both glucosamine and chondroitin showed a trend toward a measurable improvement.[89,90]

Glucosamine and chondroitin appear to be safe, with mild side effects that include headache, edema, leg pain, and GI upset. However, glucosamine, which is isolated from the exoskeleton of shellfish, has the potential to produce an allergic reaction in sensitive individuals. Whether glucosamine affects blood glucose levels in patients with type II diabetes is unclear, but caution should be exercised regarding these patients. Several case reports have shown that glucosamine increased the international normalized ratio or bruising/bleeding in patients taking warfarin.[91] Chondroitin may cause bleeding in persons with bleeding disorders or in those using blood thinners. Glucosamine and chondroitin should be stopped 2 weeks before surgery and not resumed until anticoagulant therapy is completed.

Review of the clinical trial literature suggests that (1) glucosamine sulfate, with or without chondroitin, is likely effective for reducing the pain of OA of the knee and hip; (2) chondroitin alone may reduce pain in OA, but the evidence is less robust than for glucosamine; (3) both glucosamine and chondroitin are well tolerated, safe, and have fewer side effects than NSAIDs; and (4) glucosamine alone, chondroitin alone, or the two in combination may reduce the progression of OA.[92-98] Further study investigating the use of glucosamine and chondroitin in fracture healing is necessary.

NUTRACEUTICALS

The term nutraceuticals is often applied to a large number of products that include isolated nutrients, dietary supplements, alternative medication, and herbal products. Glucosamine sulfate and chondroitin are typically grouped within this broad category and have already been discussed. The role of nutraceuticals in fracture healing has not been investigated. Future research is necessary to determine the role of alternative medications and herbal supplementation in fracture healing.

SUMMARY

Fracture repair is a complex and highly regulated process that is influenced by physiological, cellular, molecular, and genetic factors. Given the prevalence of malnutrition in orthopaedic patients and the impact on outcomes of orthopaedic procedures, the surgeon should assess the preoperative markers for malnutrition as described above. Although not always possible or practical in a trauma setting, delaying surgical intervention for an elective orthopaedic procedure until a patient's nutritional status has improved is recommended. Nutrition is an important adjunctive therapy and has been shown to have a positive effect on fracture healing. We advocate a postoperative regimen of calcium and vitamin D for all patients recovering from fracture fixation. Continued research is necessary to determine additional modalities that may be of benefit to a patient with a healing fracture.

REFERENCES

1. Giganti MG, Tresoldi I, Masuelli L, et al. Fracture healing: from basic science to role of nutrition. *Front Biosci (Landmark Ed)*. 2014;19:1162-1175.
2. Cross MB, Yi PH, Thomas CF, Garcia J, Della Valle CJ. Evaluation of malnutrition in orthopaedic surgery. *J Am Acad Orthop Surg*. 2014;22(3):193-199.
3. Jaberi FM, Parvizi J, Haytmanek CT, Joshi A, Purtill J. Procrastination of wound drainage and malnutrition affect the outcome of joint arthroplasty. *Clin Orthop Relat Res*. 2008;466(6):1368-1371.
4. Smith TK. Nutrition: its relationship to orthopedic infections. *Orthop Clin North Am*. 1991;22(3):373-377.
5. World Health Organization:WHO, N.E.T.A.o.M.A.a.h.w.w.i.n.p.a.o.m .e.A.
6. Via M. The malnutrition of obesity: micronutrient deficiencies that promote diabetes. *ISRN Endocrinol*. 2012;2012:103472.
7. Greene KA, Wilde AH, Stulberg BN. Preoperative nutritional status of total joint patients. Relationship to postoperative wound complications. *J Arthroplasty*. 1991;6(4):321-325.
8. Beiner JM, Grauer J, Kwon BK, Vaccaro AR. Postoperative wound infections of the spine. *Neurosurg Focus*. 2003;15(3):E14.
9. Guo JJ, Yang H, Qian H, Huang L, Guo Z, Tang T. The effects of different nutritional measurements on delayed wound healing after hip fracture in the elderly. *J Surg Res*. 2010;159(1):503-508.
10. Font-Vizcarra L, Lozano L, Ríos J, Forga MT, Soriano A. Preoperative nutritional status and post-operative infection in total knee replacements: a prospective study of 213 patients. *Int J Artif Organs*. 2011;34(9):876-881.
11. Pratt WB, Veitch JM, McRoberts RL. Nutritional status of orthopedic patients with surgical complications. *Clin Orthop Relat Res*. 1981;155:81-84.
12. Jensen JE, Jensen TG, Smith TK, Johnston DA, Dudrick SJ. Nutrition in orthopaedic surgery. *J Bone Joint Surg Am*. 1982;64(9):1263-1272.
13. Rai J, Gill SS, Kumar BR. The influence of preoperative nutritional status in wound healing after replacement arthroplasty. *Orthopedics*. 2002;25(4):417-421.
14. Puskarich CL, Nelson CL, Nusbickel FR, Stroope HF. The use of two nutritional indicators in identifying long bone fracture patients who do and do not develop infections. *J Orthop Res*. 1990;8(6):799-803.
15. Ozkalkanli MY, Ozkalkanli DT, Katircioglu K, Savaci S. Comparison of tools for nutrition assessment and screening for predicting the development of complications in orthopedic surgery. *Nutr Clin Pract*. 2009;24(2):274-280.
16. Zorrilla P, Gómez LA, Salido JA, Silva A, López-Alonso A. Low serum zinc level as a predictive factor of delayed wound healing in total hip replacement. *Wound Repair Regen*. 2006;14(2):119-122.
17. McPhee IB, Williams RP, Swanson CE, Factors influencing wound healing after surgery for metastatic disease of the spine. *Spine (Phila Pa 1976)*. 1998;23(6):726-732. discussion 732-733.
18. Gherini S, Vaughn BK, Lombardi AV Jr, Mallory TH. Delayed wound healing and nutritional deficiencies after total hip arthroplasty. *Clin Orthop Relat Res*. 1993;293:188-195.
19. Beck FK, Rosenthal TC. Prealbumin: a marker for nutritional evaluation. *Am Fam Physician*. 2002;65(8):1575-1578.
20. Cereda E, Pusani C, Limonta D, Vanotti A. The association of geriatric nutritional risk index and total lymphocyte count with short-term nutrition-related complications in institutionalised elderly. *J Am Coll Nutr*. 2008;27(3):406-413.
21. Murphy MC, Brooks CN, New SA, Lumbers ML. The use of the Mini-Nutritional Assessment (MNA) tool in elderly orthopaedic patients. *Eur J Clin Nutr*. 2000;54(7):555-562.
22. Rainey-Macdonald CG, Holliday RL, Wells GA, Donner AP. Validity of a two-variable nutritional index for use in selecting candidates for nutritional support. *JPEN J Parenter Enteral Nutr*. 1983;7(1):15-20.
23. Guigoz Y, The Mini Nutritional Assessment (MNA) review of the literature – What does it tell us? *J Nutr Health Aging*, 2006;10(6):466-485. discussion 485-487.
24. Li Y, Glotzbecker M, Hedequist D. Surgical site infection after pediatric spinal deformity surgery. *Curr Rev Musculoskelet Med*. 2012;5:111-119.
25. Jevsevar DS, Karlin LI. The relationship between preoperative nutritional status and complications after an operation for scoliosis in patients who have cerebral palsy. *J Bone Joint Surg Am*. 1993;75(6):880-884.
26. Sponseller PD, LaPorte DM, Hungerford MW, Eck K, Bridwell KH, Lenke LG. Deep wound infections after neuromuscular scoliosis surgery: a multicenter study of risk factors and treatment outcomes. *Spine (Phila Pa 1976)*. 2000;25(19):2461-2466.
27. Friedman ND, Sexton DJ, Connelly SM, Kaye KS. Risk factors for surgical site infection complicating laminectomy. *Infect Control Hosp Epidemiol*. 2007;28(9):1060-1065.
28. Olsen MA, Nepple JJ, Riew KD, et al. Risk factors for surgical site infection following orthopaedic spinal operations. *J Bone Joint Surg Am*. 2008;90(1):62-69.
29. Pull ter Gunne AF, Cohen DB. Incidence, prevalence, and analysis of risk factors for surgical site infection following adult spinal surgery. *Spine (Phila Pa 1976)*. 2009;34(13):1422-1428.
30. Bozic KJ, Lau E, Kurtz S, Ong K, Berry DJ. Patient-related risk factors for postoperative mortality and periprosthetic joint infection in medicare patients undergoing TKA. *Clin Orthop Relat Res*. 2012;470(1):130-137.
31. Malinzak RA, Ritter MA, Berend ME, Meding JB, Olberding EM, Davis KE. Morbidly obese, diabetic, younger, and unilateral joint arthroplasty patients have elevated total joint arthroplasty infection rates. *J Arthroplasty*. 2009;24(6 suppl):84-88.
32. Chesney D, Sales J, Elton R, Brenkel IJ. Infection after knee arthroplasty a prospective study of 1509 cases. *J Arthroplasty*. 2008;23(3):355-359.
33. Dowsey MM, Choong PF. Obese diabetic patients are at substantial risk for deep infection after primary TKA. *Clin Orthop Relat Res*. 2009;467(6):1577-1581.
34. Jamsen E, Nevalainen P, Eskelinen A, Huotari K, Kalliovalkama J, Moilanen T. Obesity, diabetes, and preoperative hyperglycemia as predictors of periprosthetic joint infection: a single-center analysis of 7181 primary hip and knee replacements for osteoarthritis. *J Bone Joint Surg Am*. 2012;94(14):e101.
35. Iorio R, Williams KM, Marcantonio AJ, Specht LM, Tilzey JF, Healy WL. Diabetes mellitus, hemoglobin A1$_C$, and the incidence of total joint arthroplasty infection. *J Arthroplasty*. 2012;27(5):726-729.e1.

36. Bozic KJ, Lau E, Kurtz S, et al. Patient-related risk factors for periprosthetic joint infection and postoperative mortality following total hip arthroplasty in Medicare patients. *J Bone Joint Surg Am.* 2012;94(9):794-800.

37. Jamsen E, Nevalainen P, Kalliovalkama J, Moilanen T. Preoperative hyperglycemia predicts infected total knee replacement. *Eur J Intern Med.* 2010;21(3):196-201.

38. Peersman G, Laskin R, Davis J, Peterson M. Infection in total knee replacement: a retrospective review of 6489 total knee replacements. *Clin Orthop Relat Res.* 2001;392:15-23.

39. Seibert DJ. Pathophysiology of surgical site infection in total hip arthroplasty. *Am J Infect Control.* 1999;27(6):536-542.

40. Marzocchella L, Fantini M, Benvenuto M, et al. Dietary flavonoids: molecular mechanisms of action as anti-inflammatory agents. *Recent Pat Inflamm Allergy Drug Discov.* 2011;5(3):200-220.

41. Masuelli L, Marzocchella L, Focaccetti C, et al. Resveratrol and diallyl disulfide enhance curcumin-induced sarcoma cell apoptosis. *Front Biosci (Landmark Ed).* 2012;17:498-508.

42. Byun CH, Koh JM, Kim DK, Park SI, Lee KU, Kim GS. Alpha-lipoic acid inhibits TNF-alpha-induced apoptosis in human bone marrow stromal cells. *J Bone Miner Res.* 2005;20(7):1125-1135.

43. Masuelli L, Morzocchella L, Quaranta A, et al. Apigenin induces apoptosis and impairs head and neck carcinomas EGFR/ErbB2 signaling. *Front Biosci (Landmark Ed).* 2011;16:1060-1068.

44. Renis M, Calandra L, Scifo C, et al. Response of cell cycle/stress-related protein expression and DNA damage upon treatment of CaCo2 cells with anthocyanins. *Br J Nutr.* 2008;100(1):27-35.

45. Masuelli L, Benvenuto M, Fantini M, et al. Curcumin induces apoptosis in breast cancer cell lines and delays the growth of mammary tumors in neu transgenic mice. *J Biol Regul Homeost Agents.* 2013;27(1):105-119.

46. Benvenuto M, Fantini M, Masuelli L, et al. Inhibition of ErbB receptors, Hedgehog and NF-kappaB signaling by polyphenols in cancer. *Front Biosci (Landmark Ed).* 2013;18:1290-1310.

47. Scalbert A, Manach C, Morand C, Rémésy C, Jiménez L. Dietary polyphenols and the prevention of diseases. *Crit Rev Food Sci Nutr.* 2005;45(4):287-306.

48. Tanumihardjo SA. Vitamin A and bone health: the balancing act. *J Clin Densitom.* 2013;16(4):414-9.

49. Sheweita SA, Khoshhal KI. Calcium metabolism and oxidative stress in bone fractures: role of antioxidants. *Curr Drug Metab.* 2007;8(5):519-25.

50. Mohan S, Kapoor A, Singgih A, et al. Spontaneous fractures in the mouse mutant sfx are caused by deletion of the gulonolactone oxidase gene, causing vitamin C deficiency. *J Bone Miner Res.* 2005;20(9):1597-1610.

51. Sarisozen B, Durak K, Dinçer G, Bilgen OF. The effects of vitamins E and C on fracture healing in rats. *J Int Med Res.* 2002;30(3):309-313.

52. Binkley N, Krueger D. Hypervitaminosis A and bone. *Nutr Rev.* 2000;58(5):138-144.

53. Bei R, Frigiola A, Masuelli L, et al. Effects of omega-3 polyunsaturated fatty acids on cardiac myocyte protection. *Front Biosci (Landmark Ed).* 2011;16:1833-1843.

54. Masuelli L, Trono P, Marzocchella L, et al. Intercalated disk remodeling in delta-sarcoglycan-deficient hamsters fed with an alpha-linolenic acid-enriched diet. *Int J Mol Med.* 2008;21(1):41-48.

55. Fiaccavento R, Carotenuto F, Minieri M, et al. Alpha-linolenic acid-enriched diet prevents myocardial damage and expands longevity in cardiomyopathic hamsters. *Am J Pathol.* 2006;169(6):1913-1924.

56. Das UN. Essential fatty acids and osteoporosis. *Nutrition.* 2000;16(5):386-390.

57. Sabour H, Larijani B, Vafa MR, et al. The effects of n-3 fatty acids on inflammatory cytokines in osteoporotic spinal cord injured patients: a randomized clinical trial. *J Res Med Sci.* 2012;17(4):322-327.

58. Lerner UH. Inflammation-induced bone remodeling in periodontal disease and the influence of post-menopausal osteoporosis. *J Dent Res.* 2006;85(7):596-607.

59. Watkins BA, Li Y, Seifert MF. Dietary ratio of n-6/n-3 PUFAs and docosahexaenoic acid: actions on bone mineral and serum biomarkers in ovariectomized rats. *J Nutr Biochem.* 2006;17(4):282-289.

60. Yamaguchi M. Nutritional factors and bone homeostasis: synergistic effect with zinc and genistein in osteogenesis. *Mol Cel Biochem.* 2012;366(1-2):201-221.

61. Kuiper GG, Larijani B, Vafa MR, et al. Comparison of the ligand binding specificity and transcript tissue distribution of estrogen receptors alpha and beta. *Endocrinology.* 1997;138(3):863-870.

62. Yamaguchi M. Regulatory mechanism of food factors in bone metabolism and prevention of osteoporosis. *Yakugaku Zasshi.* 2006;126(11):1117-1137.

63. Hsieh HS, Navia JM. Zinc deficiency and bone formation in guinea pig alveolar implants. *J Nutr.* 1980;110(8):1581-1588.

64. Igarashi A, Yamaguchi M. Increase in bone protein components with healing rat fractures: enhancement by zinc treatment. *Int J Mol Med.* 1999;4(6):615-620.

65. Uchiyama S, Yamaguchi M. Genistein and zinc synergistically enhance gene expression and mineralization in osteoblastic MC3T3-E1 cells. *Int J Mol Med.* 2007;19(2):213-220.

66. Choi MJ, Park EJ, Jo HJ. Relationship of nutrient intakes and bone mineral density of elderly women in Daegu, Korea. *Nutr Res Pract.* 2007;1(4):328-334.

67. Sakuma M, Endo N, Oinuma T, et al. Vitamin D and intact PTH status in patients with hip fracture. *Osteoporos Int.* 2006;17(11):1608-1614.

68. Patton CM, Powell AP, Patel AA. Vitamin D in orthopaedics. *J Am Acad Orthop Surg.* 2012;20(3):123-129.

69. Norman AW. From vitamin D to hormone D: fundamentals of the vitamin D endocrine system essential for good health. *Am J Clin Nutr.* 2008;88(2):491S-499S.

70. Holick MF. Vitamin D deficiency. *N Engl J Med.* 2007;357(3):266-281.

71. DeLuca HF. Overview of general physiologic features and functions of vitamin D. *Am J Clin Nutr.* 2004;80(6 suppl):1689S-1696S.

72. Thomas MK, Lloyd-Jones DM, Thadhani RI, et al. Hypovitaminosis D in medical inpatients. *N Engl J Med.* 1998;338(12):777-783.

73. Bischoff-Ferrari HA, Can U, Staehelin HB, et al. Severe vitamin D deficiency in Swiss hip fracture patients. *Bone.* 2008;42(3):597-602.

74. Brinker MR, O'Connor DP. Outcomes of tibial nonunion in older adults following treatment using the Ilizarov method. *J Orthop Trauma.* 2007;21(9):634-642.

75. Bogunovic L, Kim AD, Beamer BS, Nguyen J, Lane JM. Hypovitaminosis D in patients scheduled to undergo orthopaedic surgery: a single-center analysis. *J Bone Joint Surg Am.* 2010;92(13):2300-2304.

76. Robertson DS, Jenkins T, Murtha YM, et al. Effectiveness of vitamin D therapy in orthopaedic trauma patients. *J Orthop Trauma.* 2015;29:e451-e453.

77. Brinker MR, O'Connor DP, Monla YT, Earthman TP. Metabolic and endocrine abnormalities in patients with nonunions. *J Orthop Trauma.* 2007;21(8):557-570.

78. Tosi LL, Gliklich R, Kannan K, Koval KJ. The American Orthopaedic Association's "own the bone" initiative to prevent secondary fractures. *J Bone Joint Surg Am.* 2008;90(1):163-173.

79. Sanders KM, Stuart AL, Williamson EJ, et al. Annual high-dose oral vitamin D and falls and fractures in older women: a randomized controlled trial. *J Am Med Assoc.* 2010;303(18):1815-1822.

80. Hathcock JN, Shao A, Vieth R, Heaney R. Risk assessment for vitamin D. *Am J Clin Nutr.* 2007;85(1):6-18.

81. Institute of Medicine Committee to Review Dietary Reference Intakes for Vitamin, D. and Calcium, The National Academies Collection: Reports funded by National Institutes of Health. In: Ross AC, Taylor CL, Yaktine AL, Del Valle HB, eds. *Dietary Reference Intakes for Calcium and Vitamin D.* Washington, DC: National Academies Press (US) National Academy of Sciences; 2011.

82. Hanley DA, Cranney A, Jones G, et al. Vitamin D in adult health and disease: a review and guideline statement from Osteoporosis Canada. *CMAJ.* 2010;182(12):E610-E618.

83. Dawson-Hughes B, Mithal A, Bonjour JP, et al. IOF position statement: vitamin D recommendations for older adults. *Osteoporos Int.* 2010;21(7):1151-1154.

84. Browne JE, Branch TP. Surgical alternatives for treatment of articular cartilage lesions. *J Am Acad Orthop Surg.* 2000;8(3):180-189.

85. Buckwalter JA. Articular cartilage injuries. *Clin Orthop Relat Res.* 2002;402:21-37.

86. Jackson DW, Scheer MJ, Simon TM. Cartilage substitutes: overview of basic science and treatment options. *J Am Acad Orthop Surg.* 2001;9(1):37-52.

87. Rispler DT, Sara J. The impact of complementary and alternative treatment modalities on the care of orthopaedic patients. *J Am Acad Orthop Surg.* 2011;19(10):634-643.

88. Maxine A, Papadakis SJM, Rabow MW. *Current Medical Diagnosis & Treatment 2015.* Lange; 2015

89. Clegg DO, Reda DJ, Harris CL, et al. Glucosamine, chondroitin sulfate, and the two in combination for painful knee osteoarthritis. *N Engl J Med.* 2006;354(8):795-808.

90. Sawitzke AD, Shi H, Finco MF, et al. The effect of glucosamine and/or chondroitin sulfate on the progression of knee osteoarthritis: a report from the glucosamine/chondroitin arthritis intervention trial. *Arthritis Rheum.* 2008;58(10):3183-3191.

91. Knudsen JF, Sokol GH. Potential glucosamine-warfarin interaction resulting in increased international normalized ratio: case report and review of the literature and MedWatch database. *Pharmacotherapy.* 2008;28(4):540-548.

92. Greenlee H, Crew KD, Shao T, et al. Phase II study of glucosamine with chondroitin on aromatase inhibitor-associated joint symptoms in women with breast cancer. *Support Care Cancer.* 2013;21(4):1077-1087.

93. Henrotin Y, Lambert C. Chondroitin and glucosamine in the management of osteoarthritis: an update. *Curr Rheumatol Rep.* 2013;15(10):361.

94. Henrotin Y, Mobasheri A, Marty M. Is there any scientific evidence for the use of glucosamine in the management of human osteoarthritis?. *Arthritis Res Ther.* 2012;14(1):201.

95. Hochberg M, Chevalier X, Henrotin Y, Hunter DJ, Uebelhart D. Symptom and structure modification in osteoarthritis with pharmaceutical-grade chondroitin sulfate: what's the evidence? *Curr Med Res Opin.* 2013;29(3):259-267.

96. Reginster JY, Neuprez A, Lecart MP, Sarlet N, Bruyere O. Role of glucosamine in the treatment for osteoarthritis. *Rheumatol Int.* 2012;32;10:2959-2967.

97. Zegels B, Crozes P, Uebelhart D, Bruyère O, Reginster JY. Equivalence of a single dose (1200 mg) compared to a three-time a day dose (400 mg) of chondroitin 4&6 sulfate in patients with knee osteoarthritis. Results of a randomized double blind placebo controlled study. *Osteoarthritis Cartilage.* 2013;21(1):22-27.

98. Wildi LM, Raynauld JP, Martel-Pelletier J, et al. Chondroitin sulphate reduces both cartilage volume loss and bone marrow lesions in knee osteoarthritis patients starting as early as 6 months after initiation of therapy: a randomised, double-blind, placebo-controlled pilot study using MRI. *Ann Rheum Dis.* 2011;70(6):982-989.

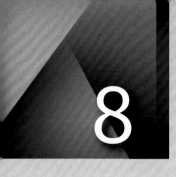

8

Special Considerations in Geriatric Fracture Healing and Rehabilitation

Carmen E. Quatman
Catherine Quatman-Yates
Deborah Kegelmeyer
Laura Phieffer

Approximately one in three elderly patients fall each year, resulting in more than 1.5 million fragility fractures annually in the United States.[1,2] Osteoporotic fractures, in particular hip fractures, often lead to permanent impairments in physical function and loss of independence and have a 15% to 30% risk for mortality within 1 year of fracture.[3-6] The socioeconomic impact of caring for geriatric fractures is profound when accounting for the financial costs associated with treatments, hospitalization, and rehabilitation needs for these patients.[7] Estimated annual associated healthcare costs for fragility fractures in the United States are over 17 billion dollars.[8] In addition, prior fragility fracture is one of the strongest predictors for future fracture risk.[9,10] The treatment approaches for geriatric fracture patients often differ significantly from those for younger patients as expectations, disease management, quality of life, and overall approach to the health of the patient may be quite different depending on each patient.[11,12]

One central tenet of the aging process is the concept of deterioration in strength, mobility, and agility over time. In particular, decreased muscle mass and strength, decreased bone density, and loss of skeletal height are common musculoskeletal manifestations of the aging process. These musculoskeletal changes, coincident with age-related alterations in gait, balance, and posture as well as sensory losses in vision, hearing, vestibular function, and proprioception, make elderly patients at high risk for falls and fragility fractures.[11] It is critical that practitioners who treat elderly fractures have a basic understanding of the fundamentals of aging and musculoskeletal and sensory changes that occur in older adults in order to provide the best rehabilitation strategies. It is also important to recognize how these aging concepts

impact fracture prevention, but to also recognize that these risks do not go away in the treatment phase. If anything, they are intensified in the early treatment period. In addition, 5% of patients who are 65 years of age or older present with multiple fractures, which can make the rehabilitation process even more difficult.[13]

The healing capacity of fractures slows down through all phases of fracture healing with increasing chronological age. Age-related changes in cartilage and bone formation, osteochondral stem cells, callus mineralization, and callus ossification significantly impact geriatric patients' recovery after fractures.[14] These fracture healing concepts have been a driving force for surgical fracture treatment innovations for the past 30 years. Implant innovations such as locking plate technology, bone augmentation methods, and cellular enhancement techniques have created new domains of treatment for geriatric fractures. In addition, we have a growing body of literature on pharmaceutical options such as anticatabolic, antiresorptive, and anabolic medications that may enhance fracture healing potential and reduce osteoporotic fracture risk.[7,15-18]

Although surgical and medical treatment options are expanding, several underlying rehabilitation and service delivery strategies are also pivotal to the outcome of patients: (1) mobility, (2) medical optimization, and (3) optimized care transitions. Recently, an "APGAR SCORE" checklist was developed to help enhance the quality of life for geriatric hip fracture patients, but perhaps it could have a wider scope approach to all geriatric fracture patients. As part of the "APGAR SCORE," there is emphasis of Alimentation (and nutrition) Polypharmacy Gait, Advance care planning, addressing Reversible cognitive impairment, maximizing Social support, remediating Cataracts (or other visual impairments), addressing Osteoporosis, and ensuring Referrals for multidisciplinary care and safe Environments after discharge.[19] Much of the APGAR SCORE mentality for hip fracture patients encompasses the biopsychosocial needs that should be addressed in order for geriatric fracture patients to have the best outcomes. The following sections below discuss in detail rehabilitation strategies for geriatric fracture patients with emphasis on mobility, medical optimization, and safe care transitions.

MOBILIZATION

In the early recovery stages, focused strategies around optimization of mobility, medical care, and discharge planning/transition of care are critical for patient outcomes (**Table 8.1**) and often must be tailored to patient needs, expected outcomes, and goals for recovery.[20] Many older patients require hospitalization to help with safe risk stratification of medical, caregiving, and mobilization needs including appropriate safe discharge destination, physical therapy, speech therapy, occupational therapy, pain control, and/or surgical treatment. Multidisciplinary care for elderly fracture patients often leads to improvements in quality measures of length of stay, avoidance of hospital readmissions, and improvements in overall morbidity and mortality.[21,22]

EARLY RECOVERY PHASE

Rehabilitation strategies in elderly patients should focus on early mobilization, balance training, fall prevention, muscle strengthening, and overall endurance for activities of daily living (ADLs).[23,24] It is also important to recognize that injuries and falls in elderly patients are associated with fear of falling, loss of self-confidence, and self-imposed or caregiver-imposed restricted ambulation.[11] Historically, common rehabilitation strategies for fracture care have been immobilization and protected weight bearing to allow for biological fracture healing.[25] However, limited weight bearing for an elderly patient can lead to significant disability, loss of independence, higher risk for falls, second fractures, and mortality.[4,26] Instead, focused rehabilitation with emphasis on safe mobilization strategies can considerably improve fracture outcomes for older patients. While it is becoming more common to allow hip fracture patients to "weight bear as tolerated," evidence about weight bearing for other fracture sites remains limited.[25,27-30]

Evaluation of patient mobility and self-care limitations of fracture patients helps create an understanding of care needs for hospitalized patients and helps with discharge destination plans. The Activity Measure for Post-Acute Care (AM-PAC) instrument and the AM-PAC "6-click" are tools that assess functional measures of basic mobility, daily activities, and applied cognition that predict hospital discharge destination and help facilitate communication among colleagues and different disciplines. In general, the tools may

TABLE 8.1 Important Care Elements in Geriatric Fracture Patients

Inpatient/Early Recovery:
- Pain control
- Delirium (prevention, recognition, treatment)
- Early mobilization (first day if possible)
- Patient comprehension of post-op restrictions (ie, weight bearing, hip precautions)
- Medical optimization of chronic conditions
- Treatment of anemia
- Optimized nutrition (including vitamin D, calcium)
- Appropriate bowel regimen
- Multidisciplinary care (treatment and communication)
- Optimized discharge planning and transition of care communication

Postdischarge Skilled Nursing/Rehabilitation:
- Pain control
- Safe mobilization (address fear of falling as well)
- Build confidence in activities of daily living
- Balance and strength training
- Nutrition optimization (including bone health pharmaceutical options)
- Optimized discharge planning and transition of care communication

Post Discharge to Home:
- Safe home environment (remove fall hazards)
- Safe mobilization (address fear of falling as well)
- Build confidence in activities of daily living
- Balance and strength training
- Nutrition optimization (including bone health pharmaceutical options)
- Optimized transition of care (awareness of a patient's success of return)

Long Term:
- Lifelong safe mobilization
- Lifelong balance and strength maintenance
- Lifelong nutrition optimization
- Lifelong safe home environment (remove fall hazards)

oversimplify a patient's overall function and access to social support and may not be helpful alone for clinical decision-making about discharge plans.[31] However, interprofessional mobility measures, such as the AM-PAC, may help facilitate care transitions and decision-making for geriatric fracture patients overall.

Deconditioning due to immobility can result in debilitating consequences for patients. Prolonged periods of bed rest are associated with increased length of stay, increased risk of falls, functional decline, delirium, pneumonia, thromboembolisms, need for extended care facility placement, and many other adverse outcomes.[32-37] Despite these known adverse outcomes associated with immobility, low mobility of hospitalized patients is common due to the competing initiatives between promoting mobility and preventing falls.[38-40] In response to increased societal awareness of medical errors, federal policy and hospital culture have recently prioritized fall prevention in the hospital, which has resulted in a resurgence of physical restraints and decreased overall mobility in patients.

The problem of immobility in hospitalized patients and the effects it can have on healthcare outcomes are becoming increasingly recognized worldwide. In fact, the Nottingham University Hospital started a social media campaign called "End PJ Paralysis" that focuses on getting hospitalized patients out of their nightwear, out of bed, and into their normal clothes.[41] This effort has gained much attention and has been successfully embraced in other institutions worldwide. Connecting mobilization strategies to daily activities such as dressing and eating creates a daily schedule of normalcy and promotes physical and emotional well-being in hospitalized patients.

There is also increasing evidence that patients who mobilize with just a few steps on the first day in the hospital can lead to significant improvement in patient confidence, endurance, and improved patient outcomes (**Table 8.2**).[23,24,34] In particular, hip fracture patients are at high risk for pressure sores, with greater than 30% of hip fracture patients developing sores due to prolonged periods of immobility.[42,43] As a result, many hospital initiatives have focused on mobilizing patients safely, even in the sickest of patients such as ventilated intensive care unit patients and transplant patients.[44,45] Inpatient mobilization protocols have significantly improved patient outcomes for hospitalized patients.[46-48] Barriers to safe mobilization after injury are often tied to the challenge of behavioral and cultural challenges for patients, families, and care providers (**Table 8.3**).[45,49,50] In addition, appropriate

pain control for physical therapy and mobility needs after fracture can significantly improve early postoperative pain, chronic pain, hospital length of stay, postoperative mobility, and long-term function.[51,52]

Research demonstrates that increased minutes of physical therapy per day can increase patient function at discharge from hospitals.[53] However, simply increasing the frequency and length of physical therapy sessions can be a costly burden and may be difficult to implement across a healthcare system. Additionally, the minutes used should be used to focus on functional mobility tasks, rather than just minutes in therapy. Instead, Drolet et al demonstrated that nursing-driven protocols have successfully increased patient ambulation in the first 72 hours of a hospital stay. As part of the "Move to Improve" initiative by Drolet et al, a multidisciplinary team effectively developed and implemented a mobility order set that had an algorithm to guide assessment of mobility potential and implement mobilization strategies for patients in the hospital.[54] The algorithm has been endorsed by the Agency for Healthcare Research and Quality (AHRQ) for Mobilizing Patients as part of the Prevention of Falls in Hospitals Toolkit.[55] The "Move to Improve" study successfully improved ambulation of patients in intermediate care settings by 70%. Specifically for hip fracture patients, delays in getting a patient out of bed are associated with poor outcomes at 2 and 6 months post hip fracture.[56] Mobility after fracture evidenced by

---

TABLE 8.2 Benefits of Early Mobilization

Prevents:
- Functional decline
- Pneumonia
- Pressure ulcers
- Delirium
- Depression
- Muscle wasting

Reduces:
- Length of stay
- Need for extended care facilities
- Fall risks
- Readmissions
- Mortality risk

Improves:
- Patient confidence in mobilization over time
- Patient sense of "normalcy"
- Physical and emotional well-being
- Digestion/heart burn symptoms
- Caregiver engagement/interaction

TABLE 8.3 Examples of Organizational Barriers to Mobilization

Patients:
- Pain
- Fatigue
- Physical limitations
- Delirium/dementia
- Depression
- Planned procedures/imaging/tests
- Unaware of benefits of mobility

Family:
- Fear of patient moving safely
- Worry about patient's pain
- Unaware of benefits of mobility

Physicians/Service Team:
- Unaware of benefits of mobility
- Physical limitation orders (ie, weight bearing)
- Unaware that championing/coaching can improve patient confidence and willingess

Nursing/Staff:
- Unaware of benefits of mobility
- Fear of falling event (fall prevention initiatives)
- Not confident in ability to safely move patient
- Not enough equipment
- Not enough resources/people

ability to stand, sit down, or walk 2 weeks after surgery is a strong predictor for mortality within 1 year after fracture.[4] Instead early ambulation after fracture can accelerate functional recovery and is associated with more discharges to home and less need for transitional care at institutions for recovery.[57,58]

Many nursing-driven initiatives have led to great results in improving patient mobility in hospitalized patients. Phelan et al, Pearson et al, and Moore et al, published reports on the most common barriers to mobilizing hospitalized patients.[44,45,50] Strategies to improve patient mobility often include providing knowledge about the importance of mobilization, building staff confidence in how to safely mobilize patients, promotion of mobilization to patients and families as part of the recovery process, proper equipment needs for patient safe mobility readily available, improved documentation about mobility, and regular staff audits about patient mobility. Establishing a culture of safe mobility by engaging multiple teams to improve actionable, team-oriented results to achieve mobility for patients may have an important impact on patient-centered outcomes as well as quality of life and level of independence at discharge for geriatric fracture patients.

MID-RECOVERY PHASE

Mobility after discharge from the hospital has been postulated to be a physical biomarker of overall health and risk of 30-day readmission for elderly patients.[35] For geriatric patients with fractures specifically, safe mobility after hospital discharge remains an important part of the recovery. The Timed "Up and Go" (TUG) test, a common geriatric physical function assessment, is a sensitive measure for identifying patients at high risk for falls after hip fracture. In a study by Kristensen et al, 32% of patients with hip fractures reported falls in the 6 months post injury, with 21% of the patients who reported a fall experiencing a second hip fracture. The TUG test performed at discharge from the hospital for these patients was a significant predictor of falls, with 95% of patients that had TUG times of >24 seconds experiencing falls.[59] In addition, persistent pain may occur after hip fracture treatment, with greater than 60% of patients reporting moderate to severe pain 3 months after hip fracture treatment.[60] Pain control remains an important part of helping patients safely mobilize, even after hospital discharge.

Mobility remains an important focus, even for patients with cognitive impairments. Patients with dementia fall more frequently, often receive less physical therapy, and have poorer mobility and functional outcomes than patients who do not have permanent cognitive impairment.[61-66] However, patients with mild to moderate dementia who receive rehabilitation can have similar gains in function to patients without dementia including improved ambulation and decreased risk of falls.[67] Thus, regardless of a patient's cognitive abilities, rehabilitation

with a focus on physical and occupational therapy can improve ADLs and mobility, while also reducing fall risks in older fracture patients.

Rehabilitation after discharge from the hospital is important after fracture in geriatric patients, and structured exercise after discharge can significantly improve mobility.[68] Mortality at 1 year can be predicted by functional status as early as 2 weeks after hip fracture. Heinonen et al demonstrated that the inability to stand, sit down, or walk 2 weeks after hip fracture surgery is a strong predictor for mortality. The authors concluded that more intensive rehabilitation in the early postoperative period may significantly alter outcomes for fracture patients.[4] Progressive resistance exercise can significantly improve physical function, lower extremity strength, and overall mobility in hip fracture patients and should be considered part of the short-term and long-term rehabilitation strategy.[69,70] In fact, progressive resistance exercise can counteract muscle weakness, improve ADLs, and prevent falls even in very frail, elderly patients.[71-74] Several clinical trials for hip fracture mobility have found improved mobility with weight-bearing programs in the first 2 weeks, quadriceps strengthening exercises, and electrical stimulation from pain.[75] Intensive home-based physical therapy and strength training have also demonstrated improvements in overall mobility and function; however, adherence for home-based therapy may be relatively low.[76] Collectively, most literature supports continued physical and occupational therapy and exercise programs, both immediately after and for up to 1 year after discharge from the hospital for geriatric fracture. Thus, mobility and physical function remain a fundamental strategy throughout the continuum of care for geriatric patients with fractures.

LATE RECOVERY PHASE

Mobility after fragility fracture, particularly lower extremity fracture, remains a challenge long-term for many patients. Vochteloo et al found that nearly 20% patients with hip fractures may be bedridden 1 year after hip fracture surgery. In addition, more than half of patients with hip fractures do not regain their prefracture mobility by 1 year after fracture, with dementia, living in institutionalization, and delirium during hospital admission identified as significant risk factors for loss of prefracture mobility.[77] Many geriatric patients have persistent strength and mobility deficits after fractures, despite rehabilitation in a care facility. Often patients are discharged once they achieve independent ambulation, but they continue to have residual disability and difficulty with ADLs.[78] However, extended outpatient rehabilitation for 6 months after hip fracture has been shown to significantly improve physical function and quality of life, while also reducing overall disability.[79] Significant strength and functional gains in mobility can be achieved even after discharge from traditional rehabilitation programs with higher exercise training intensity.[80] In addition, home-based physical therapy for 6 months after hip fracture significantly improves physical function with improved results persisting greater than 9 months after fracture.[81]

MEDICAL OPTIMIZATION

EARLY RECOVERY PHASE

In the early recovery phase, medical optimization (addressing medical comorbidities) both for chronic and acute conditions can improve the patient's ability to recover and mobilize, as well as lower the risks for complications. "Geriatric giants" of impairment are important considerations in the recovery period for geriatric fracture patients. These impairments, which may be present at baseline, include immobility, instability, incontinence, and impaired memory/intellect, which often lead to loss of independence, higher risk for falls, and increased frailty.[11] Optimal medical care strategies that address geriatric impairments are important for outcomes in geriatric fracture patients.

Acutely, many elderly patients may be anemic, due to either fracture hematoma or surgical intervention, which may be exacerbated by age-related anemia at baseline.[82,83] Anemia can lead to weakness, fatigue, and disability ultimately impacting a patient's ability to participate in rehabilitation care. The threshold for transfusion in geriatric fracture patients remains somewhat controversial, but it is increasingly recognized that lower hemoglobin thresholds (8-9.5 g dl) do not result in significant differences in mortality, hospital stay, mobility, or complications.[84,85] Clinical judgment is necessary to determine transfusion needs by accounting for patient symptoms as well as hemoglobin levels.

Delirium is the most common medical complication for hospitalized hip fracture patients and can have a significant impact on recovery after geriatric fractures.[86,87] Delirium, characterized as a serious disturbance in cognition and defined as an acute disorder of attention and cognition, can be distressing and a terrifying experience for patients and relatives.[88,89] Although delirium can be life threatening, it is often preventable and early recognition can significantly improve outcomes for patients.[90] In particular, delirium intervention (prevention, early recognition, and treatment) can lower the risk of delirium in geriatric hip fracture patients and decrease complications of decubitus ulcers, urinary tract infections, nutritional complications, sleeping problems, and falls while also improving overall mobility.[91] Multicomponent interventions to prevent delirium should be instituted for older patients, such as early mobilization, patient orientation, addressing visual and hearing needs, sleep enhancement, medication review and optimization, hydration, pain management, nutrition, and addressing bowel and bladder functions.[89] Rehabilitation with emphasis on modifiable delirium prevention strategies can significantly improve outcomes for geriatric fracture patients.

At the same time, malnutrition is a very real concern and a risk factor that must be addressed in the care of the geriatric fracture patients.[92] Elderly patients often fail to meet nutritional requirements due to loss of smell and taste, hormonal changes (insulin, leptin, and ghrelin), malabsorption and anorexia, reduced appetite, living in isolation, and many other conditions that impede nutritional optimization.[11] Approximately 50% of patients with hip fractures are reportedly malnourished at presentation.[93] Nutrition is essential for recovery after fracture, as it is important for wound healing, strength, endurance, and fracture healing.[26] Patients are often asked to refrain from eating and drinking in preparation for anesthesia and surgery. Nutritional deficits can be exacerbated if patients have a delay to surgery, if they experience delirium post-op, develop an ileus, and have swallowing restrictions and many other complications that may result in further "NPO" (nothing by mouth) status.

Malnutrition in hospitalized patients has also been reported to be between 20% and 40%, with malnourished patients having lower scores on basic mobility tests such as the "TUG" test, steps performed in the hospital, and balance tests. It is reported that 33% of patients in the hospital who are classified as malnourished may experience a fall in the hospital and malnourished patients with hip fracture often suffer from greater than 25% losses in ADLs.[94] Hospital mortality rates are 27% for malnourished hip fracture patients compared with well-nourished patients who have a reported 7% inpatient mortality after a hip fracture.[95,96] Thus, optimized nutrition for geriatric patients with fractures can significantly improve outcomes and is a critical element of care during the recovery process.[97]

MID-RECOVERY PHASE

Nearly 70% of people over the age of 65 require assisted living, nursing home healthcare, or long-term care.[98] In cases of geriatric fracture, 40% to 70% of patients may discharge to inpatient rehabilitation or to a skilled nursing facility after injury.[99,100] Hospital readmissions from nursing homes after hip fracture and all lower extremity fractures are reported to be approximately 8% to 15%.[101-103] Older patients who sustain fragility fractures have a high risk for readmission even after they have complete care at a rehabilitation facility. Ottenbacher et al demonstrated that 9% of patients who were discharged from the hospital after fragility fracture and complete a postacute rehabilitation may still be readmitted to the hospital within 30 days of discharge from the rehabilitation stay. Pneumonia is the leading cause of admission after hip fracture, and hospital costs for readmission after hip fracture ranges from $14,000 to upward of $25,000.[102,104] Thus, in the early phases of recovery, medical optimization is an important component of the rehabilitation process.

LATE RECOVERY PHASE

Nearly one-third of patients are readmitted to the hospital within 6 months of initial hospital discharge after hip fracture, with 8% having multiple readmissions.[105] Readmission after a hip fracture leads to abysmal results with approximately 20% of readmitted hip fracture patients dying during hospital readmission and 52% dying within 1 year if they had a hospital readmission.[103,106,107] Approximately 80% of hospital readmissions after hip fracture are from medical complications, with nearly 15% of readmissions felt to be preventable.[107] Medical optimization remains a critical component of the recovery process for geriatric fracture patients, even after they discharge from the hospital and within the first year of recovery.

Malnutrition may also continue to impact outcomes after discharge from the hospital. One-year mortality for malnourished patients with hip fracture is 46% compared to 17% for well-nourished patients.[95,96] In addition, osteopenia and osteoporosis are often only recognized after a fragility fracture, and despite sustaining a fragility fracture, treatment for osteoporosis remains low.[2,26] More than 50% of hip fracture patients may fall at least once during the first year after fracture, with nearly 30% of patients experiencing recurrent falls.[3-6] Prior fragility fracture is one of the strongest predictors of sustaining a fragility fracture.[6] However, despite the high risk for secondary fracture and well-established literature demonstrating the effectiveness of pharmaceutical agents for fracture reduction, less than 20% of fragility fracture patients receive pharmacological treatment for prevention of second fracture.[108-110] Long-term guidance to patients about important nutritional strategies including vitamin D and calcium supplementation through diet, emphasis on weight-bearing exercise, and balance training could have significant impact on helping prevent secondary fractures.

CARE COORDINATION AND TRANSITIONS IN CARE

EARLY RECOVERY PHASE

Caring for patients with geriatric fractures necessitates effective coordination, cooperation, and communication among the many care providers that may be involved in treatments for these patients. Coordinated care teams across the continuum of care (hospital, transitional care, and home care can significantly improve clinical outcomes by reducing hospital readmissions, reducing mortality, and improving functional recovery after fracture.[111] Patients with hip fractures, in particular, may experience 2 to 10 care transitions over the course of 6 months following surgical treatment.[112,113] Older adults may be particularly vulnerable to transitions in care, with communication barriers, cognitive difficulties, unintended errors in transitions, and overall medical complexities associated with aging often impacting safe care transitions.[113,114] Unintended errors such as inadvertent medication errors in the type of medication, frequency, dosage and end dates, failure to include pertinent information in discharge summaries, failure to arrange follow-up studies and appointments, and incomplete handoffs can occur

when transferring patients from hospitals to discharge destinations.[115] Involvement of patients and caregivers in the care transition is critical for the success of care transition since many transition errors are caught by patients and caregivers.[113-115] Fragmentation in care after geriatric fractures can lead to hospital readmissions, patient dissatisfaction with care, and overall poor outcomes. Instead, integrated care pathways across the entire continuum of care for geriatric fracture patients that emphasize communication, particularly the most vulnerable elderly patients, could significantly improve patient outcomes.[114,116]

MID-RECOVERY PHASE

Fragmented care in the mid-recovery phase after geriatric fracture remains a difficult problem. Geriatric patients with fractures may have significant barriers to care once they are discharged from the hospital, regardless of the discharge destination. Travel to physician visits and healthcare needs can be a significant disruption to a patient's environment and daily routines, leading to unintended consequences such as missed medication doses; delirium; costs for transportation; and dependence on family members for transportation, communication, and cognitive needs. The disruptions in routine can also lead to significant loss of time at work and financial hardships for family members if patients have to rely heavily on support from family to attend therapy visits, physician visits, and overall care.[12]

Falls among older adults that lead to significant injury or death often occur at home.[117] Mitigating fall risks within homes is paramount for a successful return to independent living after geriatric fracture. Understanding a patient's home environment is critical for safe mobility within the home, including known risk factors for falls such as poor vision, balance and gait disturbances, and need for proper ambulation aids. Other risk factors for falls within a home include pets, poor lighting, inadequate railings, uneven floors, unsafe footwear (slippers), uneven sidewalks, bathroom hazards, loose rugs, and electrical cords.[118,119] Regular exercise and balance training, environmental modifications to reduce fall hazards in the home, use of assistive devices such as gait aids, medication checks, and optimization, and providing interventions to address vision problems can help prevent falls within a home environment and should be implemented prior to a patient returning to independent living after a fragility fracture.[120]

LONG-TERM RECOVERY PHRASE

Long-term goals after fragility fracture often include returning home or back to baseline activity prior to fracture. However, it is under-recognized that many fragility patients have a high prevalence of disability prior to presentation with an injury.[121] More than 40% of patients with hip fracture demonstrate debility (need for assistance in ADLs) prior to their injury.[121] Although understanding a patient's debility prior to injury can help with goal planning and expectations of recovery for patients, this can be a challenge as many patients are not aware or willing to acknowledge that they have difficulties with ADLs.[121]

With an average of 3.5 care transitions for hip fracture patients within 12 months of discharge from the hospital, care transitions remain an essential part of the long-term care process for geriatric fracture patients.[112,113] After a hip fracture, 15% to 45% of patients are unable to regain functional abilities well enough to return to home and need additional support through assisted living or a long-term care nursing home. Factors associated with need for a change in residency status from independent living after a fragility fracture include unmarried status, bowel or bladder incontinence, low mental status scores, and dependence in ambulation. Although changes in residence are often unwanted by patients, it is important to help facilitate the necessary care transitions if needed, through family planning and patient engagement along all phases of care in order to help patients and families understand long-term expectations and outcomes.

SUMMARY

Older orthopaedic patients require a rehabilitation strategy that accounts for the complex needs that accompany the aging process, including priorities focused on safe mobility, nutrition, and medical optimization across the entire spectrum of care. Teams that focus on seamless transitions in care can help safely mobilize patients and provide the best evidence-based medical care during the recovery process, while also helping prevent second fragility fractures. Through excellent care coordination, optimized medical care, and robust rehabilitation programs for older patients with fractures, clinicians can maximize the quality of care and bridge the unique needs of geriatric orthopaedic patients to help all patients have the best quality of life possible at all stages in life.

REFERENCES

1. Chang JT, Morton SC, Rubenstein LZ, et al. Interventions for the prevention of falls in older adults: systematic review and meta-analysis of randomised clinical trials. *BMJ*. 2004;328:680.
2. Office of the Surgeon GReports of the Surgeon General. *Bone Health and Osteoporosis: A Report of the Surgeon General*. Rockville, MD: Office Surgeon General (US); 2004.
3. Cooper C. The crippling consequences of fractures and their impact on quality of life. *Am J Med*. 1997;103:12S-17S. discussion 7S-9S.
4. Heinonen M, Karppi P, Huusko T, Kautiainen H, Sulkava R. Postoperative degree of mobilization at two weeks predicts one-year mortality after hip fracture. *Aging Clin Exp Res*. 2004;16:476-480.
5. Jacobsen SJ, Goldberg J, Miles TP, Brody JA, Stiers W, Rimm AA. Race and sex differences in mortality following fracture of the hip. *Am J Public Health*. 1992;82:1147-1150.
6. Magaziner J, Simonsick EM, Kashner TM, Hebel JR, Kenzora JE. Survival experience of aged hip fracture patients. *Am J Public Health*. 1989;79:274-278.
7. Bouxsein ML, Kaufman J, Tosi L, Cummings S, Lane J, Johnell O. Recommendations for optimal care of the fragility fracture patient to reduce the risk of future fracture. *J Am Acad Orthop Surg*. 2004;12:385-395.
8. Cosman F, de Beur SJ, LeBoff MS, et al. Clinician's guide to prevention and treatment of osteoporosis. *Osteoporos Int*. 2014;25:2359-2381.
9. Klotzbuecher CM, Ross PD, Landsman PB, Abbott TA III, Berger M. Patients with prior fractures have an increased risk of future fractures: a summary of the literature and statistical synthesis. *J Bone Miner Res*. 2000;15:721-739.
10. van Staa TP, Leufkens HG, Cooper C. Does a fracture at one site predict later fractures at other sites? A British cohort study. *Osteoporos Int*. 2002;13:624-629.
11. Kane RL, Ouslander JG, Abrass IB. *Essentials of Clinical Geriatrics*. 3rd ed. New York, NY: McGraw-Hill; 1994.
12. Quatman CE, Switzer JA. Geriatric orthopaedics: a new paradigm for management of older patients. *Curr Geriatr Rep*. 2017;6:15-19.
13. Clement ND, Aitken S, Duckworth AD, McQueen MM, Court-Brown CM. Multiple fractures in the elderly. *J Bone Joint Surg Br*. 2012;94:231-236.
14. Clark D, Nakamura M, Miclau T, Marcucio R. Effects of aging on fracture healing. *Curr Osteoporos Rep*. 2017;15:601-608.
15. Bawa HS, Weick J, Dirschl DR. Anti-osteoporotic therapy after fragility fracture lowers rate of subsequent fracture: analysis of a large population sample. *J Bone Joint Surg Am*. 2015;97:1555-1562.
16. Chevalley T, Hoffmeyer P, Bonjour JP, Rizzoli R. An osteoporosis clinical pathway for the medical management of patients with low-trauma fracture. *Osteoporos Int*. 2002;13:450-455.
17. Koh A, Guerado E, Giannoudis PV. Atypical femoral fractures related to bisphosphonate treatment: issues and controversies related to their surgical management. *Bone Joint J*. 2017;99-B:295-302.
18. Saito T, Sterbenz JM, Malay S, Zhong L, MacEachern MP, Chung KC. Effectiveness of anti-osteoporotic drugs to prevent secondary fragility fractures: systematic review and meta-analysis. *Osteoporos Int*. 2017;28:3289-3300.
19. Bernstein J, Weintraub S, Hume E, Neuman MD, Kates SL, Ahn J. The new APGAR SCORE: a checklist to enhance quality of life in geriatric patients with hip fracture. *J Bone Joint Surg Am*. 2017;99:e77.
20. Hung WW, Egol KA, Zuckerman JD, Siu AL. Hip fracture management: tailoring care for the older patient. *J Am Med Assoc*. 2012;307:2185-2194.
21. Gosch M, Hoffmann-Weltin Y, Roth T, Blauth M, Nicholas JA, Kammerlander C. Orthogeriatric co-management improves the outcome of long-term care residents with fragility fractures. *Arch Orthop Trauma Surg*. 2016;136:1403-1409.
22. Sabharwal S, Wilson H. Orthogeriatrics in the management of frail older patients with a fragility fracture. *Osteoporos Int*. 2015;26:2387-2399.
23. Hulsbaek S, Larsen RF, Troelsen A. Predictors of not regaining basic mobility after hip fracture surgery. *Disabil Rehabil*. 2015;37:1739-1744.
24. Morri M, Forni C, Marchioni M, Bonetti E, Marseglia F, Cotti A. Which factors are independent predictors of early recovery of mobility in the older adults' population after hip fracture? A cohort prognostic study. *Arch Orthop Trauma Surg*. 2018;138:35-41.
25. Kubiak EN, Beebe MJ, North K, Hitchcock R, Potter MQ. Early weight bearing after lower extremity fractures in adults. *J Am Acad Orthop Surg*. 2013;21:727-738.
26. Mears SC, Kates SL. A guide to improving the care of patients with fragility fractures, edition 2. *Geriatr Orthop Surg Rehabil*. 2015;6:58-120.
27. Arazi M, Ogun TC, Oktar MN, Memik R, Kutlu A. Early weight-bearing after statically locked reamed intramedullary nailing of comminuted femoral fractures: is it a safe procedure? *J Trauma*. 2001;50:711-716.
28. Brumback RJ, Toal TR Jr, Murphy-Zane MS, Novak VP, Belkoff SM. Immediate weight-bearing after treatment of a comminuted fracture of the femoral shaft with a statically locked intramedullary nail. *J Bone Joint Surg Am*. 1999;81:1538-1544.
29. Koval KJ, Friend KD, Aharonoff GB, Zukerman JD. Weight bearing after hip fracture: a prospective series of 596 geriatric hip fracture patients. *J Orthop Trauma*. 1996;10:526-530.
30. Koval KJ, Sala DA, Kummer FJ, Zuckerman JD. Postoperative weight-bearing after a fracture of the femoral neck or an intertrochanteric fracture. *J Bone Joint Surg Am*. 1998;80:352-356.
31. Dewhirst RC, Ellis DP, Mandara EA, Jette DU. Therapists' perceptions of application and implementation of AM-PAC "6-Clicks" functional measures in acute care: qualitative study. *Phys Ther*. 2016;96:1085-1092.

32. Brown CJ, Friedkin RJ, Inouye SK. Prevalence and outcomes of low mobility in hospitalized older patients. *J Am Geriatr Soc.* 2004;52:1263-1270.
33. Chase JD, Lozano A, Hanlon A, Bowles KH. Identifying factors associated with mobility decline among hospitalized older adults. *Clin Nurs Res.* 2018;27:81-104.
34. Fisher SR, Graham JE, Ottenbacher KJ, Deer R, Ostir GV. Inpatient walking activity to predict readmission in older adults. *Arch Phys Med Rehabil.* 2016;97:S226-S231.
35. Fisher SR, Kuo YF, Sharma G, et al. Mobility after hospital discharge as a marker for 30-day readmission. *J Gerontol A Biol Sci Med Sci.* 2013;68:805-810.
36. Fried LP, Bandeen-Roche K, Chaves PH, Johnson BA. Preclinical mobility disability predicts incident mobility disability in older women. *J Gerontol A Biol Sci Med Sci.* 2000;55:M43-M52.
37. Hoenig HM, Rubenstein LZ. Hospital-associated deconditioning and dysfunction. *J Am Geriatr Soc.* 1991;39:220-222.
38. Growdon ME, Shorr RI, Inouye SK. The tension between promoting mobility and preventing falls in the hospital. *JAMA Intern Med.* 2017;177:759-760.
39. Inouye SK, Brown CJ, Tinetti ME. Medicare nonpayment, hospital falls, and unintended consequences. *N Engl J Med.* 2009;360:2390-2393.
40. King B, Pecanac K, Krupp A, Liebzeit D, Mahoney J. Impact of fall prevention on nurses and care of fall risk patients. *Gerontologist.* 2018;58(2):331-340.
41. Oliver D. David Oliver: fighting pyjama paralysis in hospital wards. *BMJ.* 2017;357:j2096.
42. Baumgarten M, Margolis DJ, Orwig DL, et al. Pressure ulcers in elderly patients with hip fracture across the continuum of care. *J Am Geriatr Soc.* 2009;57:863-870.
43. Berry SD, Samelson EJ, Bordes M, Broe K, Kiel DP. Survival of aged nursing home residents with hip fracture. *J Gerontol A Biol Sci Med Sci.* 2009;64:771-777.
44. Pearson JA, Mangold K, Kosiorek HE, Montez M, Smith DM, Tyler BJ. Registered nurse intent to promote physical activity for hospitalised liver transplant recipients. *J Nurs Manag.* 2018;26:442-448.
45. Phelan S, Lin F, Mitchell M, Chaboyer W. Implementing early mobilisation in the intensive care unit: an integrative review. *Int J Nurs Stud.* 2018;77:91-105.
46. Liu B, Moore JE, Almaawiy U, et al. Outcomes of Mobilisation of Vulnerable Elders in Ontario (MOVE ON): a multisite interrupted time series evaluation of an implementation intervention to increase patient mobilisation. *Age Ageing.* 2018;47:112-119.
47. Roach KE, Ally D, Finnerty B, et al. The relationship between duration of physical therapy services in the acute care setting and change in functional status in patients with lower-extremity orthopedic problems. *Phys Ther.* 1998;78:19-24.
48. Wood W, Tschannen D, Trotsky A, et al. A mobility program for an inpatient acute care medical unit. *Am J Nurs.* 2014;114:34-40; quiz 1-2.
49. Dubb R, Nydahl P, Hermes C, et al. Barriers and strategies for early mobilization of patients in intensive care units. *Ann Am Thorac Soc.* 2016;13:724-730.
50. Moore JE, Mascarenhas A, Marquez C, et al. Mapping barriers and intervention activities to behaviour change theory for Mobilization of Vulnerable Elders in Ontario (MOVE ON), a multi-site implementation intervention in acute care hospitals. *Implement Sci.* 2014;9:160.
51. Morrison RS, Flanagan S, Fischberg D, Cintron A, Siu AL. A novel interdisciplinary analgesic program reduces pain and improves function in older adults after orthopedic surgery. *J Am Geriatr Soc.* 2009;57:1-10.
52. Morrison RS, Magaziner J, McLaughlin MA, et al. The impact of post-operative pain on outcomes following hip fracture. *Pain.* 2003;103:303-311.
53. Peiris CL, Taylor NF, Shields N. Extra physical therapy reduces patient length of stay and improves functional outcomes and quality of life in people with acute or subacute conditions: a systematic review. *Arch Phys Med Rehabil.* 2011;92:1490-1500.
54. Drolet A, DeJuilio P, Harkless S, et al. Move to improve: the feasibility of using an early mobility protocol to increase ambulation in the intensive and intermediate care settings. *Phys Ther.* 2013;93:197-207.
55. Agency for Healthcare Research and Quality. *Preventing Falls in Hospitals: A Toolkit for Improving Quality of Care.* Rockville, MD: Agency for Healthcare Research and Quality; 2013.
56. Siu AL, Penrod JD, Boockvar KS, Koval K, Strauss E, Morrison RS. Early ambulation after hip fracture: effects on function and mortality. *Arch Intern Med.* 2006;166:766-771.
57. Kimmel LA, Edwards ER, Liew SM, Oldmeadow LB, Webb MJ, Holland AE. Rest easy? Is bed rest really necessary after surgical repair of an ankle fracture? *Injury.* 2012;43:766-771.
58. Oldmeadow LB, Edwards ER, Kimmel LA, Kipen E, Robertson VJ, Bailey MJ. No rest for the wounded: early ambulation after hip surgery accelerates recovery. *ANZ J Surg.* 2006;76:607-611.
59. Kristensen MT, Foss NB, Kehlet H. Timed "up & go" test as a predictor of falls within 6 months after hip fracture surgery. *Phys Ther.* 2007;87:24-30.
60. Herrick C, Steger-May K, Sinacore DR, Brown M, Schechtman KB, Binder EF. Persistent pain in frail older adults after hip fracture repair. *J Am Geriatr Soc.* 2004;52:2062-2068.
61. Beaupre LA, Cinats JG, Jones CA, et al. Does functional recovery in elderly hip fracture patients differ between patients admitted from long-term care and the community? *J Gerontol A Biol Sci Med.* 2007;62:1127-1133.
62. Bellelli G, Frisoni GB, Pagani M, Magnifico F, Trabucchi M. Does cognitive performance affect physical therapy regimen after hip fracture surgery? *Aging Clin Exp Res.* 2007;19:119-124.
63. Crotty M, Miller M, Whitehead C, Krishnan J, Hearn T. Hip fracture treatments – What happens to patients from residential care? *J Qual Clin Pract.* 2000;20:167-170.
64. Frances Horgan N, Cunningham JC. Impact of cognitive impairment on hip fracture outcome in older people. *Br J Ther Rehabil.* 2003;10:228-232.
65. Tinetti ME, Doucette JT, Claus EB. The contribution of predisposing and situational risk factors to serious fall injuries. *J Am Geriatr Soc.* 1995;43:1207-1213.
66. van Doorn C, Gruber-Baldini AL, Zimmerman S, et al. Dementia as a risk factor for falls and fall injuries among nursing home residents. *J Am Geriatr Soc.* 2003;51:1213-1218.
67. Allen J, Koziak A, Buddingh S, Liang J, Buckingham J, Beaupre LA. Rehabilitation in patients with dementia following hip fracture: a systematic review. *Physiother Can.* 2012;64:190-201.
68. Diong J, Allen N, Sherrington C. Structured exercise improves mobility after hip fracture: a meta-analysis with meta-regression. *Br J Sports Med.* 2016;50:346-355.
69. Lee SY, Yoon BH, Beom J, Ha YC, Lim JY. Effect of lower-limb progressive resistance exercise after hip fracture surgery: a systematic review and meta-analysis of randomized controlled studies. *J Am Med Dir Assoc.* 2017;18:1096.e19-1096.e26.
70. Overgaard J, Kristensen MT. Feasibility of progressive strength training shortly after hip fracture surgery. *World J Orthop.* 2013;4:248-258.
71. Fiatarone MA, O'Neill EF, Ryan ND, et al. Exercise training and nutritional supplementation for physical frailty in very elderly people. *N Engl J Med.* 1994;330:1769-1775.
72. Latham N, Anderson C, Bennett D, Stretton C. Progressive resistance strength training for physical disability in older people. *Cochrane Database Syst Rev.* 2003;2:CD002759.
73. Liu CJ, Latham NK. Progressive resistance strength training for improving physical function in older adults. *Cochrane Database Syst Rev.* 2009;3:CD002759.
74. Sinaki M. Exercise for patients with osteoporosis: management of vertebral compression fractures and trunk strengthening for fall prevention. *PM R.* 2012;4:882-888.
75. Handoll HH, Sherrington C, Mak JC. Interventions for improving mobility after hip fracture surgery in adults. *Cochrane Database Syst Rev.* 2011:CD001704.
76. Turunen K, Salpakoski A, Edgren J, et al. Physical activity after a hip fracture: effect of a multicomponent home-based rehabilitation program – A secondary analysis of a randomized controlled trial. *Arch Phys Med Rehabil.* 2017;98:981-988.
77. Vochteloo AJ, Moerman S, Tuinebreijer WE, et al. More than half of hip fracture patients do not regain mobility in the first postoperative year. *Geriatr Gerontol Int.* 2013;13:334-341.
78. Visser M, Harris TB, Fox KM, et al. Change in muscle mass and muscle strength after a hip fracture: relationship to mobility recovery. *J Gerontol A Biol Sci Med.* 2000;55:M434-M440.
79. Binder EF, Brown M, Sinacore DR, Steger-May K, Yarasheski KE, Schechtman KB. Effects of extended outpatient rehabilitation after hip fracture: a randomized controlled trial. *J Am Med Assoc.* 2004;292:837-846.
80. Host HH, Sinacore DR, Bohnert KL, Steger-May K, Brown M, Binder EF. Training-induced strength and functional adaptations after hip fracture. *Phys Ther.* 2007;87:292-303.

81. Latham NK, Harris BA, Bean JF, et al. Effect of a home-based exercise program on functional recovery following rehabilitation after hip fracture: a randomized clinical trial. *J Am Med Assoc.* 2014;311:700-708.

82. Foss NB, Kehlet H. Hidden blood loss after surgery for hip fracture. *J Bone Joint Surg Br.* 2006;88:1053-1059.

83. Penninx BW, Pahor M, Woodman RC, Guralnik JM. Anemia in old age is associated with increased mortality and hospitalization. *J Gerontol A Biol Sci Med.* 2006;61:474-479.

84. Marcantonio ER, Flacker JM, Wright RJ, Resnick NM. Reducing delirium after hip fracture: a randomized trial. *J Am Geriatr Soc.* 2001;49:516-522.

85. Parker MJ. Randomised trial of blood transfusion versus a restrictive transfusion policy after hip fracture surgery. *Injury.* 2013;44:1916-1918.

86. Brauer C, Morrison RS, Silberzweig SB, Siu AL. The cause of delirium in patients with hip fracture. *Arch Intern Med.* 2000;160:1856-1860.

87. Edlund A, Lundstrom M, Brannstrom B, Bucht G, Gustafson Y. Delirium before and after operation for femoral neck fracture. *J Am Geriatr Soc.* 2001;49:1335-1340.

88. Duppils GS, Wikblad K. Patients' experiences of being delirious. *J Clin Nurs.* 2007;16:810-818.

89. Oh ES, Fong TG, Hshieh TT, Inouye SK. Delirium in older persons: advances in diagnosis and treatment. *J Am Med Assoc.* 2017;318:1161-1174.

90. Oberai T, Laver K, Crotty M, Killington M, Jaarsma R. Effectiveness of multicomponent interventions on incidence of delirium in hospitalized older patients with hip fracture: a systematic review. *Int Psychogeriatr.* 2018:30:481-492.

91. Lundstrom M, Olofsson B, Stenvall M, et al. Postoperative delirium in old patients with femoral neck fracture: a randomized intervention study. *Aging Clin Exp Res.* 2007;19:178-186.

92. Avenell A, Smith TO, Curtain JP, Mak JC, Myint PK. Nutritional supplementation for hip fracture aftercare in older people. *Cochrane Database Syst Rev.* 2016;11:CD001880.

93. Bell JJ, Bauer JD, Capra S, Pulle RC. Quick and easy is not without cost: implications of poorly performing nutrition screening tools in hip fracture. *J Am Geriatr Soc.* 2014;62:237-243.

94. Vivanti A, Ward N, Haines T. Nutritional status and associations with falls, balance, mobility and functionality during hospital admission. *J Nutr Health Aging.* 2011;15:388-391.

95. Goisser S, Schrader E, Singler K, et al. Malnutrition according to mini nutritional assessment is associated with severe functional impairment in geriatric patients before and up to 6 months after hip fracture. *J Am Med Dir Assoc.* 2015;16:661-667.

96. van Wissen J, van Stijn MF, Doodeman HJ, Houdijk AP. Mini nutritional assessment and mortality after hip fracture surgery in the elderly. *J Nutr Health Aging.* 2016;20:964-968.

97. Avenell A, Handoll HH. Nutritional supplementation for hip fracture aftercare in older people. *Cochrane Database Syst Rev.* 2010;1:CD001880.

98. Long Term Care. U.S. Department of Health and Human Services. 2018. Available at https://longtermcare.acl.gov/.

99. Cameron ID, Lyle DM, Quine S. Cost effectiveness of accelerated rehabilitation after proximal femoral fracture. *J Clin Epidemiol.* 1994;47:1307-1313.

100. Jette AM, Harris BA, Cleary PD, Campion EW. Functional recovery after hip fracture. *Arch Phys Med Rehabil.* 1987;68:735-740.

101. Basques BA, Bohl DD, Golinvaux NS, Leslie MP, Baumgaertner MR, Grauer JN. Postoperative length of stay and 30-day readmission after geriatric hip fracture: an analysis of 8434 patients. *J Orthop Trauma.* 2015;29:e115-e120.

102. Kates SL, Shields E, Behrend C, Noyes KK. Financial implications of hospital readmission after hip fracture. *Geriatr Orthop Surg Rehabil.* 2015;6:140-146.

103. Lizaur-Utrilla A, Serna-Berna R, Lopez-Prats FA, Gil-Guillen V. Early rehospitalization after hip fracture in elderly patients: risk factors and prognosis. *Arch Orthop Trauma Surg.* 2015;135:1663-1667.

104. Ali AM, Gibbons CE. Predictors of 30-day hospital readmission after hip fracture: a systematic review. *Injury.* 2017;48:243-252.

105. Boockvar KS, Halm EA, Litke A, et al. Hospital readmissions after hospital discharge for hip fracture: surgical and nonsurgical causes and effect on outcomes. *J Am Geriatr Soc.* 2003;51:399-403.

106. Jencks SF, Williams MV, Coleman EA. Rehospitalizations among patients in the medicare fee-for-service program. *N Engl J Med.* 2009;360:1418-1428.

107. Kates SL, Behrend C, Mendelson DA, Cram P, Friedman SM. Hospital readmission after hip fracture. *Arch Orthop Trauma Surg.* 2015;135:329-337.

108. Balasubramanian A, Tosi LL, Lane JM, Dirschl DR, Ho PR, O'Malley CD. Declining rates of osteoporosis management following fragility fractures in the U.S., 2000 through 2009. *J Bone Joint Surg Am.* 2014;96:e52.

109. Benzvi L, Gershon A, Lavi I, Wollstein R. Secondary prevention of osteoporosis following fragility fractures of the distal radius in a large health maintenance organization. *Arch Osteoporos.* 2016;11:20.

110. Iba K, Dohke T, Takada J, et al. Improvement in the rate of inadequate pharmaceutical treatment by orthopaedic surgeons for the prevention of a second fracture over the last 10 years. *J Orthop Sci.* 2018;23:127-131.

111. Kristensen PK, Thillemann TM, Soballe K, Johnsen SP. Are process performance measures associated with clinical outcomes among patients with hip fractures? A population-based cohort study. *Int J Qual Health Care.* 2016;28:698-708.

112. Boockvar KS, Litke A, Penrod JD, et al. Patient relocation in the 6 months after hip fracture: risk factors for fragmented care. *J Am Geriatr Soc.* 2004;52:1826-1831.

113. Popejoy LL, Dorman Marek K, Scott-Cawiezell J. Patterns and problems associated with transitions after hip fracture in older adults. *J Gerontol Nurs.* 2013;39:43-52.

114. Killington M, Walker R, Crotty M. The chaotic journey: Recovering from hip fracture in a nursing home. *Arch Gerontol Geriatr.* 2016;67:106-112.

115. Eslami M, Tran HP. Transitions of care and rehabilitation after fragility fractures. *Clin Geriatr Med.* 2014;30:303-315.

116. Smith TO, Hameed YA, Cross JL, Henderson C, Sahota O, Fox C. Enhanced rehabilitation and care models for adults with dementia following hip fracture surgery. *Cochrane Database Syst Rev.* 2015;6:CD010569.

117. Deprey SM, Biedrzycki L, Klenz K. Identifying characteristics and outcomes that are associated with fall-related fatalities: multi-year retrospective summary of fall deaths in older adults from 2005-2012. *Inj Epidemiol.* 2017;4:21.

118. Medical Advisory Secretariat. Prevention of falls and fall-related injuries in community-dwelling seniors: an evidence-based analysis. *Ont Health Technol Assess Ser.* 2008;8:1-78.

119. Satariano WA, Wang C, Kealey ME, Kurtovich E, Phelan EA. Risk profiles for falls among older adults: new directions for prevention. *Front Public Health.* 2017;5:142.

120. Rimland JM, Abraha I, Dell'Aquila G, et al. Effectiveness of non-pharmacological interventions to prevent falls in older people: a systematic overview. The SENATOR Project ONTOP Series. *PLoS One.* 2016;11:e0161579.

121. Smith AK, Cenzer IS, John Boscardin W, Ritchie CS, Wallhagen ML, Covinsky KE. Increase in disability prevalence before hip fracture. *J Am Geriatr Soc.* 2015;63:2029-2035.

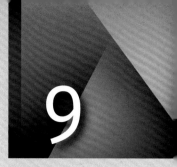

9

Rehabilitation Principles

Bronwyn Spira

WEIGHT BEARING STATUS TERMINOLOGY

Weight bearing status refers to the amount of body weight (BW) that a patient can put on his/her affected leg following injury or surgery. This is often determined by the surgeon and is based on the degree of injury, healing stage, and type of surgery. The following weight bearing categories are universally recognized by physicians and rehabilitation specialists.

NON–WEIGHT BEARING

Non–weight bearing means that the affected leg does not touch the ground during standing or walking. For example, a patient using an assistive device, such as crutches or a walker, will keep the affected leg in the air during ambulation.

TOE-TOUCH WEIGHT BEARING OR TOUCH-DOWN WEIGHT BEARING

This refers to applying a minimal amount of BW through the front part of the foot (toes) while walking. This allows the patient to have some degree of balance while still avoiding significant weight bearing through the affected leg. An assistive device, such as a walker or two crutches, is used.

PARTIAL WEIGHT BEARING

The patient can place a percentage of his/her BW through the affected leg. Typically, the percentages are 25%, 50%, and 75%. A bathroom scale can be used as a simple but accurate tool to help patients appreciate the appropriate amount of weight bearing during stance before initiating walking. A walker, single crutch, two crutches, or a cane can be used depending on the degree of partial weight bearing (PWB) allowed.

WEIGHT BEARING AS TOLERATED

Weight bearing as tolerated refers to applying as much weight through the affected leg under the condition that the patient does not experience intolerable pain. Although some discomfort is allowed, care should be taken to ensure that the patient is walking with acceptable mechanics. As with PWB, a walker, single crutch, two crutches, or a cane may be used.

FULL–WEIGHT BEARING

Full–weight bearing (FWB) entails placing 100% of BW through the affected leg during stance or while walking. Again, it is important to walk with acceptable mechanics even though some discomfort may exist during walking. No assistive device is used under FWB status.

MOTION TERMINOLOGY

PASSIVE RANGE OF MOTION

Passive range of motion (PROM) is a movement of a joint or limb within the unrestricted range of motion (ROM) that is produced entirely by an external force. External force may be produced by gravity, machine/pulley system, another person, or another part of the individual's own body. The muscles that usually move that body part do none of the work. The goals of PROM are to maintain joint and connective tissue mobility, increase circulation, prevent joint contractures or adhesions, and reduce pain, all of which are potential complications following surgery, injury, or prolonged immobilization. Adhesions are fibrous bands that form between tissues. They may be thought of as internal scar tissue that adheres to tissues and often have a whitish "spider web" appearance. The following are examples of common types of PROM. A patient uses pulleys to raise the left arm. The right arm pulls down and does all the work, whereas the left arm relaxes and is raised up. As another example, a therapist moves a patient's ankle through its available ROM without the patient's help. Finally, a patient uses his uninjured arm to bend his injured elbow following surgery. PROM is not synonymous with **stretching** which is a more intense form of exercise where the goal is to improve the plasticity (change in length) or flexibility of connective tissue.

Research has shown that an improvement in flexibility is due to an increase in the length of fasciae, a connective tissue that is attached to the muscles, tendons, ligaments, nerves, and bone. Interestingly, research has shown that it is unlikely that stretching can increase the length of the actual muscles.

ACTIVE RANGE OF MOTION

Active range of motion (AROM) is a movement of a joint or limb within the unrestricted ROM that is produced by the muscle or muscles crossing the joint. Typically, AROM is performed against gravity, although it may be performed in a gravity-eliminated position. For example, if a person raises their arm while standing, this is AROM against gravity, whereas if performed in side lying, this would qualify as AROM in a gravity-eliminated position. AROM does not involve any external resistance, except for gravity in some cases as noted above. In addition to sharing the same goals of PROM, AROM is used to minimize muscle atrophy, to provide sensory feedback to the neuromusculoskeletal system, and to develop motor skill and coordination.

ACTIVE ASSISTIVE RANGE OF MOTION

Active assistive range of motion (AAROM) is a movement of a joint or limb in which assistance is provided by an outside force, either manually or mechanically. It is used to bridge the gap between the available PROM and what the patient can achieve actively (AROM). AAROM is used when a patient has weak musculature and is unable to move a joint through the desired range, usually against gravity. An example of AAROM is when a physical therapist helps a patient tries to raise their arm after shoulder surgery using their own strength but requires the assistance of the therapist to complete the motion. AAROM can be performed against gravity or in a gravity-eliminated position. In addition, the amount of assistance supplied by the therapist can range from slight assistance, where the therapist does most of the work, to maximal assistance.

BIOMECHANICS AND JOINT REACTION FORCES

Biomechanics is defined as the study of mechanics as they apply to biological and physiological systems. Kinesiology, synonymous with biomechanics, is a more global term that refers to the study of movement. Within "mechanics" there are two subfields of study: statics, which is the study of systems that are in a state of constant motion either at rest (with no motion) or moving with a constant velocity; and dynamics, which is the study of systems in motion in which acceleration is present, which may involve **kinematics** and **kinetics**.

Kinetics is the study of forces acting on a body. Kinematics is the study of motion of a body without consideration of the actual forces that may cause the motion. Two subbranches of kinematics include **osteokinematics** and **arthrokinematics**. Osteokinematics refers to the movement between the bones.

For example, flexion of the shoulder may be described as the cranial movement of the humerus with respect to the body. Osteokinematics, on the other hand, is the movement between opposing joint surfaces. Using the previous example, the osteokinematics of shoulder flexion involves the humeral head translating inferiorly on the glenoid fossa.

Joint reaction force is defined as the force generated within a joint, specifically the net forces acting on the joint surfaces. The net forces on a joint surface are produced by the body (BW), gravity, and muscular tension. Newtons are used to quantify forces, based on the International Systems of Units. One Newton is equal to 0.225 pounds. Or stated another way, 1 pound is equal to 4.4 Newtons. Using the hip joint as an example, the joint reaction force caused by performing a supine straight leg raise is approximately twice the BW of the individual. This force is primarily caused by the muscle contractions of the hip flexors (rectus femoris and iliopsoas), which compress the femoral head against the acetabulum. The hip joint reaction forces are increased when standing on the involved side leg (3xBW), walking (5xBW), and running (10xBW) (**Figure 9.1**). In these instances, progressively greater hip muscle activity (gluteal muscles), gravitational forces, and BW contribute to the higher net joint reaction force. As supported by the previous example, the joint reaction can be greatly magnified by adding external resistance. This is especially true for the shoulder and hip, as these joints have long lever arms.

This has important implications for the rehabilitation of specific joint-related injuries and/or surgeries. For example, a patient with advanced hip arthritis may not be able to tolerate standing on one leg because of the high compressive forces on the hip joint. In the shoulder, the glenohumeral joint reaction forces during shoulder abduction are greatest at 90° of abduction, where values reach about 50% BW. For a 180-pound individual, performing shoulder abduction while holding a 5-pound weight increases the joint reaction forces to 100% BW. Finally, the knee joint reaction force increases during resisted knee extension at greater angles of knee flexion. In the rehabilitation of patients with knee joint disorders, such as "runner's knee" (anterior knee pain), performing an isometric knee extension contraction at 0° creates less force on the knee joint as compared with performing this exercise with the knee flexed.

There are two general types of muscle contractions: **isometric and isotonic**. An isometric muscular contraction occurs when there is no change in the muscle length or the joint angle. Conversely, an isotonic contraction will change the length of the muscle. There are two subtypes of isotonic contractions: **eccentric and concentric**. During eccentric contractions, the muscle lengthens as it develops tension. When weight exceeds the force developed by the muscle, as in an eccentric muscle action, the exercise is referred to as negative work because the muscle is absorbing energy in this loaded position. Eccentric contractions use less energy, even though they create more force than concentric actions. An example of an eccentric muscle contraction is the lengthening action of the biceps during

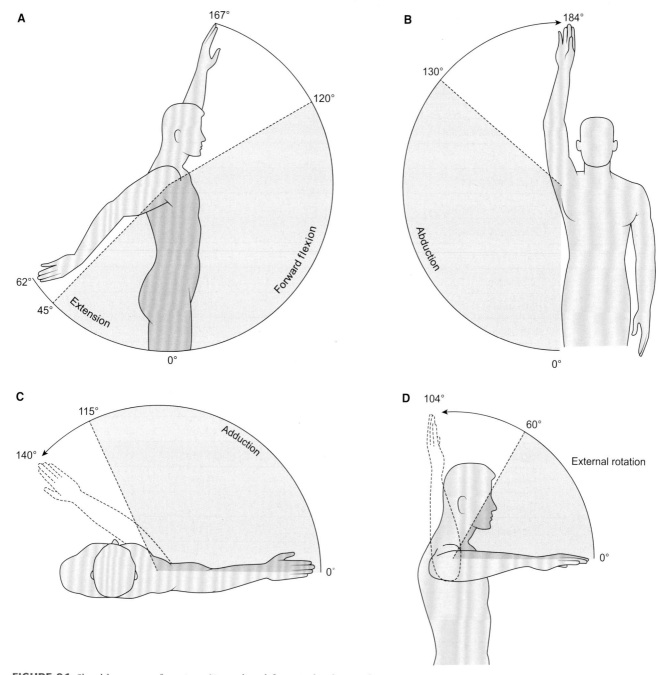

FIGURE 9.1 Shoulder range of motion. (Reproduced from Richard B, Kathy S, James C, Jane L, Joshua N, Joan S. *Fleisher & Ludwig's Textbook of Pediatric Emergency Medicine*. 8th ed. Wolters Kluwer Health; 2020.)

the "negative" (lowering or returning to the starting position) phase of the biceps curl exercise. Another example is the eccentric contraction of the gluteal muscles during the descent phase of the squat or the landing phase of a jump. A concentric contraction is a type of muscle contraction in which the muscles shorten while generating force, overcoming resistance. For example, when lifting a heavy weight, a concentric contraction of the biceps would cause the arm to bend at the elbow, lifting the weight toward the shoulder. Using the previous squat example, the hip flexors contract concentrically during the descent phase, while the gluteal muscles are lengthening thereby working eccentrically to control the descending motion.

GONIOMETRY

SAGITTAL, FRONTAL, TRANSVERSE, AND ROTATION SYSTEM

The sagittal, frontal, transverse, and rotation system involves the following set of rules for measuring joint ROM (**Table 9.1**). All joint motions are measured from the anatomical position. In this position, the subject is standing erect, with the face directed forward, the arms at the sides, and the palms of the hands facing forward. All joint motions and positions are recorded in

TABLE 9.1 Joint Range of Motion with Variances

Joint	Movement	Range of Motion (Start to End)	Variation in End Ranges of Motion
Shoulder	Extension-flexion	0°-180°	150°-180°
	Hyperextension	0°-45°	40°-60°
	Adduction-abduction	0°-180°	150°-180°
	Lateral rotation	0°-90°	80°-90°
	Medial rotation	0°-90°	70°-90°
	Horizontal abduction	30°	–
	Horizontal adduction	135°	–
Elbow	Extension-flexion	0°-145°	120°-160°
Forearm	Supination	0°-90°	80°-90°
	Pronation	0°-80°	70°-90°
Wrist	Extension	0°-70°	65°-70°
	Flexion	0°-90°	75°-90°
	Radial deviation	0°-20°	15°-25°
	Ulnar deviation	0°-30°	25°-40°
Thumb CMC	Abduction	0°-70°	50°-80°
	Flexion	0°-45°	15°-45°
	Extension	20°	0°-20°
	Opposition	Tip of thumb to tip of #5	–
Thumb MCP	Extension-flexion	0°-45°	40°-90°
Thumb IP	Extension-flexion	0°-90°	80°-90°
#2-5 finger MCP	Flexion	0°-90°	–
	Hyperextension	0°-30°	30°-45°
	Adduction-abduction	0°-20°	–
#2-5 finger PIP	Extension-flexion	0°-100°	100°-120°
#2-5 finger DIP	Extension-flexion	0°-90°	80°-90°
Hip	Extension-flexion	0°-120°	110°-125°
	Hyperextension	0°-15°	10°-45°
	Abduction	0°-45°	45°-50°
	Adduction	0°-20°	10°-30°
	Lateral rotation	0°-45°	36°-60°
	Medial rotation	0°-35°	33°-45°
Knee	Extension-flexion	0°-135°	125°-145°

TABLE 9.1 Joint Range of Motion with Variances   (Continued)

Joint	Movement	Range of Motion (Start to End)	Variation in End Ranges of Motion
Ankle	Dorsiflexion	0°-15°	10°-30°
	Plantar flexion	0°-45°	45°-65°
Subtalar joint	Inversion	0°-30°	30°-52°
	Eversion	0°-15°	15°-30°
MTP	Extension-flexion	0°-40°	30°-45°
	Hyperextension	0°-80°	50°-90°
IP	Extension-flexion	0°-60°	50°-80°

refers to the number of the finger "digit" (as in fingers 1 though 5).
CMC, carpometacarpal; DIP, distal interphalangeal; IP, interphalangeal; MCP, metacarpophalangeal; MTP, metatarsophalangeal; PIP, proximal interphalangeal.
From Shultz S, Houglum P, Perrin D. *Examination of Musculoskeletal Injuries.* *4th ed., p. 78. Human Kinetics, Inc.; 2015.*

the three basic planes (sagittal, frontal, and transverse). The motion of turning toward or away from the starting posture is considered rotation. All motions are recorded with three numbers. Motions leading away from the body are recorded first, and motions leading toward the body are recorded last. The starting position is recorded in the middle and is usually 0. For example, an elbow that can hyperextend 10° and flex 140° would be recorded as S 10-0-140. The S indicates motion in the sagittal plane.

Functional Range of Motion

Functional ROM measures whether a patient will be able to effectively function in his/her environment. Normal ROM may not be necessary to complete wanted, needed, or expected tasks.

Shoulder flexion
"Can you raise your arms above your head?"
Used to determine
Can they reach into the top shelf of the pantry?
Can they shut the window blinds?

Shoulder abduction/external rotation
"Can you place your hands behind your head?"
Used to determine
Can they wash and comb their hair?
Can they put on an overhead shirt?
Can they scratch their back?

Shoulder abduction/extension
"Can you touch your hands behind your back?"
Used to determine
Can they tuck in their shirt?
Can they put a belt through the loops?
Can they perform personal hygiene?

Shoulder flexion/elbow extension
"Can you hold your hands straight out in front of you?"
Used to determine
Can they wash the dishes?
Can they carry objects in front of them?
Can they go waterskiing?

Wrist pronation/supination
"Can you turn your hands palm up…palm down?"
Used to determine
Can they turn a doorknob?
Can they turn a key in the ignition?

Wrist extension/flexion
"Can you wave your hands up and down?"
Used to determine
Can they tie their shoes?
Can they type on a keyboard?

Elbow flexion
"Can you touch your mouth?"
Used to determine
Can they eat?
Can they brush their teeth?

Thumb opposition
"Can you touch your fingers to your thumb?"
Used to determine
Can they pick up change on the table?
Can they hold a pencil?

SUGGESTED READINGS

Bergmann G, Graichen F, Rohlmann A. Hip joint loading during walking and running, measured in two patients. *J Biomech.* 1993;26(8):969-90.

Gerhardt JJ, Rondinelli RD. Goniometric techniques for range-of-motion assessment. *Phys Med Rehabil Clin N Am.* 2001;12(3):507-527.

Giarmatzis G, Jonkers I, Wesseling M, Van Rossom S, Verschueren S. Loading of hip measured by hip contact forces at different speeds of walking and running. *J Bone Miner Res.* 2015;30(8):1431-1440.

Nordin M, Frankel V. *Basic Biomechanics of the Musculoskeletal System.* 3rd ed. Philadelphia, PA: Lippincott Williams & Wilkins; 2001.

10

Assistive Modalities Used in Rehabilitative Medicine

Elisabeth McGee

Sabrina Wang

John Layne

INTRODUCTION

The epidemiology of adult fractures is changing quickly. An analysis of 5953 fractures reviewed in a single orthopaedic trauma unit in 2000 showed that there are eight different fracture distribution curves into which all fractures can be placed.[1] These fractures lead to an economic loss between 3 and 6 billion dollars every year. The common symptoms associated with acute fractures are pain, swelling, bruising, discoloration of skin and the surrounding area, and difficulty moving the injured area. The signs and symptoms of a fracture, however, vary according to the location and severity of injury as well as the patient's age and general health. As a consequence of these factors, the fracture problem today must be considered as having two aspects: a biomedical aspect, which includes the recognition, reduction, and stabilization of fractures immediately after the injury, and a biopsychosocial aspect, which includes the biological, psychological, and social factors unique to each individual during the rehabilitation process.[2]

Successful operative management of any fracture is crucial for the optimization of postinjury mobility and the functional recovery of the patient.[3] Rehabilitation after fracture is also a critical component for any patient attempting to reach ultimate functional outcomes. The rehabilitation provided by physical or occupational therapists is a patient goal-oriented process. The focus is on providing therapeutic interventions that help the patient/client reach optimal physical, mental, and social functional outcomes, as well as prevent possible long-term disability due to the injury. The prevalence and excessive cost of pain after injury and surgery, especially when the pain becomes chronic, can remain a major healthcare problem.[4]

The scope of practice for physical therapists and occupational therapists in treating patients with postfracture injuries includes identifying and maximizing movement potential, within the spheres of promotion, prevention, and treatment. Common intervention methods such as manual therapy, therapeutic exercises, and neuromuscular reeducation have proven to be effective treatments in improving patient mobility and functional levels. In addition, palliative interventions are often used to assist in improving treatment and activity tolerance. Therapeutic modalities are often categorized into palliative intervention strategies. Palliative intervention strategies include the administration of thermal, mechanical, electromagnetic, and light energies for a specific therapeutic effect.[4] The intended therapeutic effects include decreased pain, increased range of motion, improved tissue healing, and improved muscle recruitment.[5]

TYPES OF THERAPEUTIC MODALITIES

Therapeutic modalities are generally categorized into thermal agents (cold and heat), electromagnetic waves (electrotherapy, diathermy, and ultraviolet and infrared light), or mechanical forms (ultrasound, traction, and compression). Often the specific therapeutic effects are aimed at decreasing pain, improving tissue healing, increasing range of motion, and/or improving muscle recruitment.

THERMAL MODALITIES: CRYOTHERAPY AND THERMOTHERAPY

Cryotherapy

Cryotherapy is the use of cold agents to elicit therapeutic and physiological responses in the tissue resulting from a decrease in tissue temperature. There are numerous techniques and methods of applying cold agents to tissue including cold or ice packs, ice massage, cold bath/whirlpool, cold compression units, and vapocoolant sprays (**Table 10.1**).

TABLE 10.1 Cryotherapy Methods

Type of Cryotherapy	Convection	Conduction	Evaporation
Cold pack/ice pack		X	
Ice massage		X	
Cold whirlpool	X		
Ice towels		X	
Vapocoolant sprays			X

The transmission of cooling effects occurs through the primary mechanisms of conduction, convection, and evaporation. Conduction is involved when there is an exchange of thermal energy between two materials in physical contact. Convection is the transfer of thermal energy through the circulation of a specific medium consisting of a different temperature. Evaporation occurs when a liquid is changed to gas, which requires the body to expend thermal energy.

Therapeutic Effects

The application of a cold agent may have hemodynamic, neuromuscular, and metabolic effects that may be beneficial in fracture rehabilitation. Both physiological and clinical evidence suggest that cold application can reduce nerve conduction velocity,[6] decrease local blood flow,[7-9] and suppress cellular metabolic rate.[10] These effects reduce the inflammatory reaction to trauma,[11] lessen pain,[12,13] decrease edema,[14] and reduce secondary hypoxic injury.[15] Temperature change of the target tissue is directly related to the time of exposure of the cryotherapy application (**Figures 10.1** and **10.2**).[15,16] The therapeutic effect of cryotherapy produces a physiological change in the tissues up to 2 cm in depth.[5,15,16]

Clinical Indications and Contraindications

A patient with impaired sensation will not have appropriate sensory feedback; therefore, the application of cryotherapy must be used with caution. If protective sensation is absent, this modality should be contraindicated (**Table 10.2**). In individuals with underlying loss of the vascular system, the response to cryotherapy can be extremely atypical leading to excessive vasoconstriction, which increases the risk of developing frostbite. Tissue and nerve injuries are most common when cold and compression are applied simultaneously. Compromised circulation should be assessed by a capillary refill test to ensure blood flow to the treatment site is not limited. Applying cryotherapy over a regenerating superficial nerve may cause ischemia and therefore may delay regeneration. The application of cold after a superficial nerve injury may produce a burning sensation, reduce nerve conduction velocity, and may result in further nerve injury.

Thermotherapy

The therapeutic application of heat has existed for thousands of years. It provides a variety of benefits including facilitation of tissue healing, relaxation of the skeletal muscles, pain modulation, preparation for soft-tissue stretching and mobilization, and most importantly increasing blood flow for tissue regeneration and repair.[17,18]

There are several clinical methods of therapeutic heat application (**Table 10.3**). Heat can be transferred to a tissue through radiation, conduction, or convection.[5,19] Therapeutic ultrasound and diathermy are considered deep heating agents. Superficial heating agents include the following: moist hot packs, heating pads, fluidotherapy, infrared, and paraffin baths.

Therapeutic Effects

Superficial heating agents produce a variety of positive clinical effects. This includes allowing the patients to manage their pain and muscle guarding through inducing a sense of analgesia.[20,21] The heating process will also increase blood

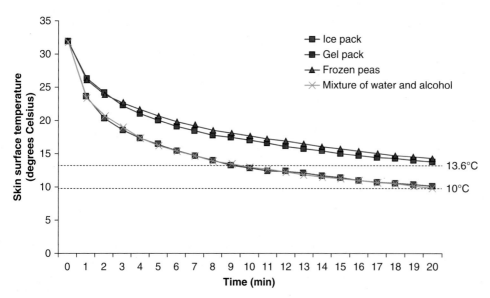

FIGURE 10.1 Mean skin surface temperature during the application of the ice pack, gel pack, frozen peas, and mixture of water and alcohol for 20 minutes (from 0 to 20 minutes) (*N* = 50). (Redrawn from Rotsalai K, Prawit J. Comparison of skin surface temperature during the application of various cryotherapy modalities. Copyright. Elsevier. 2005:1411-1415. © 2005 American Congress of Rehabilitation Medicine and the American Academy of Physical Medicine and Rehabilitation. Published by Elsevier Inc. All rights reserved.)

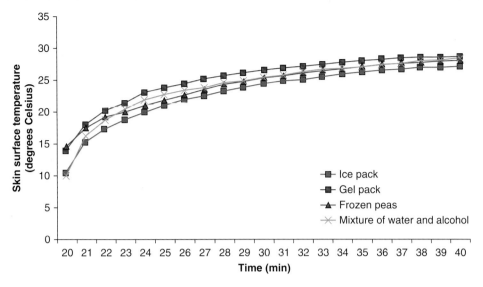

FIGURE 10.2 Mean skin surface temperature after the application of the ice pack, gel pack, frozen peas, and mixture of water and alcohol for 20 minutes (from 20 to 40 minutes) (*N* = 50). (Redrawn from Rotsalai K, Prawit J. Comparison of skin surface temperature during the application of various cryotherapy modalities. Copyright. Elsevier. 2005:1411-1415. © 2005 American Congress of Rehabilitation Medicine and the American Academy of Physical Medicine and Rehabilitation. Published by Elsevier Inc. All rights reserved.)

flow to facilitate an influx of increased oxygen, nutrients, and antibodies to the treatment region. When there is an increase in body temperature, there will be an increase in cellular metabolic activity facilitating the release of histamines, prostaglandins, and bradykinins. This results in increased vasodilation and increased vascular perfusion, which may enable pain relief and tissue repair. Heat can improve superficial collagen extensibility and may facilitate soft-tissue elongation when combined with a stretch.

Clinical Indications and Contraindications

Heating modalities are often used to assist in the reduction of pain and stiffness, alleviate muscle spasms, increase range of motion, and improve tissue healing by increasing blood flow and nutrients to the area. Mild heating usually elevates temperature at the site of pathology to less than 104°F and may be thought of as having a soothing, counterirritant effect.[5,22,23] As seen in **Table 10.4**, heating modalities have several precautions and contraindicators that should be considered prior to application. Superficial heating agents should not be used when the patient is unable to provide accurate sensory feedback. In the absence of normal sensory feedback, the risk that a patient may be burned and develop permanent tissue damage is increased. It is recommended to avoid the use of heat directly over very superficial metal implants (staples in the skin, percutaneous pins). Metals have high thermal conductivity; therefore, there is increased risk injury from tissues surrounding these metal implants. Internal hardware covered by intact skin and subcutaneous tissue can receive superficial heating agents with normal precautions.

Therapeutic Ultrasound

Ultrasound utilizes acoustic energy to produce mechanical vibrations that transmit energy and may produce thermal and nonthermal effects.[24,25] Ultrasound waves are transmitted by the flow of an alternating current across a piezoelectric crystal. The electrical energy causes the crystal to vibrate and creates high-energy sound waves. Therapeutic ultrasound can elevate tissue temperatures as well as produce nonthermal cellular healing effects based on the parameters utilized (**Table 10.5**). The optimal therapeutic ultrasound frequencies for physical and occupational therapy are 1.0 to 3.0 MHz. A frequency of 1.0 MHz (1 million hertz) will

TABLE 10.2 Cryotherapy Precautions and Contraindications

Precautions	Contraindications	Adverse Effects
Cold pack on >20 min	Cold hypersensitivity	Tissue death
Superficial branch peripheral nerve	Cold intolerance	Frostbite
Open wound	Cryoglobulinemia	Nerve damage
Diminished sensation	Raynaud phenomenon	Unwanted vasodilation (hunting response
Limited cognition	Regenerating peripheral nerve	if cold applied for >20 min)
Poor skin integrity	Circulatory compromise or repair	
CRPS (formerly RSD)	Diminished/absent protective sensation	
HTN, cardiac failure	PVD	
	DVT, thrombophlebitis	

CRPS, complex regional pain syndrome; DVT, deep vein thrombosis; HTN, hypertension; PVD, peripheral vascular disease; RSD, regional sympathetic dystrophy

TABLE 10.3 Thermotherapy Methods

Type of Thermotherapy	Convection	Conduction	Radiation
Moist hot packs		X	
Heating pads		X	
Fluidotherapy	X		
Infrared			X
Paraffin		X	

provide deep penetration up to 5 cm below the tissue surface.[25] A frequency of 3.0 MHz will penetrate superficial tissues up to 2.5 cm in depth.[25]

Clinical Indications and Contraindications

Ultrasound is a form of acoustic sound energy that is often used to treat impairments associated with fractures (**Table 10.6**). When tissues absorb ultrasound waves, the kinetic energy increases which results in a heating effect between the molecules. Depending on the intensity and length of time ultrasound is applied, increased temperature may occur in tissues that are high in collagen. Draper and colleagues[26] described the heating effects of therapeutic ultrasound at various intensities on uninjured triceps surae muscles in 24 college students. The 3 MHz frequency heating rate was significantly faster than the 1 MHz frequency heating rate. Tissue temperature was dependent upon the time and intensity of the ultrasound

TABLE 10.4 Thermotherapy Precautions and Contraindications

Precautions	Contraindications
Anterior neck, carotid sinus	Inflamed or infected tissues
Pregnant women	Regions of suspected or known malignancy
Cardiac failure	DVT, thrombophlebitis
Mild-moderate edema	Impaired sensation
	Hemorrhage
	Impaired mentation
	Impaired circulation
	Heat-sensitive skin
	Poor skin integrity
	Severe edema
	Reproductive organs

TABLE 10.5 Thermal and Nonthermal Effects

Thermal	Nonthermal
Increase in collagen tissue extensibility of tendons and joint capsules	Stimulation of tissue healing and repair
Decrease in pain	Increase in cell and vascular wall permeability to calcium and sodium ions
Altered nerve conduction	Increase in protein synthesis
Increase in peripheral blood flow	Stimulation of release of histamine from mast cells accelerating the healing process
Decrease in muscle spasms	
Increase in tissue temperature	
Increase in metabolic rate	

treatment. As the ultrasound treatment time increased, the temperature of the muscle also elevated. Similarly, as the ultrasound intensity increased, the temperature within the targeted muscle also increased. Therapeutic low-frequency ultrasound has been used extensively to treat a variety of conditions because of its documented thermal and nonthermal effects.[26-31] Furthermore, 75% to 80% of ultrasound energy is reflected while the remaining portion is absorbed by the periosteum. Continuous ultrasound over a healing fracture may stimulate abnormal bone growth or demineralization of the bone.[31] Low dose pulsed ultrasound has been shown to promote osteoblastic activity to heal fractures.[31] However, the effective parameters are different from those used in therapeutic ultrasound.

TABLE 10.6 Thermal and Nonthermal Indications

Thermal	Nonthermal
Joint contracture	Tissue repair
Scar tissue	Acute injury or inflammation
Chronic conditions/inflammation	Bone healing
Tissue with limited extensibility	Open wounds, ulcers, surgical skin incisions
Pain	Pain
Muscle spasms/trigger points	Muscle spasms/trigger points

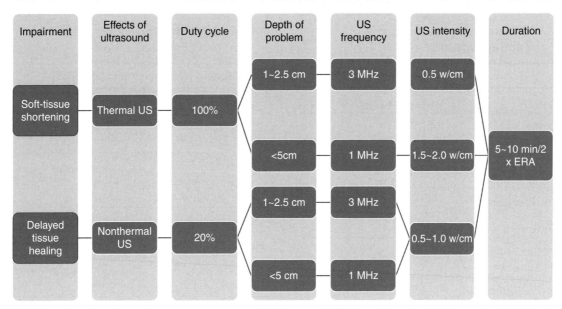

FIGURE 10.3 Thermal and nonthermal treatment parameters. US, ultrasound. (Adapted from Physical Agents in Rehabilitation. 3rd edition. Synder-Mackler L, Delitto A, Stralka SW, Bailey SL. Use of electrical stimulation to enhance recovery of quadriceps femoris muscle force production in patients following anterior cruciate ligament reconstruction. *Phys Ther.* 1994;74(10):901-907.)

Due to the heating property of continuous ultrasound, an inflamed tissue may become exacerbated resulting in increased redness, swelling, heat, and pain. Pulsed ultrasound may stimulate cellular healing to promote resolution of a prolonged inflammatory phase leading to faster tissue repair.[31] A summary of thermal and nonthermal treatment parameters is provided in **Figure 10.3**.

In summary, the use of therapeutic ultrasound has been focused on increasing connective tissue extensibility, increasing cell filtration rate, increasing local blood flow, and decreasing joint pain and stiffness. Furthermore, posttraumatic effects include decreasing inflammation and facilitating wound, muscle, fracture, articular cartilage, and peripheral nerve healing and repair.[5,32-35]

Special Considerations
As seen in **Table 10.7**, ultrasound modalities have several precautions and contraindicators that should be considered prior to application. Additional precautions and contraindications include avoiding using ultrasound over ectopic bone as it may stimulate increased unwanted bone growth, as well as over plastic and cemented implants due to these materials' high coefficient of ultrasound absorption, which may lead to loosening of an implant. It is safe to use ultrasound over internal metal implants. Caution, however, is required to avoid standing waves and unstable cavitation. Ultrasound over external metal (staples, external fixator) should be avoided. The synthetic material has a high coefficient of ultrasound absorption, which may alter the integrity of the conduit leading to poor return of the regenerating nerve. Therefore, ultrasound near postsurgical nerve repair sites with synthetic material should be carried out with caution.

ELECTRICAL STIMULATION: TENS AND NMES

Two different forms of electrical stimulation are commonly used clinically: pulsatile current and burst-modulated alternating current such as "Russian current," "interferential current," and "premodulated current." Burst-modulated alternating current stimulation is claimed to be more comfortable than PC and capable of eliciting greater muscle torque.[36-40] There are also numerous ways to utilize electrical stimulation based on therapeutic treatment goals specific to the patient's needs and impairments. Common types of clinical electrical stimulation include neuromuscular electrical stimulation (NMES) for muscular reeducation and strengthening transcutaneous electrical nerve stimulation (TENS) for pain control, high volt pulsatile current (HVPC) for pain and edema control, and direct/galvanic current to stimulate denervated musculature and deliver ionic medications.[5,41,42]

Transcutaneous Electrical Nerve Stimulation

TENS is the application of electric current (often in biphasic PC, premodulated, or interferential current) into a tissue to depolarize nerve fibers (A-beta fibers and alpha motor neurons) in order to control pain. After a trauma or a surgery, TENS can be effective in controlling pain and helping the patients reduce their amount or dependency on pain medication. It can also enable the patients to take on a more active role in their pain management, as well as improve comfort during functional movements and tasks. TENS treats the symptoms and not the cause of the impairment, so it should be used in conjunction with skilled therapeutic treatment techniques. As seen in **Table 10.8**, TENS has several precautions and contraindicators that should be considered prior to application.

TABLE 10.7 Ultrasound Precautions and Contraindications

Conditions	Nonthermal	Thermal
Active epiphysis	C	C
Healing fracture	P	C
Plastic implants		C
Over cemented implant		C
Synthetic nerve conduit		C
External hardware	C	C
Electric implant (cardiac pacemaker)	C	C
Over areas of hemorrhage	C	C
Impaired circulation	P	C
Myositis ossificans, heterotopic ossification	C	C
Thrombophlebitis, DVT	C	C
Active infection, acute inflammation	P	C
Poor skin integrity (frail, psoriasis, eczema)	P	C
Poor sensation	P	C
Poor mentation	P	C
Pregnancy	C	C
Malignancy	C	C
Over CNS	C	C
Over heart, eyes, or reproductive organs	C	C
Over area of breast implant	C	C
Over recently radiated tissues	C	C
Over anterior neck or carotid sinus	C	C
Internal metal hardware (plates, pins, screws)		P
Peripheral and regenerating nerves	P	P

C, contraindication; P, precaution.

Special Considerations
Surgical Implants
Electrical stimulation may be used on intact skin overlying implants containing metal, plastic, or cement.[43] It should not, however, be utilized over external staples or tissues treated

TABLE 10.8 TENS Precautions and Contraindications

Precautions	Contraindications
Acute pain	Cardiac instability
Postoperatively	Implanted electrical stimulator (cardiac pacemaker)
During occupational tasks when patient may "over-do it"	External hardware
Internal hardware	Epilepsy/seizures
Elderly	Over carotid sinuses or CNS
Obese (increased adipose tissue)	Infected tissues, osteomyelitis
Skin impairments (eczema, psoriasis)	PVD, impaired circulation
Active epiphysis	Recently radiated tissues
	Decreased sensation
	Decreased mentation
	Undiagnosed pain
	Pregnancy
	Poor skin integrity
	Regions of known or suspected malignancy
	Thrombophlebitis, DVT
	Areas of hemorrhage

with dressings or topical agents containing metal ions (silver, zinc).[43] There is a theory that suggests increased risk in skin irritation/burning when applying a current to skin overlying superficial metal implants.[43] There is little consensus on how superficial the implant must be in order to alter current flow.[43] The majority of literature demonstrates that the conduction of an electric current will not be influenced by most metal materials including the implants utilized in joint replacements.[43] Individuals with metal hardware and joint replacements have been successfully treated with electrical stimulation without adverse reactions.[43]

Recent Surgery, Unstable Fracture
High-intensity motor-level TENS should not be used on recent postoperative muscle/tendon/ligament repairs, skin flaps, joint replacements, or recent unstable fractures.[43] Forceful muscle contractions can cause fracture displacement, tear recent tendon and skin sutures, or disturb an incision or graft.[43] Conventional/sensory level stimulation is a more appropriate choice to help the patients manage their postoperative pain.[5]

Pain Theories and Applications

Gate Theory

This theory was initially described by Melzack and Wall in 1968.[44] They hypothesized that stimulation of non-nociceptor nerve fibers would block the transmission of a pain sensation from the nociceptors to the higher cortical areas where pain is perceived. Nociceptors (A-delta and C fibers) are small-diameter, slow conducting fibers that have little or no myelin.[44,45] These fibers transmit painful stimuli to the spinal cord and then the impulse travels to the brain to be processed and yield a perception of pain. These smaller diameter fibers can be inhibited by stimulating the large diameter, fast-conducting, highly myelinated proprioceptive sensory nerve fibers (A-beta fibers). Through stimulation of the A-beta fibers, the spinal cord is "flooded" with sensory input and "closes the gate" to the nociceptor/pain stimulation. As a result, the brain will recognize the stimulation from the TENS unit and will interpret pain relief.[44,45] The gate control phenomenon is thought to be localized in the substantia gelatinosa in specialized T-cells.[44] This type of TENS would be appropriate for the following conditions: acute pain after an injury or surgery, joint mobilization techniques, and pain with a positional or dynamic stretch. A summary of sensory-level treatment parameters is provided in **Table 10.9**.

Endogenous Opioids—Beta Endorphin and Dynorphin Release Theory

Endorphins are endogenous opioids produced by the pituitary gland and hypothalamus.[45] When released, they create a feeling of analgesia and well-being. The patient's sensation should be somewhat of an obvious muscle twitching response. This "motor-level" stimulation TENS is thought to act via descending methods of pain modulation by the release of endogenous opioids.[31,32] As this endorphin binds to the opioid receptors, it can modulate the patient's perception of pain.[44,45] The endogenous pain reliever is a neurohormone, and therefore, the analgesia duration should last for several hours. This type of TENS would be appropriate for subacute and chronic pain conditions. Since a twitch contraction is produced, caution not to disturb the tissue healing process must be considered. Possible conditions appropriate for this level of stimulation include subacute, settled, chronic pain syndromes, prior to passive stretching, before or during burn debridement or a minor surgery.[44] A summary of motor-level treatment parameters is provided in **Table 10.10**.

NEUROMUSCULAR ELECTRICAL STIMULATION

There is a strong interdependence between normal muscle activity and joint function. There can be significant muscle atrophy that occurs following a trauma, such as a fracture, to the bone and/or joint. The combination of pain, swelling, and immobilization has an inhibitory effect on muscle activity. Due to these factors, the development of muscular atrophy occurs and can be quite disabling to the patient. Recent studies have demonstrated the potential of NMES training protocols to elicit a hypertrophic response in skeletal muscle.[33,34] NMES can also be used to stimulate a muscular contraction by depolarizing peripheral nerves, which may be used to prevent disuse atrophy during immobilization or inactivity, as well as to maintain or improve ROM. Other therapeutic benefits include decreasing muscle spasms, facilitating or reeducating a muscular contraction, increasing muscle strength, facilitating tendon excursion, substituting for an orthosis, and reducing edema through a "muscle pumping" action (**Tables 10.11-10.13**). As seen in **Table 10.14**, NMES has several precautions and contraindicators that should be considered prior to application.

Special Considerations

Surgical Implants

Electrical stimulation may be used on intact skin overlying implants containing metal, plastic, or cement.[43] It

---

TABLE 10.9 Sensory-Level Parameters

Parameter	Setting
Pulse duration	50-125 μs
Pulse rate	80-150 pps
Amplitude	Sensory level: strong but comfortable tingle
Treatment duration	20-30 min
Treatment area	Bracket or directly over the painful site
Pain relief duration	Pain modulation stops when stimulus stops
Pain relief onset	Almost immediately

TABLE 10.10 Motor-Level Parameters

Parameter	Setting
Pulse rate	1-10 pps
Pulse duration	>200 μs
Amplitude	Strong but comfortable muscle twitch
Treatment duration	10-20 min
Treatment area	Over motor points in painful area
Pain relief duration	>1 h
Pain relief onset	10-20 min

TABLE 10.11 Relaxation of Subacute and Chronic Muscle Spasms

Parameter	Setting
Pulse duration (width)	200-400 µs (small muscles) 600-800 µs (large muscles)
Pulse rate (frequency)	<10 pps (muscle twitch for subacute) or >50 pps (muscle fatigue for chronic) For acute muscle spasm, use sensory level stimulation
Amplitude (intensity)	Patient tolerance for gentle contraction
Duty cycle (on:off ratio)	1:1
Waveform	Asymmetrical (small muscles) Symmetrical (large muscles)
Treatment time	10-15 min (stimulation until fatigue present)

should not, however, be utilized over external staples or tissues treated with dressings or topical agents containing metal ions (silver, zinc).[43] There is a theory that suggests increased risk in skin irritation/burning when applying a current to skin overlying superficial metal implants.[43] There is little consensus on how superficial the implant must be in order to alter current flow.[43] The majority of literature demonstrates that the conduction of an electric current will not be influenced by most metal materials including the implants utilized in joint replacements.[43] Individuals with metal hardware and joint replacements have been successfully treated with electrical stimulation without adverse reactions.[43]

TABLE 10.12 Maintaining or Increasing Active ROM and Strength

Waveform	Setting
Pulse duration (width)	200-400 µs (small muscles) 600-800 µs (large muscles)
Pulse rate (frequency)	25-50 pps
Amplitude (intensity)	Strong but comfortable contraction
Duty cycle (on:off ratio)	1:3-1:5 to allow for recovery and prevent fatigue
Waveform	Asymmetrical (small muscles) Symmetrical (large muscles)
Treatment time	10-30 min; 1-2 times/d; 3-5 d/wk

TABLE 10.13 Reduction in Edema

Parameter	Setting
Pulse duration (width)	100-400 µs
Pulse rate (frequency)	Subacute: <10 pps (twitch) Chronic: 25-50 pps (contraction)
Duty cycle (on:off ratio)	Subacute: Continuous twitch Chronic: 1:1-1:3 contraction
Waveform	Asymmetrical (small muscles) Symmetrical (large muscles)
Treatment time	10-30 min; 1-4 times/d

TABLE 10.14 NMES Precautions and Contraindications

Precautions[43-45]	Contraindications[43-45]
Internal metal hardware (pins, plates)	Patients with pacemakers
Elderly	Implanted stimulators
Obese patient (excessive adipose tissue may require higher electrical intensity which may lead to increase in skin irritation)	Over areas where movement is contraindicated (unstable fracture)
Over areas of thoracic region (interference with heart activity)	DVT or thrombophlebitis
Hypersensitive patient	Pregnant women
	Diminished sensation
	Diminished mentation
	Poor skin integrity
	External metal hardware
	Over carotid sinus
	Over areas of pathology with myelin sheath (diabetic neuropathy, MS, peripheral neuropathy)
	Over areas of pathology of the cell body (polio)
	Over areas of pathology within the muscle (muscular dystrophy)

Recent Surgery, Unstable Fracture

High-intensity NMES should not be used on recent postoperative muscle/tendon/ligament repairs, skin flaps, joint replacements, or recent unstable fractures.[43] Forceful muscle contractions can cause fracture displacement, tear recent tendon and skin sutures, or disturb an incision or graft.[43]

Common NMES Parameters[43-46]

See **Tables 10.11-10.13**.

MODALITIES USED IN TISSUE HEALING

Tissue healing has been a primary focus in patient management after traumatic injury. In addition to using modalities for decreasing inflammation and swelling, controlling post-trauma pain, and improving range of motion and strength, one of the most important reasons for modality applications may be their effectiveness in promoting tissue healing. After an injury or surgery, injured tissue typically goes through three basic wound healing phases: inflammatory, proliferation, and maturation phases. Tissue healing can become problematic at any phase. Chronic inflammation or regeneration failure can lead to even more complications and decrease in function. The following modalities have been shown to be effective in tissue healing:

LOW-FREQUENCY ULTRASOUND

Low-frequency ultrasound shares many of the same principles of conventional ultrasound at 1 and 3 MHz; however, it has a frequency in the 20,000 to 40,000 Hz range. Voigt et al[47] published a systematic review on the use of low-frequency ultrasound to promote chronic wound healing. The researcher found that in treating chronic wounds, low-frequency ultrasound showed quicker healing by both high-intensity and low-intensity ultrasound delivered at a low frequency (either via contact or noncontact techniques).[47]

ELECTRICAL STIMULATION

Foulds and Barker[48] had long described that there is a separation of charges between the interior and exterior surfaces of human skin. The skin's exterior has a negative polarity relative to the interior aspect, which is referred to as a human skin battery. When there is any disruption on the skin surface, the interior of the wound is positively charged compared with the periwound area, which potentially drives wound healing.[48] When electrical stimulation is applied to the skin, it mimics the skin battery in wound healing. The common waveforms used in this circumstance are HVPC and microcurrent. Both types are galvanotactic currents, which can attract charged cells to an electric field of opposite polarity. This type of direct current generates an electric field, which enables cell migration, DNA and protein synthesis, and calcium uptake. These processes are essential for tissue healing and regeneration.[49-53]

INFRARED ENERGY

Peripheral nerve injuries associated with fractures are not uncommon.[54-56] The current use of monochromatic infrared energy (MIRE) shows positive effects on restoring the loss of protective sensation, ranging from mild improvement to complete resolution.[57,58] Many of these studies do not address traumatic injuries. In order to better understand the treatment benefits of MIRE, well-designed clinical research with large sample sizes in traumatic nerve injuries is needed.

REFERENCES

1. Court-Brown CM, Caesar B. Epidemiology of adult fractures: a review. *Injury*. 2006;37(8):691-697. doi:10.1016/j.injury.2006.04.130.
2. Dionyssiotis Y, Dontas IA, Economopoulos D, Lyritis GP. Rehabilitation after falls and fractures. *J Musculoskelet Neuronal Interact*. 2008;8(3):244-250.
3. Koval KJ, Cooley MR. Clinical pathway after hip fracture. *Diabil Rehabil*. 2005;27:1053-1060.
4. Kumar SP, Jim A. Physical therapy in palliative care: from symptom control to quality of life. A critical review. *Indian J Palliat Care*. 2010;16(3):138-146. doi:10.4103/0973-1075.73670.
5. Michlovitz SL, Bellew JW, Nolan TP. *Modalities for Therapeutic Intervention*. Philadelphia, PA: F.A.Davis; 2012.
6. McMeeken J, Murray L, Cocks S. Effects of cooling with simulated ice on skin temperature and nerve conduction velocity. *Aust J Physiother*. 1984;30:111-142.doi:10.1016/S0004-9514(14)60682-6.
7. Cobbold AF, Lewis OJ. Blood flow to the knee joint of the dog: effect of heating, cooling and adrenaline. *J Physiol*. 1956;132:379-383.
8. Taber C, Contryman K, Fahrenbruch J, LaCount K, Cornwall MW. Measurement of reactive vasodilation during cold pack application to non-traumatized ankles. *Phys Ther*. 1992;72:294-299.
9. Weston M, Taber C, Casagranda L, Cornwall M. Changes in local blood volume during cold-gel pack application to traumatized ankles. *J Orthop Sports Phys Ther*. 1994;4:197-199.
10. Sapega AA, Heppenstall RB, Sokolow DP, et al. The bioenergetics of preservation of limbs before replantation. *J Bone Joint Surg Am*. 1988;70:1500-13.
11. Cameron MH. *Physical Agents in Rehabilitation: From Research to Practice*. Philadelphia, PA: WB Saunders; 1999.
12. Bugaj R. The cooling, analgesic, and rewarming effects of ice massage on localized skin. *Phys Ther*. 1975;55:11-19.
13. Ohkoshi Y, Ohkoshi M, Nagasaki S, Ono A, Hashimoto T, Yamane S. The effect of cryotherapy on intraarticular temperature and postoperative care after anterior cruciate ligament reconstruction. *Am J Sports Med*. 1999;27:357-362.
14. Deal DN, Tipton J, Rosencrance E, Curl WW, Smith TL. Ice reduces edema. *J Bone Joint Surg Am*. 2002;84:1573-1578.
15. Merrick MA, Rankin JM, Andres FA, Hinman CL. A preliminary examination of cryotherapy and secondary injury in skeletal muscle. *Med Sci Sports Exerc*. 1999;31:1516-1521.
16. Rotsalai K, Prawit J. Comparison of skin surface temperature during the application of various cryotherapy modalities. *Arch Phys Med Rehabil*. 2005;86:1411-1415.
17. Algafly A, George K. The Effect of cryotherapy on nerve conduction velocity, pain threshold and pain tolerance. *Br J Sports Med*. 2007;41:365-369.
18. Leung M, Cheing GJ. Effects of deep and superficial heating in the management of frozen shoulder. *Rehabil Med*. 2008;40:145-150.
19. Robertson V, Ward A, Jung P. The effect of heat on tissue extensibility: a comparison of deep and superficial heating. *Arch Phys Med Rehabil*. 2005;86:819-825.
20. Baba-Akbari Sari A, Flemming K, Cullum NA, Wollina U. Therapeutic ultrasound for pressure ulcers. *Cochrane Database Syst Rev*. 2006;3:CD001275.
21. Allen RJ. Physical agents used in the management of chronic pain by physical therapists. *Phys Med Rehabil Clin North Am*. 2006;17:315-345.
22. Nadler SF, Steiner DJ, Erasala GN, Hengehold DA, Abeln SB, Weingand KW. Continuous low-level heatwrap therapy for treating acute nonspecific low back pain. *Arch Phys Med Rehabil*. 2003;84:329-334.

23. Kitchen S. Thermal effects. In: Walson T, ed. *Electrotherapy Evidence-Based Practice*. 12th ed. Edinburgh: Churchill Livingstone Elsevier; 2008.

24. Lentell G, Hetherington T, Eagan J, Morgan M. The use of thermal agents to influence the effectiveness of a low-load prolonged stretch. *J Orthop Sports Phys Ther*. 1992;16:200-207.

25. Saini NS, Roy KS, Banasal PS, et al. A preliminary study on the effects of ultrasound therapy on the healing of surgically severed achilles tendons in five dogs. *J Vet Med A Physiol Pathol Clin Med*. 2002;49:321-328.

26. Draper DO, Castel JC, Castel D. Rate of temperature increases in human muscle during 1 MHz and 3 MHz continuous ultrasound. *J Orthop Sports Phys Ther*. 1995;22:142-150.

27. Lehmann JF, DeLateur BJ, Silverman DR. Selective heating effects of ultrasound in human beings. *Arch Phys Med Rehabil*. 1966;47:331-339.

28. Hayes BT, Merrick MA, Sandrey MA, Cordova ML. Three-MHz ultrasound heats deeper into the tissues than originally theorized. *J Athl Train*. 2204;39(3):230-234.

29. Jeremias Júnior SL, Camanho GL, Bassit AC, Forgas A, Ingham SJ, Abdalla RJ. Low-intensity pulsed ultrasound accelerates healing in rat calcaneus tendon injuries. *Orthop Sports Phys Ther*. 2011;41(7):526-531. doi:10.2519/jospt.2011.3468.

30. Takakura Y, Matsui N, Yoshiya S, et al. Low-intensity pulsed ultrasound enhances early healing of medial collateral ligament injuries in rats. *J Ultrasound Med*. 2002;21:283-288.

31. Azuma Y, Ito M, Harada Y, Takagi H, Ohta T, Jingushi S. Low-intensity pulsed ultrasound accelerates rate femoral fracture healing by acting on various cellular reactions in the fracture callus. *J Bone Miner Res*. 2001;16:671-680.

32. Katsuyuki M, Kazumori M, Takayuki F. Effect of therapeutic ultrasound on intramuscular circulation and oxygen dynamics. *J Jpn Phys Ther Assoc*. 2014;17:1-7.

33. Bierman W. Ultrasound in the treatment of scars. *Arch Phys Med Rehabil*. 1954;35:209-213.

34. Castel JC. Therapeutic ultrasound. *Rehab Ther Product Rev*. 1993:22-32.

35. Stratton SA, Heckman R, Francis RS. Therapeutic ultrasound: its effects on the integrity of a nonpenetrating wound. *J Orthop Sports Phys Ther*. 1984;3:278-281.

36. Robertson VJ, Ward AR, Low J, Reed A. *Electrotherapy Explained: Principles and Practice*. 4th ed. Oxford, U K: Butterworth Heinemann; 2006.

37. Kloth LC. Interference current. In: Nelson RM, Currier DP, eds. *Clinical Electrotherapy*. 2nd ed. East Norwalk, CT: Appleton & Lange; 1991:221-260.

38. Selkowitz DM. High-frequency electrical stimulation in muscle strengthening. *Am J Sport Med*. 1989;17:103-111.

39. Low J, Reed A. *Electrotherapy Explained Principles and Practice*. 3rd ed. Oxford, UK: Butterworth-Heinemann; 2000:94-95.

40. Siolund B, Terenius L, Eriksson M. Increased cerebrospinal fluid levels of endorphins after electroacupuncture. *Acta Physiol Scand*. 1977;100:382-384.

41. Stevens JE, Mizner RL, Synder-Mackler L. Neuromuscular electrical stimulation for quadriceps muscle strengthening after bilateral total knee arthroplasty: a case series. *J Orthop Sports Physic*. 2004;34(1):21-29.

42. Synder-Mackler L, Delitto A, Stralka SW, Bailey SL. Use of electrical stimulation to enhance recovery of quadriceps femoris muscle force production in patients following anterior cruciate ligament reconstruction. *Phys Ther*. 1994;74(10):901-907.

43. Cameron MH. *Physical Agents in Rehabilitation from Research to Practice*. St. Louis, MO: Saunders Elsevier; 2013.

44. Electrophysical Agents – Contraindications and precautions: an evidence-based approach to clinical decision making in physical therapy. *Physiother Can*. 2010;62(5):1-80. doi:10.3138/ptc.62.5.

45. Bracciano AG. *Physical Agent Modalities: Theory and Application for the Occupational Therapist*. 2nd ed. Thorofare, NJ: SLACK; 2008.

46. Prentice WE. *Therapeutic Modalities in Rehabilitation*. 2nd ed. China: McGraw-Hill Professional Publishing; 2011.

47. Voigt J, Wendelken M, Driver V, Alvarez OM. Low-frequency ultrasound (20-40kHz) as an adjunctive therapy for chronic wound healing: a systematic review of the literature and meta-analysis of eight randomized controlled trials. *Int J Low Extrem Wounds*. 2011;10(4):190-199. doi:10.1177/1534734611424648.

48. Foulds IS, Barker AT. Human skin battery potentials and their possible role in wound healing. *Br J Dermatol*. 1983;109(5):515-522.

49. Bassett C, Herrmann I. The effect of electrostatic fields on macromolecular synthesis by fibroblasts in vitro (abstract). *J Cell Biol*. 1968;39;9a.

50. Bourguignon GJ, Bourguinon LYW. Effect of high voltage pulsed galvanic stimulation on human fibroblasts in cell culture (abstract). *J Cell Biol*. 1986;103(suppl):344a.

51. Bourguignon GJ, Bourguignon LYW. Electric stimulation of protein and DNA synthesis in human fibroblasts. *FASEB J*. 1987;1(5):398-402.

52. Cheng N, Van Hoof H, Bockx E, et al. The effects of electric currents on ATP generation, protein synthesis, and membrane transport in rat skin. *Clin Orthop Relat Res*. 1982;171:264-272.

53. Zhao M, Penninger J, Isseroff RR. Electrical activation of wound-healing pathways. *Adv Skin Wound Care*. 2010;1:567-573. doi:10.1089/9781934854013.567.

54. Li Y, Ning G, Wu Q, Wu Q, Li Y, Feng S. Review of literature of radial nerve injuries associated with humeral fractures – an integrated management strategy. *PLoS ONE*. 2013;8(11):e78576. doi:10.1371/journal.pone.0078576.

55. Nelson AJ, Izzi JA, Green A, Weiss AP, Akelman E. Traumatic nerve injuries about the elbow. *Orthop Clin North Am*. 1999;30(1):91-94. doi: 10.1016/S0030-5898(05)70063-8.

56. Bennett WF, Browner B. Tibial plateau fractures: a study of associated soft tissue injuries. *J Orthop Trauma*. 1994;8(3):183-188.

57. Prendergast JJ, Miranda G, Sanchez M. Improvement of sensory impairment in patients with peripheral neuropathy. *Endocr Pract*. 2004;10(1):24-30.

58. DeLellis SL, Carnegie DH, Burke TJ. Improved sensitivity in patients with peripheral neuropathy: effects of monochromatic infrared photo energy. *J Am Podiatr Med Assoc*. 2005;28(12):2896-2900.

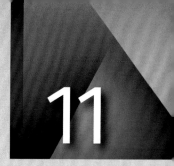

Analysis of Gait

Adam Keith Lee
Mary Kate Erdman

INTRODUCTION

Gait is simply defined as the way in which a person walks. Fractures of the lower extremity frequently impair the mechanism of gait, and a primary goal of the fracture surgeon is to restore that mechanism. To do this, the surgeon must have a thorough understanding of gait and practical knowledge of gait analysis.

The science of gait analysis has progressed in parallel with the progression of technology. Historically, gait analysis was limited to observational descriptions; however, advancements in photography, motion capture, and wireless technology added a new understanding of the nuances of normal and abnormal gait. That said, gait analysis for most orthopaedic surgeons is almost exclusively done on an observational basis in the clinical setting. Therefore, this chapter seeks to provide an overview of normal and abnormal gait concepts, which are most clinically relevant to the orthopaedic surgeon.

GAIT OVERVIEW

The five tasks of gait were defined by Winter:

1. Maintenance of support of the head, arms, and trunk, that is, preventing collapse of the lower limb.
2. Maintenance of upright posture and balance of the body.
3. Control of the foot trajectory to achieve safe ground clearance and a gentle heel or toe landing.
4. Generation of mechanical energy to maintain the present forward velocity or to increase the forward velocity.
5. Absorption of mechanical energy for shock absorption and stability or to decrease the forward velocity of the body.[1]

Gait is more than one successful step forward but the cyclic repetition of that action. The gait cycle is separated into two phases termed the stance phase and swing phase. These phases are based on the position of a single extremity, while the opposite extremity simultaneously progresses through its correlating phase of the gait cycle.

STANCE PHASE

The stance phase accounts for 60% of the gait cycle at average walking speeds and is further subdivided into five components.[2] The purpose of the stance phase is to accommodate the body weight as it shifts from one lower limb to the other while disseminating forces and maintaining forward momentum.

- *Initial contact ("heel strike")*: The stance phase starts when contact is made with the walking surface; this begins with the heel in the setting of normal gait.
- *Foot flat*: Forward momentum progresses and the foot rolls forward to conform with the ground until the entire plantar surface is engaged and flat on the surface.
- *Midstance*: The body weight shifts forward and midstance is reached when weight is directly over the supporting foot.
- *Heel-off*: As the body weight moves forward, the heel of the supporting foot rises from the ground and force is directed through the forefoot.
- *Toe-off*: The stance phase terminates when the supporting foot lifts from the walking surface and the body weight is received entirely by the opposite foot.[3]

SWING PHASE

The remaining 40% of the gait cycle, termed the swing phase, begins after toe-off of the stance phase of the ipsilateral foot and just before midstance phase of the contralateral foot.[2] As suggested by the name, the critical goal of this phase is that of ground clearance of the foot to allow forward progress of that extremity. Similar to the stance phase, the swing phase is also subdivided:

- *Early Swing/Acceleration Phase*: This phase begins at the completion of toe-off and is terminated when the extremity is directly under the body.
- *Midswing*: Following acceleration, the leg swings to be directly under body at which point the motion of the leg transitions from acceleration to deceleration.
- *Late Swing/Deceleration Phase*: Forward motion of the extremity continues, but in preparation for ground contact, muscle contraction causes deceleration to smooth the transition from the swing phase to the stance phase.

MUSCLE ACTIVITY

The successful execution of the gait cycle is dependent upon a highly coordinated muscle activity from the hip to the toes, which allows for stability and controlled motion.[4,5] Multiple muscles work in both phases of the gait cycle through both concentric and eccentric activities (**Table 11.1**).

The precise timing of each muscle group activation can be found in **Table 11.1**. Support of the body weight is maintained through hip extensors, knee extensors, and ankle plantarflexors. This grouping is intuitive if one envisions each joint collapsing toward the path of least resistance—the hip tends to collapse in flexion, the knee in flexion, and the ankle in dorsiflexion. The action of the muscle groups listed above maintains the internal moment force of each joint and balances those forces throughout the entire system. There are two main functions of the coordinated contractions: to accommodate the body weight as the limb transitions from a swing to a stance phase and to add a propulsion force from a stance phase to the next stance phase.

TABLE 11.1 Concentric and Eccentric Activity During Normal Gait

Phase	Eccentric Activity	Concentric Activity
Heel strike to foot flat	Tibialis anterior Quadriceps Gluteus maximus Hamstrings Extensor hallucis Extensor digitorum	
Foot flat to midstance	Quadriceps	
Midstance to heel-off		Triceps surae
Heel-off to toe-off	Quadriceps Gluteus medius (contralateral)	Triceps surae Tibialis anterior Peroneus longus Flexor digitorum Flexor hallucis
Toe-off to acceleration	Gluteus medius (contralateral)	Triceps surae Tibialis anterior Hamstrings
Acceleration to midswing	Gluteus medius (contralateral)	Quadriceps Iliopsoas Tibialis anterior
Midswing through deceleration	Hamstrings Gluteus medius (contralateral)	Tibialis anterior

Reprinted with permission from Hoppenfeld S, Murthy VL. *Treatment and Rehabilitation of Fractures. Philadelphia: Lippincott Williams & Wilkins;* 2000.

The accommodative forces tend to be eccentric as velocity is slowed to allow the joints to gradually load with the body's weight. The hip extensors eccentrically contract and slow the limb in the late swing phase in preparation for heel strike. At heel strike, the dorsiflexors contract eccentrically to slow the forefoot to the ground. The knee extensors counter the tendency for the knee to buckle under body weight throughout the stance phase and allow for controlled knee flexion, and similarly the hip flexors contract eccentrically to counter the hip flexion collapse. During the swing phase, the contralateral hip abductors eccentrically contract to slow the pelvic tilt caused by the unsupported limb. The exception is concentric dorsiflexion in the swing phase, which acts to clear the foot off the ground.

As the body weight shifts over the planted foot in the flatfoot segment of the stance phase, accommodative contractions transition to propulsive contractions. During the cycle, there are short bursts of muscle activity that generate the momentum required for ambulation. Dorsiflexors concentrically contract to pull the leg forward over the foot in preparation for toe-off. A concentric contraction occurs in the plantarflexors at toe-off to propel body weight forward. The hip flexors engage and shorten in the swing phase to accelerate the limb through the swing.

JOINT MOTION

Lower extremity trauma can inhibit normal joint range of motion. Periarticular bony injury can disrupt normal joint mechanics if the articular surface is involved or if the mechanical axis is altered once healed, and soft tissue injuries can lead to weakness, instability, or arthrofibrosis. Since appropriate range of motion of the hip, knee, and ankle facilitates a smooth and efficient gait pattern, adequate joint mobility is a critical concern for the traumatologist.

In the sagittal plane, normal hip range of motion in the gait cycle is 20° of extension between heel-off and toe-off to 20° of flexion, which occurs at initial contact. The knee must bend from full extension at initial contact to 60° of flexion at the midswing phase. Lastly, the ankle dorsiflexes to 7° at heel strike and plantarflexes to 25° at the completion of the stance phase (**Figure 11.1**).

The sagittal plane includes the most significant arcs of motion; however, motion also occurs in the coronal plane. The hip range of motion spans from 5° of adduction to 5° of abduction, which is reached at the end of the stance phase. Also, the ankle will evert to 5° in the early stance phase and reach maximum inversion at 15° during toe-off.[6]

PARAMETERS OF GAIT

The most commonly referenced parameters of gait can be categorized by measurements of length and time. Comparing these values between the affected and unaffected extremities typically provides more clinical utility than absolute measurements.

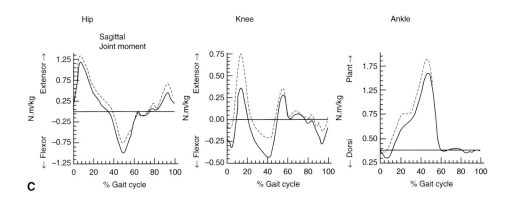

FIGURE 11.1 Free body diagram demonstrating internal net moments at each joint and ground reaction force vector (GRFV) relative to the center of pressure (CoP) through (A) heel-strike to midstance and (B) midstance to toe-off. (C) Internal joint moments in the sagittal plane throughout the progression of gait for hip, knee, and ankle. Solid lines represent mean values while dotted lines represent standard deviations. (Diagrams of internal moments redrawn from Winter DA, Eng JJ, Isshac MG. A review of kinetic parameters in human walking. In: Craik RL, Otis CA, eds. *Gait Analysis: Theory and Application.* St. Louis, MO: Mosby-Year Book; 1994:263-265, with permission from Elsevier.)

LENGTH

Step length	• The distance between sequential points of contact of the opposite foot with the ground measured in the direction of motion.
Stride length	• The distance between sequential points of contact of the *same* foot with the ground measured in the direction of motion. • Stride length comprises two step lengths.

Step width	• The distance between the medial borders of the heels of opposite feet measured perpendicular to the direction of motion. • The measurement defines the walking base or base of support. • Normal values range from 2 to 4 in.
Step angle (foot progression angle)	• The angle subtended by the vector of the direction of walking and the sagittal axis of the foot. • Normal values range from 0° to 7°.

TIME

Walking speed/ velocity	• The linear distance traveled per unit time. • This is frequently reported in miles per hour. • Walking speed is one of the simplest measurements to track clinically. • The importance of reconstituting this parameter following lower extremity fracture will be discussed later in this chapter.
Cadence	• The number of steps per unit of time. • As the cadence increases, the time of double-leg support decreases. • Eventually the time of double-leg support reached zero, at approximately 180 steps/min, and this is the delineation between walking and running. • Further aspects of running gait are beyond the scope of this chapter.
Step duration	• The time spent during a single step.[7]

DETERMINANTS OF GAIT

In 1953, Saunders et al published a work, the purpose of which was to distill the overwhelming complexities of gait analysis down to discrete, clinically relevant factors that can be assessed by an orthopaedic surgeon. They described six determinants, which optimize the efficiency of the gait cycle.[8]

PELVIC ROTATION

The pelvis rotates in the axial plane at an average of 4° in each direction during a gait cycle, and this is accomplished by relative internal and external rotation at the hip joint. Limits to this rotation may result in a difficulty transferring energy with each stride and a less efficient gait.

PELVIC TILT

In normal gait, the pelvis tilts downward at an average of 5° in relative hip adduction during the swing phase to limit vertical oscillation and energy expenditure.

PELVIC SHIFT

The hip adducts as the pelvis shifts laterally, resulting in lateral displacement of the center of mass closer to the long axis of the supporting limb. This shift yields two mechanical benefits. The moment arm on which the center of mass acts is shortened, thus reducing the work of the gluteus medius. Additionally, the shift blunts the sharp changes of direction and creates a more fluid gait.

KNEE FLEXION IN STANCE

Beginning at heel strike, the knee is locked in extension, but flexes to 15° just prior to midstance. This minimizes the vertical displacement of the center of mass as it translates forward.

KNEE MECHANICS

The fifth and sixth determinants of gait are paired because they both reference the rotational motion about the knee and ankle. Dorsiflexion and knee extension produce a functionally lengthened extremity, while plantarflexion and knee flexion functionally shorten the extremity. The modularity of the limb length produces the smooth, sinusoidal nature of gait.

FOOT MECHANICS

See above.

STAIR GAIT

Most gait resources focus on ground level walking; however, the urban and domestic terrain often demands proficiency with stair climbing. Patients are often withheld from discharge until separate physical therapy sessions targeting stair training are completed. The ability of a patient to navigate stairs has even been proposed as a method by which to determine one's gait capacity.[9,10] It is important that the orthopaedic surgeon recognizes the mechanical demands of stair climbing gait.

Normal stair ascent and descent gait patterns, like normal gait, include a stance phase and a swing phase. The components of each phase are listed below.[11]

ASCENT

• Stance phase:
  • Weight acceptance
  • Pull-up. This introduces the greatest risk of instability because body weight is shifted to a single limb in which all major lower extremity joints are braced in flexion.
  • Forward continuance
• Swing phase
  • Foot clearance
  • Foot placement

DESCENT

• Stance phase
  • Weight acceptance
  • Forward continuance
  • Controlled lowering

- Swing phase
  - Leg pull-through
  - Preparation for foot placement

REHABILITATIVE GAIT PATTERNS

Another category of gait that is pertinent to the orthopaedic surgeon is crutch-dependent gait. Ambulatory aids are prescribed to many patients after lower extremity trauma because they broaden the base of support and allow for safe ambulation in the setting of non–weight bearing or partial weight bearing restrictions. It is important to highlight the functional demands of crutch walking, particularly the great challenge this may present to elderly patients. In a study of healthy subjects with an average age of 32 years, crutch walking resulted in a 32% increase in oxygen consumption and concordant heart rate increase of 53%[12].

Crutch gait patterns can be classified either by the coordination of steps taken or by the number of support points utilized. Step-to and step-through gait patterns are differentiated by the placement of the uninjured extremity in relation to the crutches. Step-to gait occurs when the uninjured extremity is brought planted even with the crutch points, while in step-through gait, the uninjured extremity is carried past this point. Step-to gait has been shown to decrease pressure on the plantar forefoot.[13] Although this finding is referenced mostly in the management of diabetic ulcers, it may be translatable to forefoot fractures.

The classifications of crutch walking also include two-point, three-point, and four-point gait. Intuitively, with each addition of a weight bearing point, the stability of the pattern increases but the efficiency decreases.

In two-point gait, the crutches and injured extremity encompass one point and move as a unit, while the uninjured extremity is a separate point (**Figure 11.2**). A three-point gait is differentiated by the separate action of the injured extremity. In this instance, the crutches would move forward, the injured limb would then be placed forward with the crutch points, and lastly, the uninjured limb would be advanced as the third point. This pattern may be used in the event of a partial weight bearing injured extremity that can provide some support. Four-point gait, the most supportive but least efficient crutch gait pattern, is not frequently seen. This pattern involves separate forward motion of each crutch and each extremity. It is possible to use this pattern for bilateral lower extremity weight bearing restrictions but is physically challenging.[14] Alternatively, a four-point gait may be prescribed with the use of a walker, which is much more easily tolerated by the elderly population.

ELDERLY GAIT

The gait of elderly individuals deviates from that of younger age groups in specific ways. They walk with a shorter step length and spend longer time in phases of double support, resulting in slower walking speed.[15-18] These changes may be in response to reduced range of motion at the ankle, increased anterior pelvic tilt, and hip flexion contractures present in older age.[17]

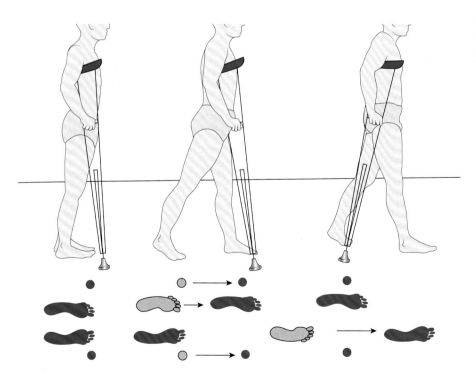

FIGURE 11.2 Diagrammatic representation of two-point gait and step-to pattern with an injured left leg.

Slower walking speed prevents elderly patients from transferring translational momentum into the next step; therefore, they require 50% more oxygen consumption at comfortable walking speeds as compared to 20- to 30-year-old healthy volunteers.[19] Despite this discrepancy, elderly persons are encouraged to remain active, and the orthopaedic surgeon should certainly strive to restore these patients as close to preinjury function as possible. A sedentary lifestyle (fewer than 5000 steps/d) and slower gait speed have been associated with significant balance deficiencies and lower quality of life.[20]

GAIT DISTURBANCE IN LOWER EXTREMITY TRAUMA

Pain-free ambulation may be something taken for granted but becomes a very critical goal following lower extremity fractures. Gait speed has been established as a correlate for disability, and the Lower Extremity Assessment Project (LEAP) Study Group[34] reported an association between self-selected walking speed and quality of life.[21-23] These findings underscore the importance of restoring the determinants of gait in patients who sustain injuries of the lower extremities. Archer et al recommended functional goals to include a reciprocal stair-climbing pattern, unilateral stance of the involved and uninvolved lower extremities for greater than 30 seconds, tandem standing balance for greater than 10 seconds, and the ability to perform more than 10 toe raises on the involved and uninvolved limbs.[22]

Lower extremity fractures can cause abnormal gait patterns for multiple reasons; pain, weakness, and restricted range of motion may all impact gait in different ways. Additionally, when assessing the gait patterns of a patient, it is important to remember that conditions independent of lower extremity fracture may be responsible for an observed gait disturbance. Gait patterns resulting from neurologic or neuromuscular conditions, rotational deformities, and amputations may impact the gait of patients with lower extremity fracture but lie beyond the scope of this text.

ABNORMAL GAIT PATTERNS

Observational gait analysis can be as simple as watching a patient walk to an exam room, but it can provide a helpful overview of a patient's functionality. Common gait disturbances after lower extremity fracture are described below.

- Antalgic Gait: The stance phase is shortened on the injured side to avoid painful weight bearing. There is a compensatory increase in the speed of the contralateral swing phase. This is the most common gait pattern seen in a fracture clinic.
- Trendelenburg Gait/Gluteus Medius Lurch: The trunk shifts over the affected side during the stance phase (gluteus medius lurch) and the pelvis sags down on the contralateral side (Trendelenburg gait). The is a compensatory mechanism to decrease the work of the hip abductor muscle group due to either abductor weakness or hip pain. This may be seen after antegrade intramedullary fixation of femur fractures.[25,26]
- Gait Compensations for Leg Length Discrepancy: Lower extremity trauma may leave a patient with a leg length discrepancy from either shortening at a fracture site or nerve injury resulting in foot drop. There are multiple compensatory mechanisms to navigate this problem, which can be categorized as "around," "over," and "through"
  - Circumduction Gait: Patients may abduct and circumduct the longer leg during the swing phase to achieve foot clearance, thus going "around" the problem foot.
  - Steppage Gait: During the swing phase, the hip and knee of the longer, injured side will be excessively flexed to clear the foot from the ground. This gait pattern is an "over" approach.
  - Vaulting Gait: In another "over" approach, a shortened extremity will maintain a plantarflexed ankle position during the stance phase to limit vertical excursion of the center of mass.
  - Toe Drag: In some cases, when the above mechanisms are not used, patients with foot drop will drag the affected foot during the swing phase in a "through" approach.
- Quadriceps Avoidance: As mentioned above, the knee extensors (quadriceps) function to accommodate the body weight in the early stance phase of gait. Either due to weakness or due to unconscious avoidance of this action (pain), patients capitalize on the osseous congruity of the knee joint in full extension or even hyperextension to prevent the knee from giving under the body's weight. The trunk leans forward to compensate for the comparative increase in leg length. This gait pattern is typically associated with patients following an anterior cruciate ligament injury.
- Gluteus Maximus Lurch: The gluteus maximus functions as a hip stabilizer when the center of mass is anterior to the hip joint. Weakness of this muscle leads patients to lean back at heel strike to keep the center of mass over the planted foot.
- No Heel Strike/Quick Heel Rise: Equinus contracture is a frequent complication following lower extremity trauma. Limited ankle dorsiflexion either prevents heel strike or quickens heel rise during the stance phase.

The literature on post-traumatic abnormal gait is limited; Archer et al performed gait analysis on 277 patients of the LEAP study and found the following gait abnormalities (incidence): uneven step length (20%), toe drag (13%), trunk asymmetry (10%), Trendelenburg gait (8%), hip hike (8%), no heel strike (7%), leg circumduction (6%), and knee hyperextension (3%).[25]

GAIT DISTURBANCE IN ANKLE FRACTURES

Following an ankle fracture, some patients will have a lower gait velocity and corresponding decrease in quality of life.[27,38] Elbaz et al reported a decreased maximum knee flexion angle during stance as well as a longer stride duration in patients treated with open reduction and internal fixation as compared to healthy controls.[30] Interestingly, in a similar cohort, there was overall gait symmetry observed; however, there was a difference in the plantar pressure of the affected extremity, suggesting that these patients have adopted a subtle compensatory mechanism.[29] Most notably, Suciu et al reported a significant difference in the gait of patients with ankle fractures before and after a 12-week course of physical therapy.[32] This finding underscores the importance of aggressive rehabilitation following ankle fracture.[37]

GAIT DISTURBANCE IN TIBIAL SHAFT FRACTURES

Tibial shaft fractures may result in gait disturbance from pain, shortening, and rotational malalignment.[31] Gait observation has even been shown to correlate with validated means by which to establish tibial shaft fracture union.[32]. Larsen et al performed gait analysis on 43 patients that sustained a tibial shaft fracture treated with an intramedullary nail and compared them to healthy controls. They found that asymmetric gait was common at the 6-month follow-up but had nearly normalized by 1-year follow-up. There was a corresponding increase in walking speed during this interval as well as nearly complete resolution of rotational asymmetry.[33]

GAIT DISTURBANCE IN TIBIAL PLATEAU FRACTURES

The literature on gait analysis in tibial plateau fractures is sparse. One prospective case-control study reported an 18% slower cadence, a shortened step length bilaterally, and a poorer quality of life in patients with operatively treated tibial plateau fractures compared to healthy controls.[35] Specifically, patients treated with a ring fixator have prevalent asymmetry with shorter step length and shorter time with single-leg support.[36]

THE FUTURE DIRECTIONS OF GAIT ANALYSIS

The field of gait study has advanced in parallel with technological development. Certain developments that make complex gait analysis accessible to any surgeon without the need for a sophisticated lab expedite reliable gait assessment in the clinical setting. These advancements include smartphone applications,[39-41] wireless pressure sensors,[42] and wearable inertial measurement sensors.[43-46] This technology has not supplanted observational gait analysis but may prove to be a useful tool in restoring the injured patient to a normal, function gait pattern. Fracture surgeons must continually strive to restore normal gait mechanics in patients with traumatized lower extremities by whatever means to improve patient function and outcomes.

REFERENCES

1. Winter DA. Biomechanics of normal and pathological gait: implications for understanding human locomotor control. *J Mot Behav.* 1989;21(4):337-355.
2. Lamoreux LW. Kinematic measurements in the study of human walking. *Bull Prosthet Res.* 1971;10(15):3-84.
3. Los Amigos Research and Education Institute, Rancho Los Amigos National Rehabilitation Center, Rancho Los Amigos Hospital Physical Therapy Department. *Observational Gait Analysis.* Downey, CA: Los Amigos Research and Education Institute, Rancho Los Amigos National Rehabilitation Center; 2001.
4. Sadeghi H. Contributions of lower-limb muscle power in gait of people without impairments. *Phys Ther.* 2000;80(12):1188-1196.
5. Sadeghi H, Sadeghi S, Allard P, Labelle H, Duhaime M. Lower limb muscle power relationships in bilateral able-bodied gait. *Am J Phys Med Rehabil.* 2001;80(11):821-830.
6. Craik R, Oatis CA. *Gait Analysis: Theory and Application.* St. Louis, MO: Mosby; 1995.
7. Levangie PK, Norkin CC. *Joint Structure and Function: A Comprehensive Analysis.* Philadelphia, PA: F.A. Davis Company; 2011.
8. Saunders JB, Inman VT, Eberhart HD. The major determinants in normal and pathological gait. *J Bone Joint Surg Am.* 1953;35-A(3):543-558.
9. Kawamura H, Fuchioka S, Inoue S, et al. Restoring normal gait after limb salvage procedures in malignant bone tumours of the knee. *Scand J Rehabil Med.* 1999;31(2):77-81.
10. Deathe B, Miller WC, Speechley M. The status of outcome measurement in amputee rehabilitation in Canada. *Arch Phys Med Rehabil.* 2002;83(7):912-918.
11. McFadyen BJ, Winter DA. An integrated biomechanical analysis of normal stair ascent and descent. *J Biomech.* 1988;21(9):733-744.
12. Waters RL, Campbell J, Perry J. Energy cost of three-point crutch ambulation in fracture patients. *J Orthop Trauma.* 1987;1(2):170-173.
13. Brown HE, Mueller MJ. A "step-to" gait decreases pressures on the forefoot. *J Orthop Sports Phys Ther.* 1998;28(3):139-145.
14. O'Sullivan SB, Schmitz TJ, Fulk G. *Physical Rehabilitation.* Philadelphia, PA: F. A. Davis Company; 2013.
15. Himann JE, Cunningham DA, Rechnitzer PA, Paterson DH. Age-related changes in speed of walking. *Med Sci Sports Exerc.* 1988;20(2):161-166.
16. Kerrigan DC, Todd MK, Della Croce U, Lipsitz LA, Collins JJ. Biomechanical gait alterations independent of speed in the healthy elderly: evidence for specific limiting impairments. *Arch Phys Med Rehabil.* 1998;79(3):317-322.
17. Oberg T, Karsznia A, Oberg K. Basic gait parameters: reference data for normal subjects, 10-79 years of age. *J Rehabil Res Dev.* 1993;30(2):210-223.
18. Winter DA. *The Biomechanics and Motor Control of Human Gait: Normal, Elderly and Pathological.* Waterloo, Ontario, Canada: University of Waterloo Press; 1991.
19. Waters RL, Mulroy S. The energy expenditure of normal and pathologic gait. *Gait Posture.* 1999;9(3):207-231.
20. Dohrn IM, Hagstromer M, Hellenius ML, Stahle A. Gait speed, quality of life, and sedentary time are associated with steps per day in community-dwelling older adults with osteoporosis. *J Aging Phys Act.* 2016;24(1):22-31.
21. Higgins TF, Klatt JB, Beals TC. Lower Extremity Assessment Project (LEAP) – The best available evidence on limb-threatening lower extremity trauma. *Orthop Clin North Am.* 2010;41(2):233-239.
22. Archer KR, Castillo RC, Mackenzie EJ, Bosse MJ. Physical disability after severe lower-extremity injury. *Arch Phys Med Rehabil.* 2006;87(8):1153-1155.
23. O'Toole RV, Castillo RC, Pollak AN, MacKenzie EJ, Bosse MJ. Determinants of patient satisfaction after severe lower-extremity injuries. *J Bone Joint Surg Am.* 2008;90(6):1206-1211.

24. Teixeira-Salmela LF, Nadeau S, McBride I, Olney SJ. Effects of muscle strengthening and physical conditioning training on temporal, kinematic and kinetic variables during gait in chronic stroke survivors. *J Rehabil Med*. 2001;33(2):53-60.

25. Archer KR, Castillo RC, Mackenzie EJ, Bosse MJ. Gait symmetry and walking speed analysis following lower-extremity trauma. *Phys Ther*. 2006;86(12):1630-1640.

26. Archdeacon M, Ford KR, Wyrick J, et al. A prospective functional outcome and motion analysis evaluation of the hip abductors after femur fracture and antegrade nailing. *J Orthop Trauma*. 2008;22(1):3-9.

27. Bain GI, Zacest AC, Paterson DC, Middleton J, Pohl AP. Abduction strength following intramedullary nailing of the femur. *J Orthop Trauma*. 1997;11(2):93-97.

28. Romkes J, Schweizer K. Immediate effects of unilateral restricted ankle motion on gait kinematics in healthy subjects. *Gait Posture*. 2015;41(3):835-840.

29. Segal G, Elbaz A, Parsi A, et al. Clinical outcomes following ankle fracture: a cross-sectional observational study. *J Foot Ankle Res*. 2014;7(1):50.

30. Elbaz A, Mor A, Segal G, et al. Lower extremity kinematic profile of gait of patients after ankle fracture: a case-control study. *J Foot Ankle Surg*. 2016;55(5):918-921.

31. Becker HP, Rosenbaum D, Kriese T, Gerngross H, Claes L. Gait asymmetry following successful surgical treatment of ankle fractures in young adults. *Clin Orthop Relat Res*. 1995;311:262-269.

32. Suciu O, Onofrei RR, Totorean AD, Suciu SC, Amaricai EC. Gait analysis and functional outcomes after twelve-week rehabilitation in patients with surgically treated ankle fractures. *Gait Posture*. 2016;49: 184-189.

33. Castillo RC, MacKenzie EJ, Archer KR, Bosse MJ, Webb LX. Evidence of beneficial effect of physical therapy after lower-extremity trauma. *Arch Phys Med Rehabil*. 2008;89(10):1873-1879.

34. Say F, Bulbul M. Findings related to rotational malalignment in tibial fractures treated with reamed intramedullary nailing. *Arch Orthop Trauma Surg*. 2014;134(10):1381-1386.

35. Macri F, Marques LF, Backer RC, Santos MJ, Belangero WD. Validation of a standardised gait score to predict the healing of tibial fractures. *J Bone Joint Surg Br*. 2012;94(4):544-548.

36. Larsen P, Laessoe U, Rasmussen S, Graven-Nielsen T, Berre Eriksen C, Elsoe R. Asymmetry in gait pattern following tibial shaft fractures – A prospective one-year follow-up study of 49 patients. *Gait Posture*. 2017;51:47-51.

37. Warschawski Y, Elbaz A, Segal G, et al. Gait characteristics and quality of life perception of patients following tibial plateau fracture. *Arch Orthop Trauma Surg*. 2015;135(11):1541-1546.

38. Elsoe R, Larsen P. Asymmetry in gait pattern following bicondylar tibial plateau fractures – A prospective one-year cohort study. *Injury*. 2017;48(7):1657-1661.

39. Furrer M, Bichsel L, Niederer M, Baur H, Schmid S. Validation of a smartphone-based measurement tool for the quantification of level walking. *Gait Posture*. 2015;42(3):289-294.

40. Nishiguchi S, Yamada M, Nagai K, et al. Reliability and validity of gait analysis by android-based smartphone. *Telemed J E Health*. 2012;18(4):292-296.

41. Yamada M, Aoyama T, Mori S, et al. Objective assessment of abnormal gait in patients with rheumatoid arthritis using a smartphone. *Rheumatol Int*. 2012;32(12):3869-3874.

42. Bamberg SJM, Benbasat AY, Scarborough DM, Krebs DE, Paradiso JA. Gait analysis using a shoe-integrated wireless sensor system. *IEEE Trans Inf Technol Biomed*. 2008;12(4):413-423.

43. Mancini M, Horak FB. Potential of APDM mobility lab for the monitoring of the progression of Parkinson's disease. *Expert Rev Med Devices*. 2016;13(5):455-462.

44. Rebula JR, Ojeda LV, Adamczyk PG, Kuo AD. Measurement of foot placement and its variability with inertial sensors. *Gait Posture*. 2013;38(4):974-980.

45. Salarian A, Russmann H, Vingerhoets FJ, et al. Gait assessment in Parkinson's disease: toward an ambulatory system for long-term monitoring. *IEEE Trans Biomedical Eng*. 2004;51(8):1434-1443.

46. Washabaugh EP, Kalyanaraman T, Adamczyk PG, Claflin ES, Krishnan C. Validity and repeatability of inertial measurement units for measuring gait parameters. *Gait Posture*. 2017;55:87-93.

47. Braddom RL. *Physical Medicine and Rehabilitation E-Book*. Philadelphia, PA: Elsevier Health Sciences; 2010.

48. Brotzman SB, Manske RC. *Clinical Orthopaedic Rehabilitation E-Book: An Evidence-Based Approach - Expert Consult*. Philadelphia, PA: Elsevier Health Sciences; 2011.

49. Inman VT, Ralston HJ, Todd F, Lieberman JC. *Human walking*. Philadelphia, PA: Williams & Wilkins; 1981.

50. Lafortune MA, Cavanagh PR, Sommer HJ III, Kalenak A. Three-dimensional kinematics of the human knee during walking. *J Biomech*. 1992;25(4):347-357.

51. Mehta AJ, Nastasi AE. Rehabilitation of fractures in the elderly. *Clin Geriatr Med*. 1993;9(4):717-730.

52. Murray MP. Gait as a total pattern of movement: including a bibliography on gait. *Am J Phys Med Rehabil*. 1967;46(1):290-333.

53. Murray MP, Drought AB, Kory RC. Walking patterns of normal men. *J Bone Joint Surg Am*. 1964;46:335-360.

54. Perry J, Burnfield JM. *Gait Analysis: Normal and Pathological Function*. Thorofare, NJ: SLACK; 2010.

55. Rose J, Gamble JG. *Human Walking*. Philadelphia, PA: Lippincott Williams & Wilkins; 2006.

56. Sutherland DH. The evolution of clinical gait analysis part l: kinesiological EMG. *Gait Posture*. 2001;14(1):61-70.

57. Sutherland DH. The evolution of clinical gait analysis. Part II kinematics. *Gait Posture*. 2002;16(2):159-179.

Fractures of the Shoulder Girdle

Sandra A. Miskiel
Edward Perez
Kenneth W. Graf
Rakesh P. Mashru

INTRODUCTION

The foundation of shoulder rehabilitation interventions centers around a comprehensive understanding of the anatomy, three-dimensional joint biomechanics, and multiple functional demands of the upper extremity at the shoulder girdle.

The shoulder girdle is composed of three osseous structures (clavicle, proximal humerus, and scapula) and three joints (glenohumeral, acromioclavicular, and sternoclavicular). The scapula and the clavicle provide support and articulation for the humerus, in addition to anchoring a variety of muscles, which help to rotate and move the humerus.[1,2] Shoulder function is dependent upon the recruitment patterns of the following muscles attaching to the scapula and arm: thoracohumeral (latissimus dorsi and pectoralis major), axioscapular (serratus anterior, levator scapulae, pectoralis minor, rhomboids, and trapezius), and scapulohumeral (deltoid, supraspinatus, infraspinatus, subscapularis, teres minor, and teres major) muscles.[2,3] Shoulder girdle motion is based on the interaction among the sternoclavicular (SC), acromioclavicular (AC), and glenohumeral (GH) joints, as well as the scapulothoracic (ST) articulation.[2-4] The largest amount of normal shoulder girdle motion occurs at the GH joint and the ST articulation, with AC and SC joint motions being component motions of the resulting ST motion.[1,2]

The coordinated, sequential activation of the muscles coupled with joint stability allows the shoulder to execute the functional task demands of the upper extremity. As Thomas Reid wrote in his *Essays on the Intellectual Powers of Man* in 1786, "a chain is no stronger than its weakest link." This idiom may be applied to the treatment and rehabilitation of the shoulder, as when there is a fracture or an injury to any one component of the shoulder girdle, it will impede the ability of the entire upper extremity to carry out the functional demands required.

This chapter will focus on the treatment and rehabilitation of fractures and joint injuries of the shoulder girdle.

PROXIMAL HUMERUS FRACTURES

INTRODUCTION

Approximately 5% of all fractures of the appendicular skeleton occur at, or proximal to, the surgical neck of the humerus. It is the most common fracture of the shoulder girdle in adults.[5] Fracture incidence increases with age, with over 70% of proximal humerus fractures occurring in patients above the age of 60, with 90% of these resulting from a fall from standing height.[2,6-9] The majority of proximal humerus fractures in this demographic are minimally displaced and may be treated nonoperatively with optimal patient-reported outcomes.[1,7,10,11] Younger patients most commonly sustain proximal humerus fractures secondary to high-energy traumas, such as a fall from height, motor vehicle collisions, electric shock, or seizures.[5,6] These injuries tend to involve more significant bony and soft-tissue disruption, thus frequently requiring surgical intervention.[6]

There are three primary loading modes resulting in fractures of the proximal humerus: (1) compressive loading of the glenoid into the head of the humerus, (2) bending forces at the surgical neck, and (3) tension forces from the rotator cuff at the greater and lesser tuberosities. The biomechanics of the fracture and patient's bone quality dictate the various fracture patterns encountered.[2]

TREATMENT

When deciding between nonoperative and operative management for proximal humerus fractures, the surgeon must take into account patient age, fracture type and displacement, bone quality, general medical condition, and functional status of the patient. In addition, any concomitant injuries may influence treatment as well.[6,12,13] With respect to surgical treatment, there is still significant debate as to which method is best for varying fracture types.[13]

Nonoperative

Nonoperative treatment is the standard of treatment for nondisplaced, and minimally displaced proximal humeral fractures.[2,14] Satisfactory patient-reported outcomes along with high union rates have been widely reported in the literature.[11,15-18] Additionally, nonoperative management is indicated in elderly patients with low functional demand and medically debilitated patients who are precluded from surgical treatment. Successful nonoperative management of two-part surgical neck fractures with greater than 50% displacement and four-part valgus fractures has also been reported.[10] Relative contraindications to nonoperative treatment are displaced fractures with a loss of bony contact.[12]

During the first phase of nonoperative treatment and rehabilitation, weeks 1 to 3 post injury, the patient is to wear a sling and swathe or fixed shoulder immobilizer at all times, except during self-care and therapeutic exercises.[19] With the pectoralis major tendon's pull on the proximal shaft segment, placement of a pad in the axilla may be recommended to assist with maintaining proper alignment of the fracture. The patient is instructed to perform active range-of-motion (AROM) exercises of the cervical spine, elbow, wrist, and hand and Codman or "Rock the Baby" exercises within tolerable limits.[20] During Codman exercises, also frequently referred to as pendulum exercises, the patient is instructed to bend at the waist, so as to be parallel to the ground, with the injured arm hanging perpendicular to the floor and the uninjured arm holding a surface. Keeping the arm and shoulder muscles relaxed, the patient moves his or her arm slowly in front-to-back, side-to-side, and circular motions clockwise and counterclockwise (**Figure 12.1A and B**).[20,21] Patients must be instructed on the correct way to perform Codman exercises, as incorrect large pendulums have been shown to elicit more than 15% maximum voluntary isometric contraction of the supraspinatus and infraspinatus muscles.[20] An alternative, safer therapeutic exercise to Codman exercises is the "Rock the Baby" exercise. Patients use the contralateral limb to support the injured arm at the elbow and slowly move the arm front-to-back, side-to-side, and in circular motions clockwise and counterclockwise (**Figure 12.2A and B**).

During Phase II, weeks 4 to 6 post injury, AROM may be initiated while simultaneously improving neuromuscular control and proprioception via proprioceptive neuromuscular facilitation (PNF) (**Table 12.1**; **Figure 12.3A-E**).[22,23]

Weeks 7 to 9 are focused on strengthening and a return to normal function. According to radiographic and clinical healing, overhead and advanced resistance exercises, such as multilevel rows, may be initiated at week 10 (**Figure 12.4A-F**). The therapist should push the patient's end ROM, in addition to optimizing GH joint mobilization via anterior, inferior, and posterior glide maneuvers.[1]

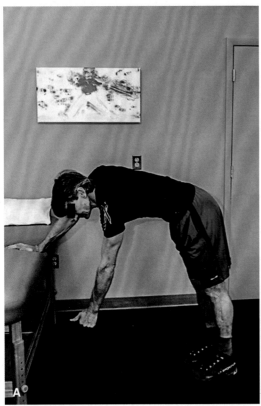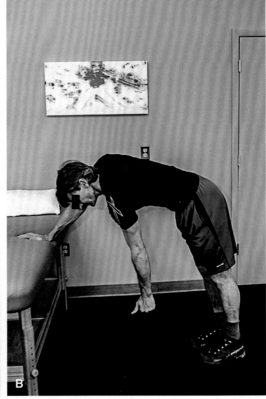

FIGURE 12.1 A and **B**, Codman exercise.

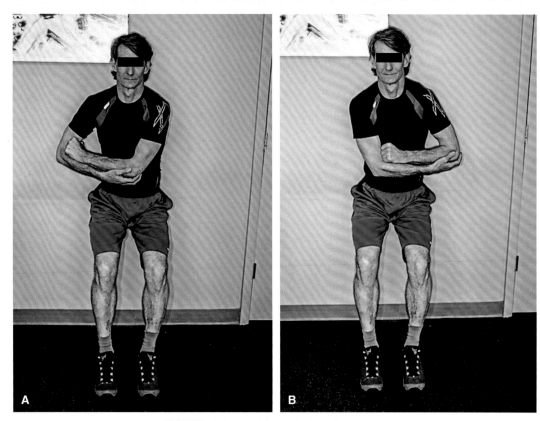

FIGURE 12.2 A and **B**, Rock the Baby exercise.

Operative

Indications for operative management of fractures of the proximal humerus include open fractures, fractures with significant neurovascular compromise, and young, high-demand patients with significant displacement.[2,12,15] In the approximately 20% to 50% of proximal humerus fractures which present significantly displaced or unstable, surgical intervention is the preferred method of treatment. Locked plate fixation and arthroplasty are the two most common methods of treatment. Locked intramedullary nailing may be used for treatment of two-part surgical neck fractures with extension into the humeral diaphysis or marked comminution and pathologic fractures.[13,14] When choosing a treatment method for the patient's fracture, bone quality and potential deforming forces must be taken into consideration. Arthroplasty is the preferred method of treatment for fracture dislocations and four-part fractures (excluding valgus-impacted) due to the high risk of humeral head necrosis.[2,16,18]

REHABILITATION[23]

Rehabilitation of the proximal humerus should be centered around the core principles of reduction of pain and inflammation, protection of healing fracture, and re-establishment of shoulder function. The ability to reduce fracture fragments and generate the necessary stabilization for early motion provides the foundation for successful rehabilitation.[15,19]

Rehabilitation protocols for operatively and nonoperatively managed fractures of the proximal humerus focus around these aforementioned principles. Nonoperative and operatively managed fractures are rehabilitated in a similar manner, with the primary difference found in phase advancement time points (**Tables 12.2** and **12.3**). The patient should be counseled on the importance of adherence to his/her rehabilitation plan, as ROM will continue to improve for up to 1 year postoperatively.[19] Assuming stable fixation, the following protocol for rehabilitation can be tailored to the individual patient's requirements.

Locking Plate Protocol[23]

Goals of rehabilitation in the initial postoperative period include pain control, protection of the fracture, and prevention of shoulder capsular contracture. An arm sling is provided postoperatively to provide comfort and protect the injured arm. Rehabilitation is performed at home during this phase. Early mobilization is encouraged as it has been reported that patients who initiate therapy earlier achieve greater functional gains and less pain than those immobilized for a longer period of time.[15] In a randomized, prospective controlled trial of minimally displaced two-part proximal humeral fractures, patients who were instructed to initiate immediate physiotherapy, versus those instructed to remain immobilized for a period of 3 weeks, mobilized earlier, had less residual pain, and had greater functional mobility of the affected limb at 16 weeks follow-up.[6]

TABLE 12.1 Joint Movements of Proprioceptive Neuromuscular Facilitation of the Upper Extremity

D1 Flexion: Flexion/Abduction/External Rotation-Straight Arm

Joint	Starting Position	Ending Position
Scapula	Posterior depression	Anterior elevation
Shoulder	Extension/abduction/IR	Flexion/adduction/ER
Forearm	Extension	Extension
Elbow	Pronation	Supination
Wrist	Extension/ulnar deviation	Flexion/radial deviation
Digits	Extension	Flexion

D1 Extension: Extension/Adduction/Internal Rotation-Straight Arm

Joint	Starting Position	Ending Position
Scapula	Anterior elevation	Posterior depression
Shoulder	Flexion/adduction/ER	Extension/abduction/IR
Forearm	Extension	Extension
Elbow	Supination	Pronation
Wrist	Flexion/radial deviation	Extension/ulnar deviation
Digits	Flexion	Extension

D2 Flexion: Flexion/Abduction/External Rotation-Straight Arm

Joint	Starting Position	Ending Position
Scapula	Anterior depression	Posterior elevation
Shoulder	Extension/adduction/IR	Flexion/abduction/ER
Forearm	Extension	Extension
Elbow	Supination	Pronation
Wrist	Flexion/ulnar deviation	Extension/radial deviation
Digits	Flexion	Extension

D2 Extension: Extension/Adduction/Internal Rotation-Straight Arm

Joint	Starting Position	Ending Position
Scapula	Posterior elevation	Anterior depression
Shoulder	Flexion/abduction/ER	Extension/adduction/IR
Forearm	Extension	Extension
Elbow	Pronation	Supination
Wrist	Extension/radial deviation	Flexion/ulnar deviation
Digits	Extension	Flexion

ER, external rotation; IR, nternal rotation.

Patients are encouraged to perform the following passive and active ROM (PROM and AROM) exercises of the cervical spine, elbow, wrist, and hand from postoperative day 1 to postoperative week 4: supine passive forward flexion, internal and external rotation to the chest/abdomen, and Codman exercises.[20] At week 4, the patient may begin therapy at an outpatient rehabilitation clinic, twice a week beginning active-assisted range-of-motion (AAROM) exercises.[17] During active-assisted motion, a patient is actively using his shoulder muscles to perform the exercise, but requires assistance completing the motion from the therapist, equipment, or his contralateral arm (**Figures 12.5** and **12.6A, B**). During weeks 6 to 8, the patient continues twice-weekly visits with his physical therapist with the primary aim to continue progression of his ROM and prevention of muscle atrophy. The therapist may incorporate therapeutic exercises utilizing an overhead pulley.[1] Strengthening via isometric deltoid and rotator cuff exercises are commenced at week 8. At week 10, the patient may progress to an at-home strengthening program, continuing deltoid and rotator cuff

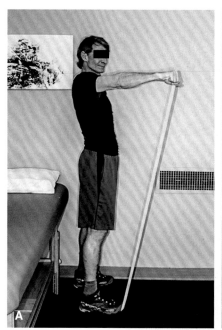
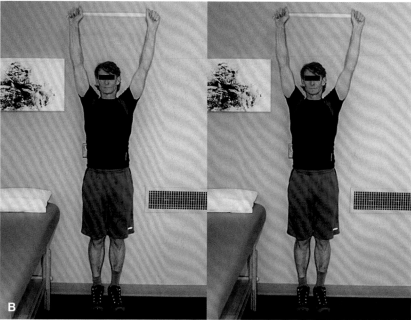
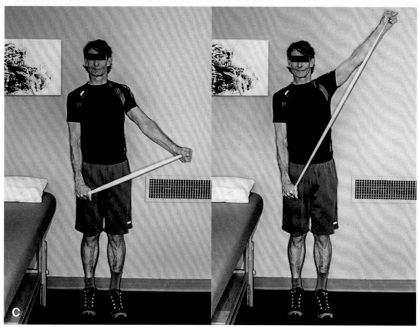

FIGURE 12.3 Proprioceptive neuromuscular facilitation: flexion (**A**), extension (**B**), abduction (**C**), internal rotation (**D**), and external rotation (**E**).

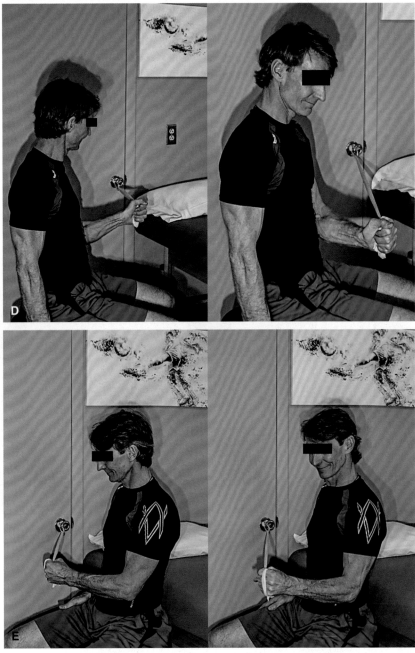

FIGURE 12.3 Cont'd

strengthening exercises. At 6 months postoperatively, over-head heavy lifting and manual labor may be slowly reini-tiated, should the patient have reached optimal goals with ROM and strengthening exercises.

Arthroplasty[23]

The rehabilitation of patients surgically managed with arthroplasty is similar to that of plate fixation, using the same therapeutic exercises; however, an important difference is that safe ranges are narrower and phase transitions slower. Postoperatively, the injured arm is placed into a sling, with the patient instructed to continue sling and swathe usage for 2 to 4 weeks postoperative when at home and for up to 6 to 8 weeks in public settings.[12]

The amount of initial motion performed postoperatively is individual to the patient and additionally dependent on safe ROM attained in the operating room. Typically, safe ranges include 130° of flexion and 30° of external rota-tion.[1,24] Should there be a concern for the quality of fixation, safe ranges are 90° of flexion and 0° of external rotation.[24] These suggestions may be adjusted accordingly, dependent upon tuberosity fixation stability obtained in the operating

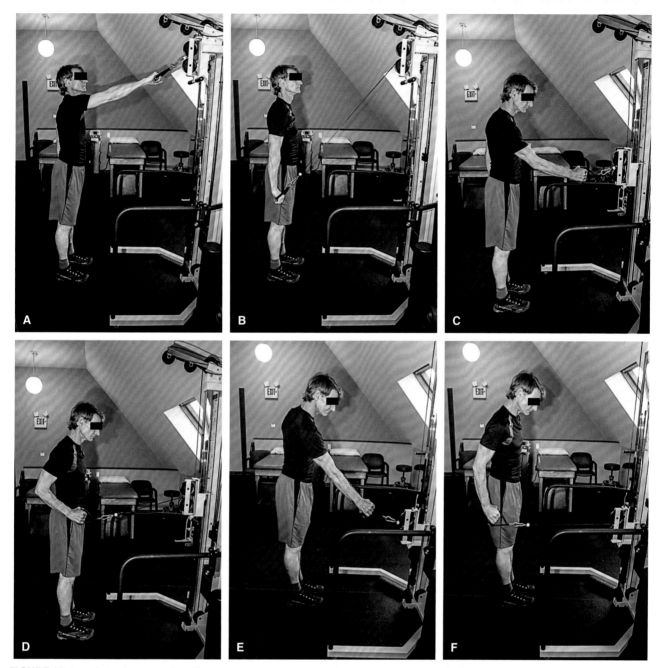

FIGURE 12.4 Multilevel rows with pulley. Patient initiates exercise by stretching out arm of affected limb while maintaining the pulley handle (**A**, **C**, **E**). Patient is then instructed to pull the arm back, simultaneously retracting and depressing the scapula (**B**, **D**, **F**).

room.[17,25] ROM guidelines are to be tailored to each patient individually, taking into account whether the patient has achieved optimal function at each time point. Should there be a loss of ROM, patient should regain degrees of motion and advance accordingly.

At 4 to 6 weeks postoperatively, PROM may be advanced to include forward flexion and external rotation; at 6 to 8 weeks, patient may initiate AAROM with an overhead pulley and passive stretching. Full AROM is initiated at 10 to 12 weeks postoperatively, with strengthening exercises initiated at 12 to 14 weeks postoperatively.[1,12]

CLAVICLE

INTRODUCTION

The clavicle is an S-shaped bone, prismatic in shape medially and progressively flattening laterally. It is anchored to the scapula via the AC and coracoclavicular (CC) ligaments and to the trunk via the SC ligaments.[3,23,26] Fractures of the clavicle constitute approximately 2.6% to 4.0% of all fractures in adults.[27] The most frequent demographic in which these fractures occur are young males. The mechanism of

TABLE 12.2 Author's Preferred Rehabilitation Protocol for Nonoperative Management of Proximal Humerus Fractures

Weeks Post Injury	Goals	Motion	Strengthening
• 1-3	• Pain control • Inflammation control • Protection of fracture • Prevention of shoulder capsular contracture • Early mobility	• AROM, AAROM, and PROM of cervical spine, elbow, wrist, and hand • Codman or "Rock the Baby" exercise • Supine passive forward flexion • ER and IR to chest/abdomen • Scapular retractions • Repeat above motions 7 d/wk, four times per day	• No initiation of strengthening
• 4-6	• Same as above • Initiate AROM	• Continue above therapeutic exercises • Supine AAROM: forward flexion and ER • Submaximal isometric deltoid and rotator cuff exercises • Scapular PNF techniques • Repeat above motions 7 d/wk, two times per day	• Postural correction • Grip strengthening

• 7-9	• Strength and function
	• Restore full AROM
		• Continue above therapeutic exercises
		• Pulleys with eccentric lowering of injured limb
		• Progress shoulder AROM in all planes, supine first then standing, with subsequent incorporation of weights
		  • Flexion, extension, abduction, IR, and ER
		• Repeat above motions 7 d/wk, two times per day
			• Same as above
			• Rotator cuff and periscapular strengthening
			• Resistance band exercises:
			  • initially isotonic exercises and incorporate weights at week 8

• 10+	• Return to normal function
	• Continue strengthening of:
	  • rotator cuff/deltoid
	  • scapular rotators
	• Optimize scapulohumeral rhythm
		• Advanced progressive resistance exercises
		• Progress to overhead exercises
		• Overhead/throwing athletes: plyometrics program
		• Glenohumeral joint mobilization
		• Repeat above motions 7 d/wk, two times per day
			• Same as above
			• Isometric deltoid/rotator cuff strengthening
			• Periscapular strengthening
			• Resistance band/pulley exercises:
			  • ER, IR
			  • Multilevel rows
			• Dynamic:
			  • Side lying ER
			  • Prone row
			  • Prone extension
			  • "Ys": horizontal abduction with external rotation
			  • "Ts": prone horizontal extension with the arm at 100° of shoulder abduction
			  • "Ws": prone scapular retraction with downward rotation
			  • Standing scaption
			  • Isotonic biceps curl
			  • Serratus punch

AAROM, active-assisted range of motion; AROM, active range of motion; ER, external rotation, IR, internal rotation; PNF, proprioceptive neuromuscular facilitation; PROM, passive range of motion.

TABLE 12.3 Author's Preferred Rehabilitation Protocol for Operative Management of Fractures of the Proximal Humerus

Postoperative Weeks	Goals	Motion	Strengthening
• Weeks 1-4 • Weeks 1-6	• Pain control • Inflammation control • Protection of fracture • Prevention of shoulder capsular contracture	• AROM, AAROM, and PROM of cervical spine, elbow, wrist, and hand • Codman or "Rock the Baby" exercise • Supine passive forward flexion • ER and IR to chest/abdomen • Repeat above motions 7 d/wk, four times per day	• No initiation of strengthening
• Weeks 4-6 • Weeks 6-8	• Same as above • Minimize deconditioning • Maintain muscle flexibility and neuromuscular pattern • Normalize scapulohumeral kinematics	• Same as above • AAROM, PROM of shoulder in all planes • Initiate scapular retraction • Repeat above motions 7 d/wk, two times per day	• Postural correction • Grip strengthening
• Weeks 6-8 • Weeks 8-10	• Same as above • Prevent muscle atrophy • Regain ROM	• Same as above • Initiate use of overhead pulley • Repeat above motions 7 d/wk, two times per day	• Same as above
• Weeks 8-10 • Weeks 10-12	• Same as above • Initiate strengthening	• Same as above • AROM of shoulder in all planes • Posterior scapular stretching program • Repeat above motions 7 d/wk, two times per day	• Same as above • Initiate isometric deltoid/rotator cuff strengthening • Periscapular strengthening

• Weeks 10-12
• Weeks 12-14
	• Same as above
	• Continue strengthening of:
	  • rotator cuff/deltoid
	  • scapular rotators
	• Optimize scapulohumeral rhythm
		• Same as above
		• AROM/AAROM/PROM of shoulder in all planes
		• Repeat above motions 7 d/wk, two times per day
			• Same as above
			• Resistance band/pulley exercises:
			  • ER, IR
			  • Multilevel rows
			• Dynamic:
			  • Side lying ER
			  • Prone row
			  • Prone extension
			  • "Ys": horizontal abduction with external rotation
			  • "Ts": prone horizontal extension with the arm at 100° of shoulder abduction
			  • "Ws": prone scapular retraction with downward rotation
			  • Standing scaption
			  • Isotonic biceps curl
			  • Serratus punch

AAROM, active-assisted range of motion; AROM, active range of motion; ER, external rotation, IR, internal rotation; PROM, passive range of motion; ROM, range of motion.

injury in clavicular fractures is a direct, compressive force applied to the shoulder, commonly seen in patients presenting after a significant fall or motor vehicle collision.[26,28] Clavicular fractures are also commonly seen in athletes participating in contact sports. The majority of fractures occur at the midshaft of the clavicle (69%-82%), followed by the distal third (12%-26%), and finally the proximal third (2%-6%).[28] The increased incidence of shaft fractures is in part due to the proximal and distal aspects of the clavicle being strongly secured by ligaments and musculature, rendering it less vulnerable to trauma; in midshaft fractures displacement and shortening occurs due to the combined forces of

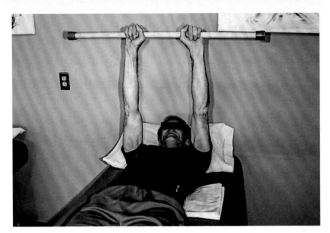

FIGURE 12.5 Supine active-assisted forward flexion. Utilizing the contralateral limb, the patient is instructed to elevate the affected limb with cane assistance.

the sternocleidomastoid muscle pulling the medial fragment superiorly and posteriorly and the pectoralis major muscle, deltoid muscle, and gravity pulling the lateral fragment inferiorly and anteriorly.[3,28,29]

TREATMENT

Treatment goals for clavicular fracture include restoration of pain-free shoulder ROM and fracture healing with acceptable deformity. The surgeon must take into account displacement, comminution, associated injuries, and patient factors when deciding an optimal treatment plan.

Nonoperative

Indications for nonoperative treatment include nondisplaced or minimally displaced midshaft, proximal, and distal fractures.[30] Typically, proximal third fractures present nondisplaced or minimally displaced and on rare occasion involve the SC joint. Treatment of midshaft fractures is a topic of much debate as optimal functional outcomes have been cited in the literature supporting both operative

and nonoperative treatments. Conservative management of fractures with greater than 1.5 to 2 cm of shortening, or greater than 100% displacement, has been shown to lead to decreased shoulder function and worse clinical outcomes. Thus, surgical intervention has been recommended for these fracture types.

For nonoperatively managed fractures, the involved arm is immediately placed into a sling and swathe and early PROM is encouraged.[28] Period of immobilization ranges from 2 to 6 weeks, dependent upon patient's comfort, with gradual progression from PROM to full AROM. Contact sports are generally prohibited for a minimum of 4 months.[28] The author's preferred rehabilitation protocol for clavicular fractures is discussed further in this chapter.

Operative

Generally, fracture-specific indications supporting operative treatment are open fractures, fractures associated with skin compromise and/or neurovascular injury, displacement or shortening >2 cm, segmental fractures (combined midshaft and proximal fracture or midshaft with distal fracture), increasing comminution (greater than three fragments), and scapular malposition. Patient motivation for rapid return to full function, especially in elite athletes, is an additional surgical indication.[28]

Open reduction and internal plate fixation is the most commonly used operative method of fixation, with a smaller number of fractures treated with intramedullary nails, pins, or wires.[26,28,31]

REHABILITATION[23]

Rehabilitation protocols for operatively and nonoperatively managed clavicle fractures utilize the same therapeutic exercises, with phase transitioning being patient-dependent (**Table 12.4**). The patient should show signs of radiographic and clinical healing, achieve phase goals, and stay within comfort limits in order to progress through the protocol phases.[3]

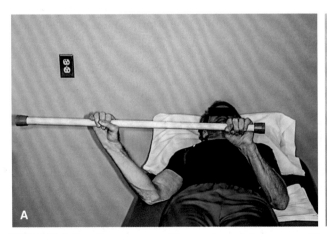
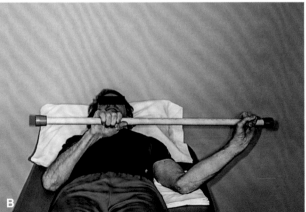

FIGURE 12.6 A and **B**, Supine active-assisted external rotation: utilizing the contralateral limb, the patient is instructed to externally rotate the affected limb with cane assistance.

TABLE 12.4 Author's Preferred Rehabilitation Protocol for Operative and Nonoperative Management of Clavicular Fractures

Postoperative Weeks	Goals	ROM/Therapeutic Exercises	Strengthening
• **Weeks 0-6**	• Pain and inflammation control • Protect healing fracture • Prevention of shoulder capsular contracture	• AROM, AAROM, and PROM of cervical spine, elbow, wrist, and hand • Codman or "Rock the Baby" exercise • Supine passive forward flexion: (limit to 90°, weeks 1-3; limit to 120°, weeks 4-6) • Supine ER • ER and IR to chest/abdomen • Scapular retractions • Repeat above motions four times per day, 7 d a week	• No initiation of strengthening

• **Weeks 7-12**	• Protect healing fracture
	• Improve ROM
	• Initiate strengthening
		• Supine cane-assisted forward flexion
		• Forward flexion in scapular plane
		• Supine and standing ER
		• Shoulder flexion and abduction, as tolerated
		  • Full flexion and abduction by week 12
		• Horizontal adduction, as tolerated
		• Scapular PNF techniques
		• Scapulohumeral rhythm exercises
		• ER at 90° abduction
		• Side lying IR at 90°
		• Standing scaption
		• Repeat above motions two times per day, 7 d a week
			• Postural correction
			• Grip strengthening
			• Resistance band exercises:
			  • IR and ER
			  • Row
			• Dynamic:
			  • Side lying ER
			  • Prone row
			  • Prone extension
			  • "Ys": horizontal abduction with external rotation
			  • "Ts": prone horizontal extension with the arm at 100° of shoulder abduction
			  • "Ws": prone scapular retraction with downward rotation
			  • Standing scaption
			  • Isotonic biceps curl
			  • Serratus punch
			• Push-ups into wall at week 8
			• Weight training at week 12

• **Weeks 13-18**	• Protect healing fracture
	• Regain full ROM
	• Continue strengthening
		• Continue as above with progression to full ROM
		• Horizontal adduction stretch
		• ER at 90° abduction stretch
		• IR—full behind back
		• Repeat above motions two times per day, 7 d a week
			• Improve scapular muscle strength
			• Resistance band exercises:
			  • Continue as above
			  • Standing "Ts"
			  • ER and IR at 90°
			  • Multilevel rows
			• Dynamic:
			  • Continue as above with increasing resistance, as tolerated
			  • Standing forward flexion
			• Add progressive resistance up to 5 lbs
			• Rhythmic stabilization and proprioceptive training drills with a physical therapist
			• Continue push-up progression
			• Progressive return to sports and recreational activities at week 18
			  • Overhead/throwing athletes: initiate plyometric program
			• Repeat above exercises 1 time per day, 7 d a week

AAROM, active-assisted range of motion; AROM, active range of motion; ER, external rotation, IR, internal rotation; PNF, proprioceptive neuromuscular facilitation; PROM, passive range of motion; ROM, range of motion.

Patients are placed into a sling and swathe for comfort for the first 2 weeks.[3] Ice and anti-inflammatories are utilized to control pain and inflammation. Cervical ROM, basic deep neck flexor activation, and active elbow, hand, and wrist ROM are started on postoperative day 1. After 6 weeks, if clinical and radiographic examinations demonstrate signs of healing, the patient may begin strengthening exercises of the involved limb. Preferred therapeutic exercises for strengthening include:[22]

- Side lying external rotation (ER) (**Figure 12.7A and B**)
- Prone row (**Figure 12.8A and B**)
- Prone shoulder extension (**Figure 12.9A and B**)
- Serratus punch (**Figure 12.10A and B**)
- "Ys"—horizontal abduction with external rotation (**Figure 12.11A and B**)
- "Ts"—prone horizontal extension with the arm at 100° of shoulder abduction (**Figure 12.12A and B**)
- "Ws"—prone scapular retraction with downward rotation (**Figure 12.13**)

Weights may be gradually introduced while performing the above exercises, starting with 1-lb weights and gradually progressing to 5-lb weights. The patient during this phase should be working to achieve full ROM, while simultaneously improving neuromuscular control and proprioception via PNFs.[23] At week 12, the patient may progressively initiate a weight-training program including seated row and machine resistance exercises. Seated bench presses may be incorporated at week 14.[22] Return to sports typically occurs between 4 and 6 months.[3,28]

SCAPULA

INTRODUCTION

Fractures of the scapula are a rare fracture type, accounting for less than 1% of all fractures and only 3% to 5% of fractures at the shoulder girdle.[32,33] The most common fracture location is at the scapular body, accounting for approximately 50% of fractures, followed by the glenoid (29%),

processes (11%), and neck (8%-10%). Scapular fractures are most commonly a result of high-energy trauma, usually occurring in polytrauma patients.[4,18,32,34,35] Scapular fractures occur predominantly in males (72%), with a mean reported age of 44 years. Most often the fracture is caused by a direct blow to the scapula, such as during a motor vehicle collision[35,36] or a fall from height.[32,37,38] Bilateral or open fractures rarely occur.[37,38] Rib fractures are the most common fracture type occurring in concomitance with scapular fractures, with incidence rates reported as high as 65%.[18,32] Additional injuries to the shoulder girdle occur in 8% to 47% of cases of scapula fractures.[2] Due to the high-energy mechanism of injury, between 80% and 95% of scapular fractures occur with additional traumatic injuries, with an associated mortality rate approaching 15%.[32,34,37] Concomitant life-threatening injuries that may occur include arterial injury, pulmonary contusion, pneumothorax, closed head injury, and splenic or liver laceration.[2,4,18,32,34,37-39]

The scapula, a triangular flat bone, is the origin of the rotator cuff muscles (supraspinatus, infraspinatus, subscapularis, and teres minor), teres major, deltoid, biceps, latissimus dorsi, coracobrachialis, and the long head of the triceps.[2] It is the site of insertion for the trapezius, levator scapulae, rhomboids, serratus anterior, and pectoralis minor, all of which stabilize the scapula against the posterior chest wall.[2] The CC ligament prevents superior migration of the distal clavicle to stabilize the AC articulation. The GH ligaments, coracohumeral ligaments, and joint capsule stabilize the GH joint as the coracoacromial (CA) ligament serves as a superior static restraint to humeral head stability.[2,4,29] Goss first described the superior shoulder suspensory complex (SSSC) to demonstrate the function the scapula serves in maintaining the normal stable relationship among the shoulder girdle, upper extremity, and the axial skeleton (**Figure 12.14**). The SSSC is a ring composed of the AC joint, acromion, CC ligaments, coracoid process, distal clavicle, and glenoid. The clavicle serves as the superior strut, and the lateral scapular body and spine serve as the inferior strut.[2,4,40] A disruption of one part of the ring will still maintain the structural integrity of the shoulder girdle with the axial

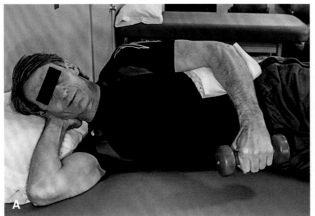
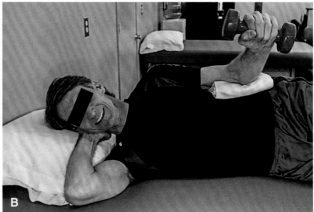

FIGURE 12.7 A and **B**, Side lying external rotation.

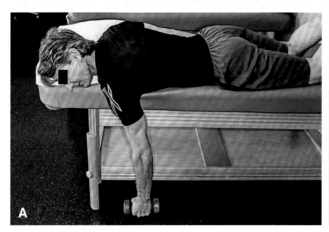 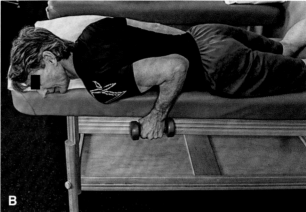

FIGURE 12.8 A and **B**, Prone rows. Patient is instructed to lie prone while holding a weight in the affected limb to lift the arm and raise the elbow to shoulder height while performing scapular retraction.

skeleton; however, a double disruption results in an unstable relationship, known as floating shoulder (**Figure 12.15**).[2,40] Of note, it has been reported in the literature that without a concomitant ligamentous disruption, pure strut injuries (ie, ipsilateral clavicle and scapular neck fractures) do not render the shoulder unstable.[2]

SCAPULOTHORACIC DISSOCIATION

ST dissociation is an avulsion injury of the musculature of the scapula, resulting in lateral displacement of the scapula. ST dissociations typically occur due to a lateral traction injury from blunt force trauma to the shoulder girdle, frequently resulting in concomitant injuries to the shoulder girdle, such as scapula/clavicle fracture, AC/SC dislocation, and severe neurovascular injuries.[4] A flail extremity results in approximately 50% of the cases, with complete loss of motor and sensory function, rendering the extremity nonfunctional. Neurologic injury occurs in up to 90% of cases, commonly due to a complete avulsion of the ipsilateral brachial plexus.[33,38] Injuries to the subclavian artery/vein are the most common vascular injuries observed, followed by an

injury to the axillary artery.[37] Emergent angiography must be performed, should a pulseless extremity be diagnosed. Following vascular repair, the SC, AC, and/or clavicle should be stabilized, with possible nerve exploration. There is a 10% mortality rate seen in patients with ST dissociations.

TREATMENT

Treatment aims include restoration of full, pain-free ROM, anatomic alignment, and prevention of complications such as malunion, nonunion, osteoarthritis at the GH joint, and chronic pain. This includes achievement of restoration of the congruency and stabilization of the GH joint in glenoid fractures, anatomical alignment of the scapular body/glenoid in scapular neck and body fractures, and prevention of malunion of the acromion or coracoid processes.[2]

Nonoperative

Indications for nonoperative treatment include nondisplaced fractures and intra- and extra-articular displaced fractures in which the patient's general condition precludes operation.[2] The majority of acromion and coracoid fractures are nondisplaced and may be treated conservatively.[4,38,41] The patient

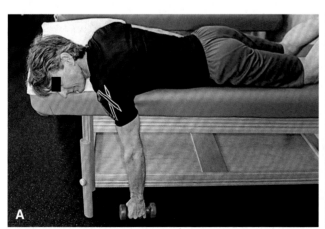 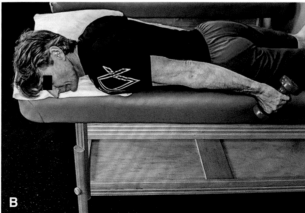

FIGURE 12.9 A and **B**, Prone shoulder extension. Patient is instructed to lie prone and to lift the affected arm in line with the body while performing scapular retraction.

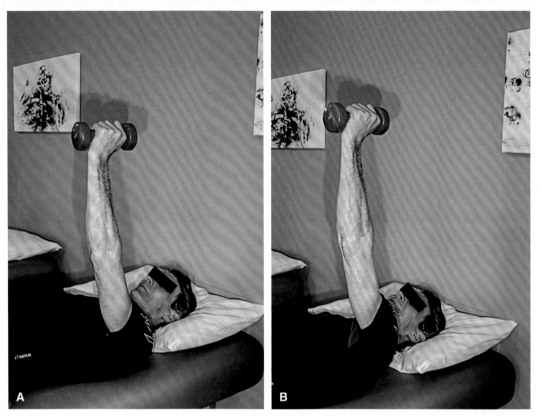

FIGURE 12.10 A and **B**, Serratus punch. While lying in the supine position, the patient is instructed to keep the elbow straight and move the arm incrementally higher toward the ceiling.

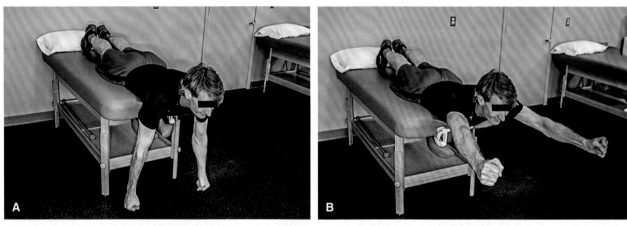

FIGURE 12.11 A and **B**, "Ys": prone horizontal abduction with external rotation.

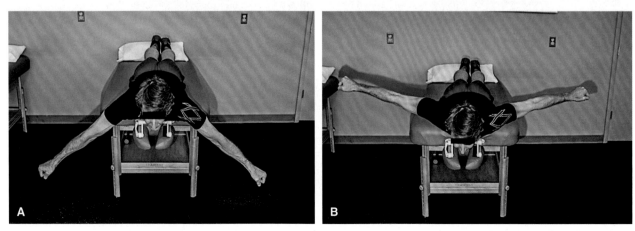

FIGURE 12.12 A and **B**, "Ts": prone horizontal extension with the arm at 100° of shoulder abduction.

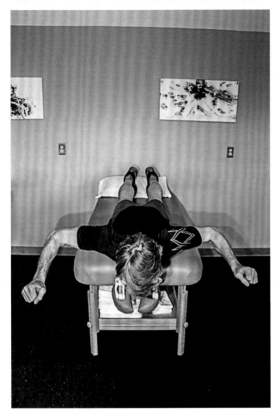

FIGURE 12.13 "Ws": prone scapular retraction with downward rotation.

is provided with a sling and swathe postoperatively and is instructed to sleep in a reclining chair. AROM exercises of the elbow, wrist, and hand are to be initiated on postoperative day 1, with Codman or Rock the Baby exercises initiated as pain begins to subside, preferably within the first few postoperative days. After 2 weeks, the patient may initiate PROM exercises, with the goal of achieving full PROM within 1 month of the injury.[2] During the second month post

injury, full AROM should be restored. Strengthening exercises for the rotator cuff and periscapular muscles are started in the third month. The potential disadvantages of nonoperative treatment include cosmetic deformity of the scapula, with incongruity and instability of the GH joint.[2]

Operative

Operative treatment is indicated for intra-articular displaced fractures of the glenoid, fractures of the neck of the scapula with significant angulation, and fractures of the acromion with concomitant impingement syndrome.[2,40] Floating shoulder is a relative indication for operative management. Open reduction internal fixation is the standard for operative treatment.[2,4,37] In the literature, arthroscopically assisted internal fixation or partial resection has been reported for treatment of glenoid and acromion fractures.[2] At present, there are a growing number of advocates for surgical management for scapular fractures, due to recent literature citing poorer patient outcomes in conservatively managed displaced fractures of the body/neck. Indications for surgical management of scapular fractures include displaced intra-articular glenoid fractures with gapping ≥3 to 10 mm and/or persistent subluxation of the humeral head.[2] Displaced glenoid rim fractures are associated with instability of the GH joint; thus, it is imperative to stabilize the GH joint and restore congruity.[2,40] With regards to floating shoulders, there are a growing number of advocates for treating these injuries nonoperatively. In the earlier literature, clavicle stabilization was thought to minimize scapular neck malunion; however, more recent papers suggest that there is no significant difference in functional outcomes between the operative and nonoperative management.[40]

REHABILITATION

Rehabilitation of operatively and nonoperatively managed scapular fractures is essentially the same, with timing and progression through therapeutic phases based upon initial

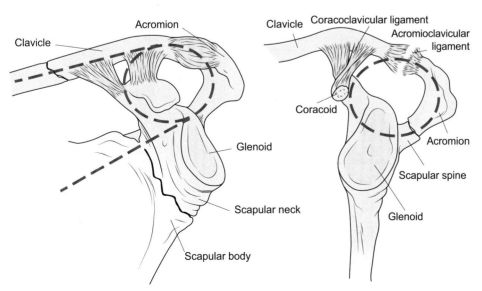

FIGURE 12.14 Oblique and lateral views of the two struts (clavicle and scapular neck) and one ring (distal clavicle, acromioclavicular ligaments, acromial process, glenoid fossa, coracoid, and coracoclavicular ligaments) of the superior shoulder suspensory complex. (Reproduced from Jeong GK, Zuckerman JD. Scapula fractures. *Musculoskeletal Key*. August 4, 2016. Accessed May 15, 2020. https://musculoskeletalkey.com/scapula-fractures-2/)

intraoperative fixation, bone quality, radiographic consolidation, clinical healing, and patient's individual pain tolerances.

A sling and swathe is provided to the patient postoperatively to secure the upper arm and forearm to the chest to achieve shoulder joint support.[34] The patient's injured side must be immobilized for the first 2 weeks postoperatively.[2] With fractures of the processes, elevation and abduction of the injured extremity with use of an abduction cushion will aid to relieve tension.

Protocol[23]

Phase I Day 1—Immobilization

It is important to maintain full mobility of the unaffected joints to reduce arm swelling and to preserve joint motion. The following exercises are recommended to initiate on the first postoperative day and continue for approximately 6 weeks[2]:

- Squeezing shoulder blades together, with shoulders relaxed.
- Flexion and extension of the elbow, wrist, and hand.
- Open and closure of the hand, with and without a stress ball.
- Supination pronation of the forearm and radial ulnar deviation of the wrist.

A continuous passive motion machine may also be utilized to assist patients with the aforementioned PROM exercises.

Phase II: Day 2 to Week 6—Mobilization

Codman/Rock the Baby exercises may be initiated as soon as pain subsides. Patient continues PROM exercises. Should PROM exercises be progressing optimally, and fracture consolidation likely (week 3-6 postop), AAROM exercises may be initiated. The recommended AAROM exercises include:

- Internal and external rotation.
- Forward flexion with arms resting on a table.
- Forward flexion and elevation of the arm with a ball on the wall.

4 weeks: Submaximal isometric exercises may be initiated. The submaximal isometric exercises recommended include:

- Internal and external rotation.
- Flexion and extension.
- Abduction.

Closed-chain exercises are optimal to initiate ROM as they unweight the limb and elicit low amounts of shoulder muscle activity (**Figure 12.16A-D**). Scapular muscle strengthening to facilitate muscle recruitment and scapular motion is achieved with closed-chain scapular exercises, such as low row and the scapular clock.[21,22,42] The scapular clock exercise facilitates the scapular motions of elevation, depression, retraction, and protraction, whereas the low-row exercise activates the lower trapezius (**Figure 12.17A and B**). A pulley may be incorporated into the patient's therapeutic protocol. With the pulley above the patient, the contralateral limb may be used to provide full passive forward flexion of the involved limb.[21,22]

Phase III: Week 6 to Week 10—Strengthening

With satisfactory progression of both PROM and AAROM exercises, and fracture consolidation observed radiographically by the surgeon, AROM and strengthening exercises of the rotator cuff and periscapular muscles may begin.[21] This will facilitate motion of the scapula and muscle recruitment. Upper extremity PNFs may be initiated at week 6.[22] By week 10, progression toward overhead exercises is made.

ACROMIOCLAVICULAR JOINT INJURIES

INTRODUCTION

AC joint injuries comprise approximately 12% of fractures of the shoulder girdle, commonly occurring in the setting of contact sports, such as football, ice hockey, rugby, and wrestling.[43] The most frequently reported mechanism of injury

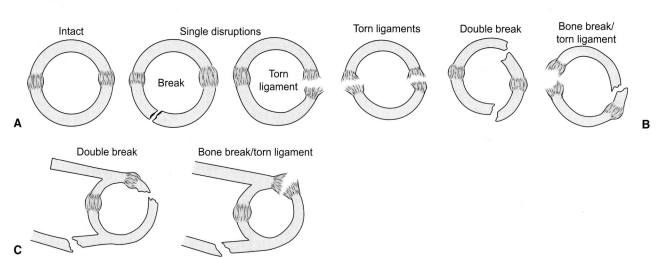

FIGURE 12.15 A-C, Intact, single, and double disruption of the shoulder suspensory complex. (Reproduced from Jeong GK, Zuckerman JD. Scapula fractures. *Musculoskeletal Key*. August 4, 2016. Accessed May 15, 2020. https://musculoskeletalkey.com/scapula-fractures-2/)

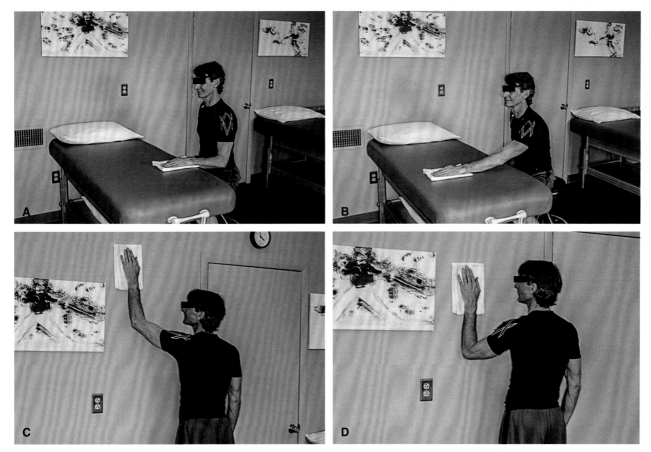

FIGURE 12.16 Closed-chain exercise for scapular stabilization. Exercises may be initiated on a flat surface (**A** and **B**), gradually progressed to an inclined surface, and finally a vertical surface (**C** and **D**).

is a fall with direct trauma to the posterosuperior aspect of the shoulder.[44,45] Injury may also occur after a fall on an outstretched adducted arm, thus driving the humeral head into the AC joint. The AC joint is a diarthrodial joint defined by the lateral clavicle articulating with the acromion process as it projects anteriorly off the scapula. The AC joint is a plane-type synovial joint, which, under normal physiological conditions, allows limited gliding movement. It attaches

the scapula to the thorax allowing for additional ROM to the scapula and assists in limb movement such as abduction and flexion of the shoulder.[44] Three primary ligaments stabilize the AC joint: the AC ligament, CC ligament, and CA ligament. The AC ligament has superior, inferior, anterior, and posterior components. The superior and posterior ligaments are the strongest ligaments, providing horizontal stability. The CC ligament complex consists of the conoid and

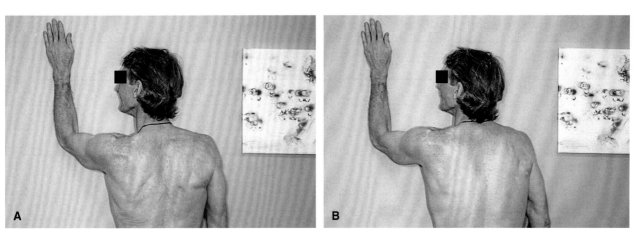

FIGURE 12.17 Scapular clocks. Retraction (adduction) (**A**) and protraction (abduction) (**B**) of the scapula. Facilitates muscle activity of the parascapular muscles and motion and control of the scapula.

trapezoid ligaments, inserting onto the posteromedial and anterolateral area of the undersurface of the distal clavicle, respectively. The CA ligament connects the coracoid process to the acromion, and, along with the CC ligament, provides vertical stability.[29,46-48]

CLASSIFICATION

AC joint separations involve varying degrees of AC and CC ligament and deltopectoral fascia injury. Injuries are classified according to the extent of injury to the AC and CC ligaments, deltotrapezial fascia, clavicular position in relation to the acromion, and radiographic findings (**Table 12.5**; **Figure 12.18**).[45]

TREATMENT

There is a paucity of high-level evidence to support definitive treatment options for patients with AC joint dislocations. There is a general consensus in the literature that Type I and II injuries are to be treated nonoperatively, Type IV-VI, operatively, and Type III may be treated nonoperatively or operatively, dependent on patient variables.[49]

Nonoperative

Indications for nonoperative management include Type I, II, and select Type III AC joint injuries.[45] Only in the case of chronic symptomatic injury is the patient treated operatively, with the intent to address one of the following possible causes of symptoms: post-traumatic arthritis, osteolysis of the clavicle, recurrent anteroposterior (AP) subluxation, torn capsular ligaments trapped within the joint, and loose pieces of articular cartilage.[49]

Nonoperative treatment involves immobilization of injured arm in a sling for 1 to 3 weeks. The sling is utilized to reduce stress placed upon the ligaments of the joint during healing.[47] Ice and analgesics are provided to the patient to reduce pain and inflammation. Early ROM exercises are encouraged. Daily activities are initiated as patient's comfort permits. Overhead use of the extremity and a course

of lifting may be initiated at week 6, with progression as tolerated. Once ROM and strength of the involved limb is equivalent to 85% of the contralateral extremity, return to sports and recreational activities may be permitted.[50]

With regards to the management of Type III injuries, there is substantial debate as to the best method of treatment. Generally, Type III injuries may be treated nonoperatively.[50,51] However, in athletes, heavy labor workers, polytrauma patients, and patients who have failed conservative treatment, operative management is recommended.

Operative

Operative indications for AC joint injuries include select Type III injuries as previously described and Type IV-VI injuries. The primary goals of surgical management for AC joint separations are to restore full pain-free ROM and strength. There are multiple surgical options available for the treatment of AC joint separation. AC joint stabilization may be achieved using Kirschner wires (K-wires), pins, or hook plates.[46] Suture anchors, endobuttons, screws, and suture loops may be utilized to stabilize the CC space. For CC reconstruction, proximally based conjoint tendon transfer may be performed.[52] For complete AC joint separation, the preferred method of treatment is open anatomic CC ligament reconstruction (ACCR).

REHABILITATION

Nonoperative Protocol[23]

Nonoperative rehabilitation, as briefly described in the treatment section, adopts the same exercises as described below in the author's preferred protocol for rehabilitation post ACCR, following the individual patient's tolerances for advancement in therapeutic motions and exercises. The primary difference between the nonoperative protocol and operative protocol is that in the nonoperative setting, early intervention centers around reducing pain and inflammation to allow for ROM and strengthening to begin. However, in the operative setting, the repair must

TABLE 12.5 Tossy-Rockwood Classification of Acromioclavicular Injuries

Type	AC Ligament	CC Ligament	Deltopectoral Fascia	Radiographic AC Appearance	Radiographic CC Distance Increase	AC Joint Reducible
I	Sprain	Intact	Intact	Normal	Normal (1.1-1.3 cm)	N/A
II	Disruption	Sprain	Intact	Widening	<25%	Yes
III	Disruption	Disruption	Disruption	Widening	25%-100%	Yes
IV	Disruption	Disruption	Disruption	Posterior clavicular displacement	Increased	No
V	Disruption	Disruption	Disruption	N/A	100%-300%	No
VI	Disruption	Disruption	Disruption	N/A	Decreased	No

AC, acromioclavicular; CC, coracoclavicular.

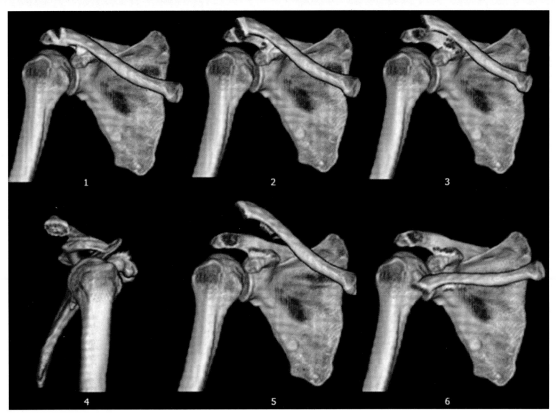

FIGURE 12.18 Rockwood classification. (Case courtesy of Dr Roberto Schubert, Radiopaedia.org, rID: 19124.)

be protected for a minimum of 6 weeks to allow for partial incorporation of the tendon graft within the bone tunnel. This allows for sufficient gains in biomechanical stability at the construct site to minimize risk of failure once rehabilitation commences.

Post-ACCR Protocol (Table 12.6)[23]

Sling

Patient must be instructed to wear a platform brace, such as the DonJoy Lerman shoulder orthosis, except during self-care and when performing therapeutic exercises. Brace is provided to prevent the gravity-dependent downward pull on the scapulohumeral complex and must be worn for 6 to 8 weeks post reconstruction.[53]

Hygiene

Patients should be counseled on fall risk while bathing. Patients should be instructed to utilize a nonslip mat in the shower/bathtub or a shower chair. The arm may be removed from the sling while showering.

Phase I: Immobilization[23,50,53]

Postoperative week 0 to 6.

Goals for Immediate Postoperative Period

1. Protection of AC joint repair.
2. Control of pain and inflammation.
3. Initiation of early shoulder ROM.
4. Prevention of shoulder stiffness.

Therapeutic Exercises and ROM

It is important to maintain full mobility of the unaffected joints to reduce arm swelling and to preserve joint motion. The following PROM exercises are recommended to initiate on the first postoperative day and continue for approximately 6 weeks:

- Squeezing shoulder blades together, with shoulders relaxed.
- Flexion and extension of the elbow, wrist, and hand.
- Open and closure of the hand, with and without a stress ball.
- Supination pronation of the forearm and radial ulnar deviation of the wrist.
- Supine internal rotation (IR) and ER.
- Shoulder abduction.

Patient must be instructed to not elevate the injured limb above 90° in any plane nor lift objects weighing over 1 to 2 pounds during Phase I.[22] Supine exercises are recommended during Phase I as lying supine neutralizes the gravitational stresses exerted on the involved joint.

Phase II: ROM Restoration and Scapular Control[23,50,53]

Postoperative week 6 to 12.

Goals

1. Protection of AC joint repair.
2. Improvement in ROM of the shoulder.
3. Beginning gentle strengthening.

TABLE 12.6 Author's Preferred Rehabilitation Protocol for Acromioclavicular Joint Reconstruction

Postoperative Weeks	Goals	Motion	Strengthening
• **Weeks 0-6**	• Pain control • Inflammation control • Protection of reconstruction • Prevention of shoulder capsular contracture	• AROM, AAROM, and PROM of cervical spine, elbow, wrist, and hand • Codman or "Rock the Baby" exercise • Supine passive forward flexion • Supine IR and ER to chest/abdomen • Scapular retraction • Repeat above motions 7 d/wk, four times per day	• No initiation of strengthening

• **Weeks 6-12**	• Same as above	• Continue as above
		• ER and IR as tolerated
		• Shoulder abduction and flexion as tolerated (full abduction and flexion by week 12)
		• Shoulder flexion in the scapular plane
		• Scapular wall slides
		• Scapular stabilization closed chain
		• Repeat above motions 7 d/wk, two times per day
			• Postural correction
			• Grip strengthening
			• Resistance band exercises:
			  • row
			  • biceps curl
			• Dynamic exercises:
			  • side lying ER
			  • prone row
			  • prone extension

• **Weeks 12-20**	• Same as above	• Continue as above • Repeat above motions 7 d/wk, two times per day	• Same as above • Multilevel rows with resistance band/pulley

• **Weeks 20-24**	• Same as above	• Continue as above	• Same as above
			• Deltoid and rotator cuff isometrics
			• Periscapular strengthening
			• Plyometric program for overhead-throwing athletes
			  • Deceleration drills with weighted ball
			  • Rebounder throws:
			    • with arm at side
			    • with weighted ball
			  • Wall dribbles:
			    • overhead
			    • at 90°
			    • circles

AAROM, active-assisted range of motion; AROM, active range of motion; ER, external rotation, IR, internal rotation; PROM, passive range of motion.

Therapeutic Exercises and ROM

- ROM closed-chain exercises, with progression to open-chain as mobility improves.
- Scapular muscle-strengthening exercises.

ROM of the involved limb is gradually initiated with closed-chain exercises, providing support to the limb and minimizing stresses to the AC joint. Supine flexion and pulley therapeutic exercises ease the patient to open-chain exercises.[52] End-range forward flexion and internal rotation behind the back increase stresses on the AC joint and must be advanced without exceeding the patient's pain tolerance. Scapular muscle strengthening to facilitate muscle recruitment and scapular motion is achieved with closed-chain scapular exercises, such as low row and the scapular clock.[22,44,54]

Phase III: Strengthening[23,50,53]

Postoperative week 12 to 20.

Goals

1. Protection of AC joint repair.
2. Regaining full ROM.
3. Continuation of strengthening progression.

Therapeutic Exercises and ROM

Isotonic strengthening exercises may be initiated at postoperative week 12. Recommended exercises to increase scapular strength are[55]:

- Prone row.
- "Ys": horizontal abduction with external rotation.[56]
- "Ts": prone horizontal extension with the arm at 100° of shoulder abduction.[56]
- "Ws": prone scapular retraction with downward rotation.
- Multilevel rowing exercises focused on combined motions with resistance band/pulley.

Phase IV: Restoration of Function[23,50,53]

Postoperative week 20 to 24.

Goals

1. Maintenance of full ROM.
2. Continuation of strengthening.
3. Return to sports and recreational activities.

Therapeutic Exercises and ROM

- Continue isotonic shoulder and scapula strengthening.
- Return to sports.
  - 4 to 5 months: Initiation of overhead throwing and swimming.
  - 6 months: Return to contact sports.
- Overhead-throwing athletes may initiate a plyometric program consisting of the following exercises[50]:
  - Deceleration drills with weighted ball.
  - Rebounder throws:
    - with arm at side.
    - with weighted ball.
  - Wall dribbles:
    - overhead.
    - at 90°.
    - circles.

STERNOCLAVICULAR JOINT

INTRODUCTION

The SC joint is a saddle-shaped synovial joint, which links the upper extremity to the axial skeleton.[57,58] It is composed of the medial end of the clavicle and the superolateral aspect of the manubrium.[58] The intra-articular disk, costoclavicular, interclavicular, and capsular ligaments of the shoulder joint support the SC joint.[58-61]

SC joint motion consists of elevation/depression around an AP axis, protraction/retraction around a vertical axis, and posterior/anterior rotation around a medial/lateral axis (**Figure 12.19**). Elevation and depression motions raise and lower the lateral aspect of the clavicle, respectively. Posterior rotation results in the anterolateral aspect of the clavicle rotating up and back, while anterior rotation results in the clavicle rotating down and forward.[58,62]

Injuries to the SC joint most commonly occur after a direct blow is applied to the shoulder, such as during a motor vehicle

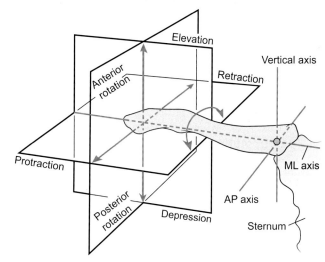

FIGURE 12.19 Sternoclavicular joint motions. (With permission from Oatis CA. *Kinesiology: The Mechanics & Pathomechanics of Human Movement.* 3 ed. Philadelphia, PA: Wolters Kluwer; 2016.)

collision or participation in contact sports.[58,61-64] Significant trauma to surrounding structures in the neck and thorax may result during SC joint injury.[60] The patient must always be evaluated for injuries to the mediastinum, especially in the setting of posterior fracture/dislocation due to the proximity of the SC joint to the mediastinum. Concomitant injuries reported in the literature include tracheal compression,[63] pneumothorax, esophageal perforation, injury to the brachial plexus and laceration/compression of the pulmonary artery, brachiocephalic vein, superior vena cava, and innominate artery.[58,65]

TREATMENT

Nonoperative

The majority of SC joint injuries are managed nonoperatively via observation or closed reduction.[58,63,65] This includes acute and chronic anterior subluxations and dislocations, acute traumatic posterior subluxations and dislocations, and acute traumatic anterior and posterior physeal injuries of the medial clavicle.[58]

In patients where observation is appropriate, the surgeon may provide with a sling for comfort and suggest a return to unrestricted activity by 3 months. Closed reductions are indicated in both acute anterior and posterior dislocations <3 weeks old.[61] If the reduction is stable, the patient may utilize a velpeau bandage for 6 weeks.[58] Most anterior dislocations are unstable; thus, a padded figure-of-eight clavicle strap to hold the shoulders back and rest the SC joint is provided.[57] The patient has to wear the harness for 1 week and should transition to a sling for one additional week. Three weeks post reduction, the patient may initiate elbow exercises, and a return to unrestricted activity is permitted at 3 months post injury.[62]

Operative

Chronic posterior dislocations and acute irreducible posterior dislocations are indications for open surgical management, so as to avoid significant complications arising from the posterior intrusion of the clavicle on the mediastinum.[58,66] Surgical techniques include plate fixation, open excision with intramedullary ligament repair, and figure-of-eight reconstruction with soft-tissue graft to reconstitute capsular ligaments.[58,59,61,66,67] Utilization of hamstring tendon graft with figure-of-eight reconstruction has been reported to be biomechanically superior to other methods when comparing graft integrity, load to failure, and translation of the medial clavicle.[58,62,64]

REHABILITATION[62]

The rehabilitation protocol for postoperative SC joint reconstruction centers around return to full, pain-free ROM of

TABLE 12.7 Author's Preferred Rehabilitation Protocol for Sternoclavicular Joint Reconstruction

Postoperative Weeks	Goals	Motion	Strengthening
• Weeks 0-6	• Pain control • Inflammation control • Protection of reconstruction • Maintain motion at elbow/wrist/hand	• AROM, AAROM, and PROM of cervical spine, elbow, wrist, and hand • Repeat above motions 7 d/wk, four times per day	• No initiation of strengthening

• Weeks 6-12	• Same as above	• Continue as above
		• Supine passive forward flexion
		• Supine external and internal rotation to chest/abdomen
		• Scapular retraction
		• Week 8: AROM as tolerated
		  • ER and IR
		  • Horizontal adduction
		  • Shoulder abduction and flexion as tolerated (full abduction and flexion by week 12)
		• Scapular wall slides
		• Scapular stabilization—closed and open chain
		• Repeat above motions two times per day, 7 d a week
			• Postural correction
			• Grip strengthening
			• Resistance band exercises:
			  • row
			  • serratus punch
			  • biceps curl
			• Dynamic exercises:
			  • side lying ER
			  • prone row
			  • prone extension

• Weeks 12-20	• Same as above	• Continue as above incorporating weights/resistance, beginning with 1 lb and incrementally increasing to 5 lb, within patient's tolerances
		• Repeat above motions two times per day, 7 days a week
			• Same as above
			• Multilevel rows with resistance band/pulley
			• Low row
			  • "Ys": horizontal abduction with external rotation
			  • "Ts": prone horizontal extension with the arm at 100° of shoulder abduction
			  • "Ws": prone scapular retraction with downward rotation

• Weeks 20-24	• Same as above	• Continue as above	• Same as above
			• Deltoid and rotator cuff isometrics
			• Periscapular strengthening
			• Plyometric program for overhead-throwing athletes
			  • Deceleration drills with weighted ball
			  • Rebounder throws:
			    • with arm at side
			    • with weighted ball
			  • Wall dribbles:
			    • overhead
			    • at 90°
			    • circles

AAROM, active-assisted range of motion; AROM, active range of motion; ER, external rotation, IR, internal rotation; PROM, passive range of motion.

the shoulder (**Table 12.7**). The patient is provided a sling to utilize for at least 6 weeks and may use ice and anti-inflammatories as needed. An initial avoidance of GH joint motions and scapular protraction, retraction, depression, and elevation are critical for the first 6 weeks post operatively.

AROM of the cervical neck, elbow, wrist, and hand may begin on postoperative day 1 and be continued for 6 weeks, after which full PROM and AAROM of the shoulder joint may commence.

Active shoulder ROM begins at 8 weeks postoperatively and focuses on strengthening of the shoulder and scapular stabilizers. The patient may focus on strengthening exercises at 12 weeks postoperatively and slowly incorporate weights and resistance into his or her existing therapeutic exercises. Return to sports is permitted once the patient demonstrates both full and painless ROM, and the strength of the involved limb is 90% equivalent to that of the contralateral limb.

REFERENCES

1. Bohsali KI, Wirth MA. *Fractures of the proximal humerus.* In: *Rockwood and Matsen's The Shoulder*: Elsevier; 2009:295-332.
2. Rockwood CA, Green DP, Bucholz RW. *Rockwood and Green's fractures in adults.* 8th ed. Philadelphia, PA: Wolters Kluwer Health/Lippincott Williams & Wilkins; 2015.
3. Craig EV. Fractures of the clavicle. In: Rockwood CA, Matsen FA, eds. *The Shoulder.* 3rd ed. Philadelphia, PA. WB Saunders; 2004.
4. Voleti PB, Namdari S, Mehta S. Fractures of the scapula. *Adv Orthop.* 2012;2012:1-7.
5. Court-Brown CM, Caesar B. Epidemiology of adult fractures: a review. *Injury.* 2006;37(8):691-697.
6. Court-Brown CM, Garg A, McQueen MM. The translated two-part fracture of the proximal humerus: epidemiology and outcome in the older patient. *J Bone Joint Surg Br Vol.* 2001;83-B(6):799-804.
7. Launonen AP, Lepola V, Saranko A, Flinkkilä T, Laitinen M, Mattila VM. Epidemiology of proximal humerus fractures. *Arch Osteoporos.* 2015;10(1):2.
8. Nordqvist A, Petersson CJ. Incidence and causes of shoulder girdle injuries in an urban population. *J Shoulder Elbow Surg.* 1995;4(2):107-112.
9. Passaretti D, Candela V, Sessa P, Gumina S. Epidemiology of proximal humeral fractures: a detailed survey of 711 patients in a metropolitan area. *J Shoulder Elbow Surg.* 2017;26(12):2117-2124.
10. Keser S, Bölükbaşı S, Bayar A, Kanatlı U, Meray J, Özdemir H. Proximal humeral fractures with minimal displacement treated conservatively. *Int Orthop.* 2004;28(4):231-234.
11. Koval KJ, Gallagher MA, Marsicano JG, Cuomo F, McShinawy A, Zuckerman JD. Functional outcome after minimally displaced fractures of the proximal part of the humerus. *J Bone Joint Surg.* 1997;79(2):203-207.
12. Jones RB. Hemiarthroplasty for proximal humeral fractures: Indications, pitfalls, and technique. *Bull Hosp Jt Dis (2013).* 2013;71 suppl 2:60-63.
13. Mittlmeier TWF, Stedtfeld HW, Ewert A, Beck M, Frosch B, Gradl G. Stabilization of proximal humeral fractures with an angular and sliding stable antegrade locking nail (Targon PH). *J Bone Joint Surg Am.* 2003;85:136-146.
14. Court-Brown CM, Cattermole H, McQueen MM. Impacted valgus fractures (B1.1) of the proximal humerus: the results of non-operative treatment. *J Bone Joint Surg Br Vol.* 2002;84-B(4):504-508.
15. Helmy N, Hintermann B. New Trends in the treatment of proximal humerus fractures. *Clin Orthop Relat Res.* 2006;442:100-108.
16. Jakob R, Miniaci A, Anson P, Jaberg H, Osterwalder A, Ganz R. Four-part valgus impacted fractures of the proximal humerus. *J Bone Joint Surg Br Vol.* 1991;73-B(2):295-298.
17. Resch H, Povacz P, Fröhlich R, Wambacher M. Percutaneous fixation of three- and four-part fractures of the proximal humerus. *J Bone Joint Surg Br Vol.* 1997;79-B(2):295-300.
18. Tucek M, Bartoníček J. Associated injuries of the scapula fractures. *Rozhl Chir.* 2010;89(5):288-292.
19. Tejani NC, Liporace F, Walsh M, France MA, Zuckerman JD, Egol KA. Functional outcome following one-part proximal humeral fractures: A prospective study. *J Shoulder Elbow Surg.* 2008;17(2):216-219.
20. Long JL, Ruberte Thiele RA, Skendzel JG, et al. Activation of the shoulder musculature during pendulum exercises and light activities. *J Orthop Sports Phys Ther.* 2010;40(4):230-237.
21. Kibler WB. Rehabilitation of rotator cuff tendinopathy. *Clin Sports Med.* 2003;22(4):837-847.
22. Escamilla RF, Yamashiro K, Paulos L, Andrews JR. Shoulder muscle activity and function in common shoulder rehabilitation exercises. *Sports Med.* 2009;39(8):663-685.
23. Green A, Hayda RA, Hecht A. *Postoperative Orthopaedic Rehabilitation.* Philadelphia, PA: Wolters Kluwer; 2017.
24. Namdari S, Yagnik G, Ebaugh DD, et al. Defining functional shoulder range of motion for activities of daily living. *J Shoulder Elbow Surg.* 2012;21(9):1177-1183.
25. Robertson DD, Yuan J, Bigliani LU, Flatow EL, Yamaguchi K. Three-dimensional analysis of the proximal part of the humerus: relevance to arthroplasty. *J Bone Joint Surg Am.* 2000;82(11):1594-1602.
26. Gangahar DM, Flogaites T. Retrosternal dislocation of the clavicle producing thoracic outlet syndrome. *J Trauma.* 1978;18(5):369-372.
27. McKee RC, Whelan DB, Schemitsch EH, McKee MD. Operative versus nonoperative care of displaced midshaft clavicular fractures: a meta-analysis of randomized clinical trials. *J Bone Joint Surg Am.* 2012;94(8):675-684.
28. van der Meijden OA, Gaskill TR, Millett PJ. Treatment of clavicle fractures: current concepts review. *J Shoulder Elbow Surg.* 2012;21(3):423-429.
29. Oatis CA. *Kinesiology: The Mechanics & Pathomechanics of Human Movement.* 3rd ed. Philadelphia, PA: Wolters Kluwer; 2016.
30. McKee MD, Pedersen EM, Jones C, et al. Deficits following nonoperative treatment of displaced midshaft clavicular fractures. *J Bone Joint Surg Am.* 2006;88(1):35-40.
31. Worman LW, Leagus C. Intrathoracic injury following retrosternal dislocation of the clavicle. *J Trauma.* 1967;7(3):416-423.
32. Baldwin KD, Ohman-Strickland P, Mehta S, Hume E. Scapula fractures: a marker for concomitant injury? A retrospective review of data in the national trauma database. *J Trauma.* 2008;65(2):430-435.
33. Thompson DA, Flynn TC, Miller PW, Fischer RP. The significance of scapular fractures. *J Trauma.* 1985;25(10):974-977.
34. Imatani RJ. Fractures of the scapula: a review of 53 fractures. *J Trauma.* 1975;15(6):473-478.
35. Weening B, Walton C, Cole PA, Alanezi K, Hanson BP, Bhandari M. Lower mortality in patients with scapular fractures. *J Trauma.* 2005;59(6):1477-1481.
36. Coimbra R, Conroy C, Tominaga GT, Bansal V, Schwartz A. Causes of scapula fractures differ from other shoulder injuries in occupants seriously injured during motor vehicle crashes. *Injury.* 2010;41(2):151-155.
37. Armstrong CP, Van der Spuy J. The fractured scapula: importance and management based on a series of 62 patients. *Injury.* 1984;15(5):324-329.
38. McGahan JP, Rab GT, Dublin A. Fractures of the Scapula. *J Trauma.* 1980;20(10):880-883.
39. Guttentag IJ, Rechtine GR. Fractures of the scapula. A review of the literature. *Orthop Rev.* 1988;17:147-158.
40. Owens BD, Goss TP. The floating shoulder. *J Bone Joint Surg Br Vol.* 2006;88-B(11):1419-1424.
41. McGinnis M, Denton JR. Fractures of the scapula: a retrospective study of 40 fractured scapulae. *J Trauma.* 1989;29(11):1488-1493.
42. Kang M-H, Oh J-S, Jang J-H. Differences in muscle activities of the infraspinatus and posterior deltoid during shoulder external rotation in open kinetic chain and closed kinetic chain exercises. *J Phys Ther Sci.* 2014;26(6):895-897.
43. Dragoo JL, Braun HJ, Bartlinski SE, Harris AHS. Acromioclavicular joint injuries in National Collegiate Athletic Association Football: data from the 2004-2005 through 2008-2009 National Collegiate Athletic Association Injury Surveillance System. *Am J Sports Med.* 2012;40(9):2066-2071.
44. Kibler W. The role of the scapula in athletic shoulder function. *Am J Sports Med.* 1998;26(2):325-327.
45. Mazzocca AD, Santangelo SA, Johnson ST, Rios CG, Dumonski ML, Arciero RA. A biomechanical evaluation of an anatomical coracoclavicular ligament reconstruction. *Am J Sports Med.* 2006;34(2):236-246.

46. Lee S, Bedi A. Shoulder acromioclavicular joint reconstruction options and outcomes. *Curr Rev Musculoskelet Med.* 2016;9(4):368-377.

47. Mazzocca AD, Arciero RA, Bicos J. Evaluation and treatment of acromioclavicular joint injuries. *Am J Sports Med.* 2007;35(2):316-329.

48. Mouhsine E, Garofalo R, Crevoisier X, Farron A. Grade I and II acromioclavicular dislocations: results of conservative treatment. *J Shoulder Elbow Surg.* 2003;12(6):599-602.

49. Beitzel K, Cote MP, Apostolakos J, et al. Current concepts in the treatment of acromioclavicular joint dislocations. *Arthroscopy.* 2013;29(2):387-397.

50. Gladstone JN, Wilk KE, Andrews JR. Nonoperative treatment ofacromioclavicular joint injuries. *Oper Tech Sports Med.* 1997;5(2):78-87.

51. Chang N, Furey A, Kurdin A. Operative versus nonoperative management of acute high-grade acromioclavicular dislocations: a systematic review and meta-analysis. *J Orthop Trauma.* 2018;32(1):1-9.

52. Jiang C, Wang M, Rong G. Proximally based conjoined tendon transfer for coracoclavicular reconstruction in the treatment of acromioclavicular dislocation. *J Bone Joint Surg Am.* 2008;90:299-308.

53. Cote MP, Wojcik KE, Gomlinski G, Mazzocca AD. Rehabilitation of acromioclavicular joint separations: operative and nonoperative considerations. *Clin Sports Med.* 2010;29(2):213-228.

54. Cooper GJ, Stubbs D, Waller DA, Wilkinson GAL, Saleh M. Posterior sternoclavicular dislocation: a novel method of external fixation. *Injury.* 1992;23(8):565-566.

55. Cools AM, Dewitte V, Lanszweert F, et al. Rehabilitation of scapular muscle balance: which exercises to prescribe? *Am J Sports Med.* 2007;35(10):1744-1751.

56. Ronai P. Prone scaption above 90 degrees in external rotation (the Prone Y). *ACSMs Health Fit J.* 2016;20(4):28-30.

57. Franck WM, Jannasch O, Siassi M, Hennig FF. Balser plate stabilization: an alternate therapy for traumatic sternoclavicular instability. *J Shoulder Elbow Surg.* 2003;12(3):276-281.

58. Rockwood CA Jr. Injuries to the sternoclavicular joint. In: Rockwood CA Jr, Green DP, eds. *Fractures in Adults.* Vol 1. 2nd ed. Philadelphia, PA: JB Lippincott; 1984.

59. Armstrong AL, Dias JJ. Reconstruction for instability of the sternoclavicular joint using the tendon of the sternocleidomastoid muscle. *J Bone Joint Surg Br Vol.* 2008;90-B(5):610-613.

60. Marcus MS, Tan V. Cerebrovascular accident in a 19-year-old patient: a case report of posterior sternoclavicular dislocation. *J Shoulder Elbow Surg.* 2011;20(7):e1-e4.

61. Martetschläger F, Warth RJ, Millett PJ. Instability and degenerative arthritis of the sternoclavicular joint: a current concepts review. *Am J Sports Med.* 2014;42(4):999-1007.

62. Logan C, Shahien A, Altintas B, Millett PJ. Rehabilitation following sternoclavicular joint reconstruction for persistent instability. *Int J Sports Phys Ther.* 2018;13(4):752-762.

63. Luhmann JD, Bassett GS. Posterior sternoclavicular epiphyseal separation presenting with hoarseness: a case report and discussion. *Pediatr Emerg Care.* 1998;14(2):130-132.

64. Petri M, Greenspoon JA, Horan MP, Martetschläger F, Warth RJ, Millett PJ. Clinical outcomes after autograft reconstruction for sternoclavicular joint instability. *J Shoulder Elbow Surg.* 2016;25(3):435-441.

65. Shuler FD, Pappas N. Treatment of posterior sternoclavicular dislocation with locking plate osteosynthesis. *Orthopedics.* 2008;31(3):1-4.

66. Spencer EE, Kuhn JE. Biomechanical analysis of reconstructions for sternoclavicular joint instability. *J Bone Joint Surg Am.* 2004;86A(1):98-105.

67. Hecox SE, Wood GW. Ledge plating technique for unstable posterior sternoclavicular dislocation. *J Orthop Trauma.* 2010;24(4):255-257.

Humeral Diaphysis or Midshaft Fractures

A. Michael Harris
L. Jared Hudspeth
Porter Young
Jennifer T. Dodson
Sabrina Wang

INTRODUCTION

Fractures of the humeral shaft are those that involve the diaphysis or midshaft and do not involve the articular or metaphyseal regions proximally or distally (**Figure 13.1**). Humeral shaft fractures are relatively common accounting for approximately 20% of all fractures.[1] Like most common orthopaedic injuries, there is a bimodal age distribution of humeral shaft fractures with a minor peak in the third decade and a major peak in the eighth decade. The incidence is approximately 14 per 100,000 persons per year with a gradually increasing age-specific incidence from the fifth decade to the ninth decade, almost reaching 60 per 100, 000 persons per year.[2] As these fractures commonly occur in the elderly, they are often a result of low-energy trauma, while younger patients are more likely to have a high-energy mechanism of injury.[2]

ANATOMY AND BIOMECHANICS

The humeral shaft extends from the proximal border of the pectoralis major insertion to the supracondylar ridge. It is cylindrical in its proximal half and becomes flattened and triangular distally. Anatomic landmarks such as the pectoralis major insertion, deltoid tuberosity, and the spiral groove have both clinical and surgical implications. The fracture location in relationship to these landmarks results in different fracture displacement patterns due to the effect of muscle forces. Fractures above the pectoralis major tendon lead to abduction and external rotation of the proximal humerus secondary to the pull of the rotator cuff muscles. Fractures below the pectoralis major insertion and above the deltoid lead to adduction of the proximal fragment (under the

influence of the pectoralis major) and proximal and lateral displacement of the distal fragment (under the influence of the deltoid). Fractures below the deltoid insertion lead to abduction of the upper fragment (under the strong influence of the deltoid).

The spiral groove, which is located on the posterior surface of the humerus, is an important landmark as it contains the radial nerve. The radial nerve, a branch of the brachial plexus arising from the posterior cord with fibers originating from C5, C6, C7, C8, and T1 roots, is the largest nerve in the upper extremity.[3] The radial nerve runs across the latissimus dorsi muscle, deep to the axillary artery, and passes through the triangular interval at the inferior border of the teres major muscle.[3] It then wraps around the proximal part of the humerus on the medial side to innervate the triceps muscle between the lateral and medial heads. At that level, two sensory branches split from the nerve to form the posterior cutaneous and inferior lateral cutaneous nerves of the arms.[3] At an average distance of 9.7 to 14.2 cm from the acromion, both the radial nerve and the deep brachial artery travel side by side in the spiral groove. The radial nerve travels adjacent to the posterior surface of the humerus for 6.5 cm exiting the spiral groove on average 12.6 cm (range, 10.1-14.8 cm) proximal to the lateral epicondyle and 18.1 to 20.7 cm proximal to the medial epicondyle.[4-7] The nerve enters the anterior compartment through the lateral intermuscular septum between the brachialis and brachioradialis at an average of 10 cm proximal to the lateral epicondyle. The close proximity of the radial nerve along the humerus puts it at risk with humeral shaft fractures (**Figure 13.2**). Furthermore, the tethering of the radial nerve as it pierces the lateral intermuscular septum is thought to account for the increased risk of nerve injury with the distal third humeral shaft fracture, aka Holstein-Lewis fracture (**Figure 13.3**).[8]

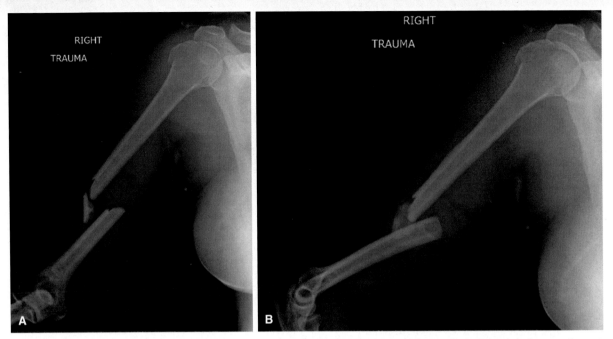

FIGURE 13.1 Anteroposterior (**A**) and lateral (**B**) radiographs of humeral shaft fracture with an ipsilateral greater tuberosity fracture after a pedestrian versus auto accident.

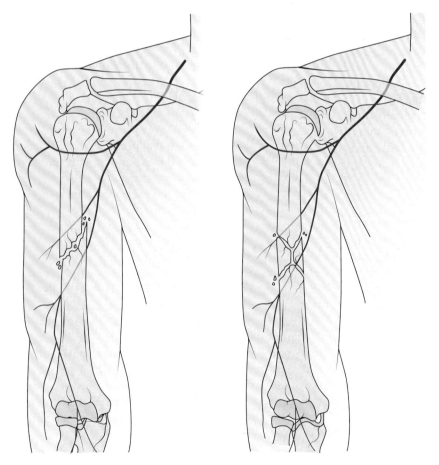

FIGURE 13.2 Oblique (**A**) and comminuted (**B**) fractures of the humerus. Note the proximity of the radial nerve at the posterior aspect of the fracture site. (Reprinted with permission from Hoppenfeld S, Murthy VL. *Treatment and Rehabilitation of Fractures.* Philadelphia: Lippincott Williams & Wilkins; 2000.)

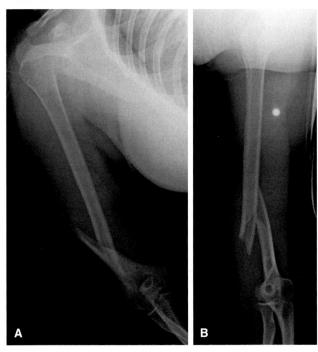

FIGURE 13.3 Anteroposterior (**A**) and lateral (**B**) radiographs of distal third humeral shaft fracture (aka Holstein-Lewis fracture).

RANGE OF MOTION

The complexity of the shoulder lies in its great mobility and dynamic control of its surrounding musculatures. Mobility at the glenohumeral joint, scapulothoracic joint, and sternoclavicular joint is critical to the shoulder complex to achieve human function. Depending on the fracture location as well as secondary trauma to the surrounding soft tissues and neurovascular structures, the patients who experience humeral shaft fractures often present with different functional limitations. The most common dysfunctions after humeral shaft fractures might be associated with altered scapulohumeral rhythm and radial nerve palsy.

One of the primary functions of the scapulothoracic articulation is to orient the glenoid fossa for optimal glenohumeral joint contact. The normal resting position of the scapula is oriented on average 2 in lateral from the midline and vertically between the second and seventh ribs.[9] The scapula, at rest, is tilted anteriorly 10° to 20°, internally rotated 30° to 35° from the coronal plane, and upwardly rotated 10° to 20° from the vertical plane.[9] The complex orientation of the scapula is integral for full ROM (range of motion) of the shoulder. With overhead activities, the coordinated movement of the scapula and arm is required to prevent subacromial impingement. Scapulohumeral rhythm is the integration of the scapulothoracic joint and glenohumeral joint contributions to overall shoulder ROM. During the initial 90° of arm abduction/elevation, the glenohumeral joint to scapulothoracic joint motion is in a 2:1 ratio. Beyond 90°, the ratio changes to 1:1 glenohumeral joint and scapulothoracic joint.[9] This is accomplished by an intricate activation pattern of the periscapular musculature. Maintaining the scapulohumeral rhythm can allow for optimal force production between the periscapular muscles to achieve normal upper extremity functional movement. Refer to **Tables 13.1** and **13.2** for the normal ROM values of the shoulder and elbow. It is important not only to understand the full normal ROM values but also to know the minimum ROM requirements of the upper extremity for functional activities of daily living (ADLs).

TREATMENT GOALS

The shoulder complex and elbow motions are very important for the human daily activities, such as eating, drinking, brushing teeth, combing hair, self-dressing, and driving. It is often very difficult for individuals to perform the basic daily function after injuries. Gopura et al conducted a study on human upper limb muscle activities during

TABLE 13.1 Shoulder Range of Motion

Motion	Normal[10]	Functional for Basic ADLs[10,11]	Associated Basic Daily Functions[11,12]
Abduction	180°	108°~120°	Reaching over head
Adduction	45°	30°	Putting earring on the opposite side
Flexion	180°	120°	Reaching over head
Extension	60°	40°	Hand to back pocket
Internal rotation with arm at side	100°	80°	Hand to back pocket
Internal rotation with arm at 90° of abduction	80°	45°	Reaching mid back
External rotation with arm at side	70°	30°	Putting earring on the same side
External rotation with arm at 90° of abduction	90°	45°	Washing or combing hair

ADLs, activities of daily living.

Data from Hoppenfeld S, Murthy VL. Treatment and Rehabilitation of Fractures. Philadelphia, PA: Lippincott Williams & Wilkins; 2000, Gates DH, Walters LS, Cowley J, Wilken JM, Resnik L. Range of motion requirements for upper-limb activities of daily living. Am J Occup Ther. 2016;70(1):7001350010p1-7001350010p10. doi:10.5014/ ajot.2016.015487, and Smith J, Dahm DL, Kaufman KR, et al. Electromyographic activity in the immobilized shoulder girdle musculature during scapulothoracic exercises. Arch Phys Med Rehabil. 2006;87(7):923-927. doi:10.1016/j.apmr.2006.03.013.

TABLE 13.2 Elbow Range of Motion

Motion	Normal[10]	Functional for Basic ADLs[10,11]	Associated Basic Daily Functions[11,12]
Flexion	135°	120°	Drinking from a cup
Extension	5°	−20° ~ −30°	Pushing off the chair
Pronation	90°	50°	Typing on the computer
Supination	90°	50°	Perineal care

ADLs, activities of daily living.
Data from Hoppenfeld S, Murthy VL. Treatment and Rehabilitation of Fractures. Philadelphia, PA: Lippincott Williams & Wilkins; 2000, Gates DH, Walters LS, Cowley J, Wilken JM, Resnik L. Range of motion requirements for upper-limb activities of daily living. Am J Occup Ther. 2016;70(1):7001350010p1-7001350010p10. doi:10.5014/ajot.2016.015487, and Smith J, Dahm DL, Kaufman KR, et al. Electromyographic activity in the immobilized shoulder girdle musculature during scapulothoracic exercises. Arch Phys Med Rehabil. 2006;87(7):923-927. doi:10.1016/j.apmr.2006.03.013.

daily functional motions.[13] According to the researchers, simple activities such as drinking from a cup involve a combination of elbow flexion, scapular protraction, shoulder internal rotation, flexion, and abduction along with forearm pronation, wrist flexion, and radial deviation.[12,13] Treatment goals for humeral shaft fractures should focus on the complete restoration of upper limb function. A team approach among orthopaedic surgeons, primary care physicians, nurse practitioners, physician assistants, and physical and occupational therapists is the key for maximizing patients' functional recovery and preventing secondary complications after the injuries.

ORTHOPAEDIC OBJECTIVES

ALIGNMENT/STABILITY

The humerus can tolerate a substantial amount of malalignment before compromising function or becoming cosmetically apparent. This is largely due to shoulder and elbow ROM, which compensates for any residual deformity.[14,15] The following parameters are the classic tolerances for humeral shaft fractures: anterior angulation of 20°, varus/valgus of 30°, rotation of 15°, and shortening of up to 3 cm. When healed, the diaphysis of the humerus should be stable in weight bearing (eg, while doing push-ups, crutches, etc). In addition, there should be shoulder and elbow ROM without motion at the fracture site.

REHABILITATION OBJECTIVES

The focus of rehabilitation following a humeral shaft fracture is on restoration of shoulder complex, elbow, wrist, and hand function. At the time of starting therapeutic interventions, rehabilitation should be designed to regain ROM at surrounding joints and articulations, improve soft tissue

and scar tissue flexibility, restore muscle strength and earlier identification of complications, such as heterotrophic ossification and radial nerve palsy, etc.

The ROM goals for the upper limbs should always be put in the context of individual functional demands during daily living (see **Tables 13.1** and **13.2**).

FUNCTIONAL GOALS

Functional goals include improving and restoring the function of the involved extremity in self-care and personal hygiene at minimum. It is important to keep in mind that small but significant ROM difference between the right and left limbs during daily functional activities might also affect patient satisfaction when addressing functional goals.[11] It is also vital to regain full muscle strength and ROM in the upper extremity for almost all sports activities. Ultimately, attempts to regain strength to five out of five in manual muscle testing should be carried out for all the major muscles given below (not limited to):

- Pectoralis major: shoulder adductor
- Deltoid: shoulder flexor, extensor, and abductor
- Biceps: elbow flexor, forearm supinator, and shoulder flexor
- Triceps: elbow extensor and shoulder adduction

NONOPERATIVE TREATMENT

The treatment of choice for the majority of humeral shaft fractures is nonoperative management. There are many methods to immobilize the humerus such as with a sling/swathe, Velpeau bandage, coaptation splint, hanging cast, and functional bracing. The most common method consists of acute stabilization of the fracture in coaptation splint followed by transition to a functional brace once swelling subsides.[16] The other methods are rarely used and will not be covered in this chapter.

COAPTATION SPLINT

A coaptation splint is a well-padded splint that starts in the axilla, travels around the elbow, and ends just above the shoulder. A valgus mold should be placed on the splint to prevent the weight of the forearm deforming the fracture into varus (**Figure 13.4**). The splint provides relative stability to the fracture while also allowing for the initial swelling of the extremity. Pay special attention to the axilla to make sure splint is well padded to avoid soft tissue breakdown. Also stress the importance of maintaining an upright or semiupright body position to aid in fracture alignment. The patient should be instructed to use only the unaffected extremity for ADLs. The splint is worn for 1 to 2 weeks or until the soft tissue swelling has subsided. Note, shoulder and elbow ROM are not possible with this splint, so transition to functional brace should occur as soon as soft tissues allow. Radiographs should be obtained before or after transitioning to a functional brace to verify the fracture is still within nonoperative limits.[17,18]

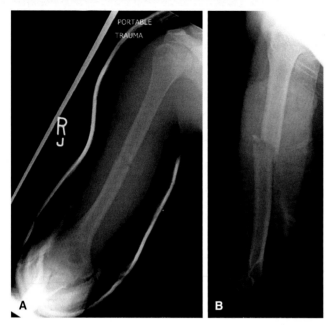

FIGURE 13.4 Anteroposterior (**A**) and lateral (**B**) radiographs of a humeral shaft in a coaptation splint. Note the valgus mold at the fracture site preventing the arm from deforming into varus. (Courtesy of Evan Rhea, MD.)

FUNCTIONAL BRACING

In 1977, Sarmiento et al described using a functional brace for the treatment of humeral shaft fractures and it is the preferred method for nonoperative treatment of these fractures.[18] The brace consists of two plastic sleeves held together with Velcro that allows for easy adjustment. The sleeves span the arm from 5 cm distal to the axilla to 5 cm proximal to the olecranon. As another option to or if prefabricated splints are not available, many occupational therapists (preferably a certified hand therapist) can make a custom thermoplastic orthosis. The patient can now begin passive and active elbow exercises. The patient is instructed to adjust the brace as needed to account for resolving soft tissue swelling. The advantage of the brace is that it allows the shoulder and elbow to remain free, thus preventing stiffness.[17] This freedom also allows the flexor and extensor muscles of the arm to exert a hydraulic force within their soft-tissue compartments on the fracture site, stabilizing the fracture for healing. The hydraulic forces exerted on the fracture by the muscles are an integral aspect of nonoperative treatment of humeral shaft fractures, hence their use is contraindicated in individuals with loss of muscle control such as brachial plexus injury or flail arm.

The brace should be worn at all times (**Figure 13.5**). Shoulder abduction is limited to 60° to 70° until callus is evident on radiographs. The brace is discontinued once the fracture has united radiographically and shoulder abduction is pain free, usually in 10 to 12 weeks.[17,18] Reported union rates with this method are 96% to 100%.[17-19] Many studies have found functional bracing to be noninferior to surgical fixation in regard to functional outcomes.[16,20,21] Reported nonunion rates range from 2% to 20.6% in closed fractures and 6% in open fractures.[17,21-24]

Collaboration and communication within the health care team is vital in fracture management. For optimal rehabilitation, the referring provider should specify the following items on the therapy orders: weight bearing status, ROM limitations to shoulder and elbow, and brace/splint wear schedule (ie, whether clients can remove it during self-care tasks or they must wear it full time). **Table 13.3** provides general rehabilitation guidelines for nonoperatively treated fractures at various stages of healing.

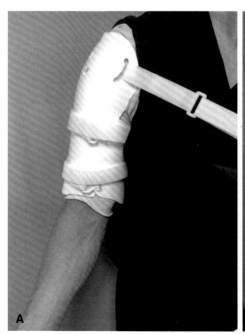
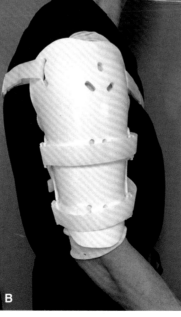

FIGURE 13.5 Anterior (**A**) and lateral (**B**) views of an example of a functional brace for humeral shaft fractures.

TABLE 13.3 Rehabilitation Guidelines for Nonoperative Treatment

	0-2 wk	2-6 wk	6-12 wk
Precautions	• Non–weight bearing • No lifting/pushing pulling with involved extremity	MD to clarify healing and if increased weight bearing and ROM to shoulder and elbow allowed	After 6 wk x-ray, MD to clarify weight bearing and lifting status
Modalities	Cold pack	Cold pack, moist heat	Continue previous as needed
Orthosis	Coaptation	Sarmiento or functional brace if fracture still within nonoperative limits	MD to determine after x-ray if further stabilization required
ROM	A/AAROM/PROM to FA, wrist, hand, scapula, cervical spine	• Continue previous • Add elbow and shoulder A/AAROM/PROM per MD clearance • Shoulder ABD limited to 60°-70°	• Continue previous • If fracture healing appropriately, full shoulder ROM
Strengthening	Grip strengthening as tolerated	• Continue previous • Light strengthening to scapula (focus on serratus anterior and low trap), see exercise examples within MD lifting restrictions • Light strengthening to wrist/FA within MD lifting restrictions	• If fracture healing progressing and MD allows increased lifting • Progress periscapular and rotator cuff strengthening • Progress wrist/FA/hand strengthening
Patient education	• ADL modifications and adaptive equipment use as needed with basic self-care • Lifting and weight bearing restrictions • Edema reduction • A/AAROM/PROM to uninvolved joints • Avoid scapular malpositioning • Role of therapy	• Continue previous • Add ROM exercises to shoulder and elbow as stated above • Educate on light use with ADLs	• HEP to emphasize full ROM if not achieved throughout involved UE • Strengthening exercises as stated above • Continue to educate of modifications to ADLs as needed within MD restrictions
Rehabilitation goals	• Decrease pain and edema • Prevent unnecessary joint contracture and muscle weakness in uninvolved areas • Maximize ADL independence within restrictions	• Progress ROM per MD orders • Progress strengthening in uninvolved joints • Progress to light use with ADLs	• Full ROM throughout entire UE • Regain strength of entire extremity • Maximize return to independent ADL status

A/AAROM, active/active assistive range of motion; ADL, activities of daily living; HEP, home exercise programs; PROM, passive range of motion; ROM, range of motion.

Special accommodations should be considered if a patient has an associated radial nerve palsy. Please refer to "Humeral Shaft Fractures Associated with Radial Nerve Palsy" section later in the chapter for complete instructions. At minimum, a wrist brace to prevent contractures as well as close monitoring of nerve recovery is required. Fabrication of a custom radial nerve orthosis by a certified hand therapist will allow functional use of the affected hand/wrist until nerve functioning returns.

OPERATIVE TREATMENT

While nonoperative treatment is successful in many humeral shaft fractures, there are situations where operative treatment is indicated. Definitive indications include loss of acceptable alignment in a brace. Open fractures with severe contamination require debridement in order to decrease the risk of infection. Skin damage that precludes bracing requires operative fixation so that skin may be exposed for wound care. Vascular injuries requiring repair necessitate fixation of the humerus in order to protect the repair.[25] Brachial plexus injuries limit the ability of the arm's musculature to provide hydraulic compression through the fracture site, thus rendering functional bracing ineffective and operative fixation is required.[26] Ipsilateral forearm fractures (floating elbow) and pathologic fracture when patient's life expectancy is greater than 6 months are other indications for surgery.[27,28] While radial nerve injury in a closed fracture is not an indication for surgery, loss of radial nerve function after closed manipulation is an indication for surgical exploration as the nerve is presumed to be entrapped in the fracture site.[29] Relative indications for surgery include polytrauma patients or those with bilateral humerus fractures in order to allow for immediate weight bearing and facilitate rehabilitation.[30]

Operative fixation in general has advantages over bracing. It helps avoid malunion in patients who will be lying recumbent for long periods of time due to other injuries. Not having to wear a splint also allows for easier nursing care and is more comfortable for the patient.[28]

PLATE FIXATION

Plate fixation is often the preferred method of surgical fixation for humeral shaft fractures. One main advantage from a rehab perspective is that open reduction internal fixation with a narrow 4.5 mm dynamic compression plate allows for immediate weight bearing with no effect on union or malunion rates.[30] Dual plating of smaller humeri with two small fragment plates also confers similar stability as larger plates.[31] Plate fixation is especially helpful in patients with additional lower extremity injuries who can now use the injured upper extremity to assist with weight bearing and transfers. In addition, the patient can now perform active ROM and avoid joint stiffness.[28]

Postoperative care includes placing the arm in a sling for support. Most surgeons will recommend starting gentle ROM 2 to 3 days after surgery. However, it is not uncommon for surgeons to limit weight bearing for 3 to 4 weeks despite recent literature supporting immediate weight bearing. If the minimally invasive plate osteosynthesis technique has been used, the surgeon may limit active rotation of the arm until callus is visible due to the instability of this construct compared to dynamic compression plating (**Figure 13.6**). Elbow flexion and extension and shoulder pendulums can still be started immediately after surgery.[32]

INTRAMEDULLARY NAIL

Proximally and distally locked intramedullary nails are another load-sharing implant that confers the same rehabilitation advantage as plates and allows for immediate weight bearing postoperatively. A unique advantage nails have over plates is that they allow for better soft tissue and blood supply preservation.[33] Multiple studies have demonstrated similar union rates and incidence of radial nerve injury when comparing nails versus plates.[34-36] However, the use of nails has recently declined.[37] This could be attributed to the higher incidence of postoperative shoulder impingement and rates of reoperation seen in antegrade humeral nails.[34-36] Shoulder pain is attributed to rotator cuff injury, which occurs when establishing the starting point for the nail. One solution for this problem is to perform retrograde nailing and avoid entering the shoulder. However, while this technique demonstrates preserved shoulder function, it is associated with worse elbow function compared to antegrade nailing.[38] Knowledge of what nailing technique was utilized can help emphasize the joints to focus on during postoperative rehabilitation.

Postoperative care for interlocked nails includes placing the patient in a sling for support (**Figure 13.7**). Pendulums and active motion of the shoulder and elbow should begin on the second postoperative day; however, some surgeons may wish to limit active external rotation until callus is visible. Patients can start using crutches when their pain allows, but full weight bearing through the extremity should not begin until signs of fracture healing are evident.[39] However,

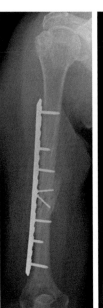
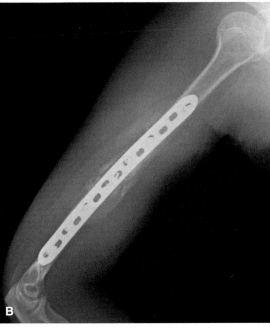

A   B

FIGURE 13.6 Anteroposterior (**A**) and lateral (**B**) radiographs of a humeral shaft fracture 11 weeks after open reduction internal fixation with a plate. Note the callous formation about the fracture site.

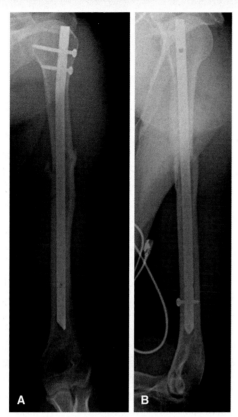

FIGURE 13.7 Anteroposterior (**A**) and lateral (**B**) radiographs of a humeral shaft fracture after antegrade intramedullary nail fixation.

if the nail is only locked on one end or completely unlocked, then active motion in all planes and weight bearing are limited until radiographic signs of healing are present, typically 3 to 4 weeks postoperatively.[40,41] These patients are allowed to start passive motion of the shoulder and elbow immediately. Some surgeons will also place a brace or plaster splint for 3 to 6 weeks postoperatively for added stability.[40]

EXTERNAL FIXATION

External fixation is utilized in cases with severe soft-tissue injury that precludes internal fixation or bracing, damage control in polytrauma patients, and for infected nonunions (**Figure 13.8**). It is mainly used as a provisional means of fracture stabilization and is the less preferred option for definitive fixation compared to the previously discussed treatment options. However, it can be used for definitive fixation when necessary and have good outcomes.[42,43]

Postoperative care includes immediate active ROM of the shoulder and elbow.[43,44] Weight bearing is typically limited until callus is evident on radiographs. Daily pin site care should be taken using a mixture of sterile saline and hydrogen peroxide to prevent infection. The skin around the pin sites should be checked daily for signs of drainage, erythema, or tenting. It may be necessary to release the skin with small incision if excessive tension from a pin is damaging the skin.[42] The external fixator is removed once the fracture has healed which usually occurs around 12 weeks postoperatively.[43]

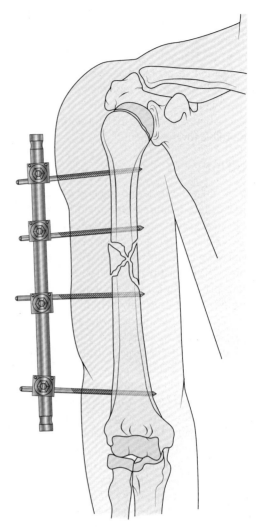

FIGURE 13.8 An external fixator used as treatment for a comminuted diaphyseal humeral fracture. Care must be taken not to injure the radial nerve when inserting the fixator pins. (From Catagni MA, Lovisetti L, Guerreschi F, et al. The external fixation in the treatment of humeral diaphyseal fractures: outcomes of 84 cases. *Injury.* 2010;41(11):1107-1111.)

POSTOPERATIVE REHABILITATION

Rehabilitation after postoperative management for humeral shaft fractures will be slightly different from nonoperative management due to the disruption of surrounding soft tissue during surgery and improved stability at the fracture sites with hardware (**Table 13.4**). Variability of incision sites might determine where and how to address related secondary soft tissue trauma after surgeries. The eight most common approaches utilized are the anterolateral approach, lateral approach, posterior approach, distal posterior approach, MIO approach, antegrade nailing approach, retrograde nailing approach, and percutaneous instrumentation.[45] The choice of surgical approaches is based on types and extensiveness of the injuries and

TABLE 13.4 Rehabilitation Guidelines After Operative Treatment

	0-2 wk	2-6 wk	6-12 wk	12 wk and up
Precautions	Non–weight bearing (NWB) or per MD	NWB or per MD	• Weight bearing at tolerance (WBAT) or per MD • No contact sports	WBAT or per MD
Modalities	Cold pack, IFC, pre-mod E-stim (see Chapter 12)	IFC, pre-mod, NMES (see Chapter 12)	Heat, NMES only if needed (see Chapter 12)	Discontinue
Orthosis	Sling	• May discontinue sling • May continue radial nerve palsy splint if needed	Discontinue sling and supportive device if it is appropriate	Discontinue
ROM	• Active/active assistive range of motion (A/AAROM) to forearm, wrist, hand as well as scapular depression, protraction, and retraction • Clarification from MD regarding ROM to GH and elbow joints depending on surgical fixation	• A/AAROM to tolerance at shoulder, elbow, wrist, and hand • Allow gentle activities of daily living (ADLs)	• Begin and progress on gentle passive range of motion (PROM) • Continue A/AAROM at shoulder complex and elbow joints	Nearly full ROM in all associated joints
Strengthening	None	Parascapular muscles and wrist and hand in open kinetic chain exercises only	Progress into resistive exercises in both closed kinetic and open kinetic chain	Progress to isotonic, plyometric exercises
Patient education	• ADL modifications and adaptive equipment use as needed with basic self-care • Lifting and weight bearing restrictions • Edema and pain reduction • A/AAROM/PROM to uninvolved joints • Avoid poor postural positioning with brace • Role of therapy	• Scar management • Basic self-care modification according to the weight bearing restriction • Edema and pain reduction • Identify and address potential emotional and psychological issues • Transportation management	• Length and nature of normal tissue healing • Progress in home exercise programs (HEPs) to reflect on weekly treatment progression	Safety and limitation before return to sports
Rehabilitation Goals	• Identifying, addressing, and preventing secondary impairments • Coordinating plan of care with providers	• Progress ROM, strength and function • Prevent secondary complications	• Gradually restore normal joint motion and muscle strength • Progress to previous level of function	Maximize functional return

surgeon's preference.[45] There is little evidence-based literature regarding optimal postoperative rehabilitation following humeral shaft fracture. **Table 13.4** includes general guidelines. Clinical decision-making should be based upon the therapist's critical reasoning skills and surgeon's preferences according to tissue healing and types of fixations. Commonly protocols or guidelines are suggested based upon the therapist's experiences and surgeon's preferences according to tissue healing and types of fixations. The secondary impairments resulted from surgical interventions will be an important rehabilitation guide, which will also significantly affect short- and long-term functional outcomes.

HUMERAL SHAFT FRACTURES ASSOCIATED WITH RADIAL NERVE PALSY

ORTHOPAEDIC CONSIDERATIONS

The incidence of radial nerve palsy in humeral shaft fractures ranges from 1.8% in proximal fractures to 23.6% in distal third fractures with an overall injury rate of 11%.

Nerve injury is more common in spiral and transverse fracture patterns.[46] It presents with inability to extend the wrist, fingers, or thumb and diminished sensation to the dorsoradial aspect of the hand in the distribution of the superficial branch of the radial nerve.

Radial nerve palsy in closed fractures is typically a transient neuropraxia due to a stretch injury or contusion.[46,47] Therefore, observation is indicated as the initial treatment of a radial nerve palsy associated with a closed humeral shaft fracture. Indications for early nerve exploration are controversial but should strongly be considered in the following scenarios: open fractures, high-energy trauma, penetrating trauma (knife), vascular injury, and/or nerve palsy after attempted closed reduction due to possible entrapment.[46,48-50] Note, radial nerve exploration is not suggested for a palsy occurring after a low velocity gunshot wound. In contrast, many would consider exploration for palsies due to high-velocity gunshot wounds.

Of radial nerve palsies associated with closed humeral shaft fractures, 70% show spontaneous recovery at an average of 7 weeks.[46] The brachioradialis is first to recover and is tested with radial deviation and wrist extension. The extensor indicis proprius is the last to recover and is tested with index finger extension. If no recovery is seen on physical examination within 2 to 3 months, then an electromyography (EMG) is performed to evaluate the status of the nerve. Repeat evaluation should occur in another 12 weeks as it can take up to 6 months to regain nerve function.[46] Clinically, recovery of nerve function can be tested with a Tinel sign. An advancing Tinel sign is a positive prognostic indicator of returning nerve activity.[50] If EMG fails to show signs of recovery at 4 to 6 months, then surgical exploration with nerve repair or grafting is indicated.[50] In the event of failed radial nerve salvage at 1 year, there are a variety of tendon transfers that can restore function of the wrist and digit extensors.[50]

The ulnar and median nerves are rarely associated with humeral shaft fractures. One study found the incidence of ulnar injury to be 2.4% and median nerve injury to be 1.3% in humeral shaft fractures.[51]

TEAM CONSIDERATIONS

The therapist may need to fabricate a custom radial nerve palsy orthosis to prevent muscle tendon lengthening/joint contractures and optimize ADL independence until nerve function returns. If the therapist is not proficient in fabricating custom orthoses, there are commercially available prefabricated radial nerve palsy orthoses. Examples of low-profile, custom-fabricated orthoses are given (**Figures 13.9** and **13.10**). The low-profile designs are more client friendly allowing increased don/doffing and aid in dressing in long sleeve shirts/jackets. To prevent metacarpophalangeal (MCP) extension contractures, patients can wear a cock-up wrist or resting hand orthosis at night. If a resting hand orthosis is chosen, the MCPs should be placed in approximately 70° of flexion and PIPs and DIPs (proximal and distal interphalangeal joints) in full extension. The thumb should be placed in palmar abduction.

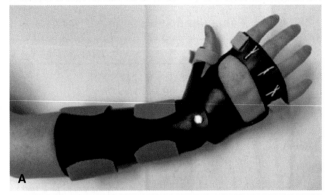

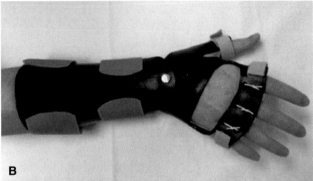

FIGURE 13.9 Radial nerve palsy orthosis. (Reproduced with permission from Peck J, Ollason J. Low profile radial nerve palsy orthosis with radial and ulnar deviation. *J Hand Ther.* 2015;28:421-424.)

The treating therapist will continue to monitor for return of nerve function, address returning muscle function deficits, and continue to modify the orthosis as needed. Ideally, joint contractures will be prevented making progression through passive and active ROM to full strengthening a smooth transition.

A home exercise program including PROM emphasizing MCP flexion, PIP/DIP extension, thumb carpometacarpal radial and palmar abduction, and wrist extension should be taught to the patient and performed three to four times a day when removing the orthosis. The orthosis can be reduced to hand based once wrist extension returns. Any other joint contractures that are noted should also be addressed and emphasized as part of the program. The home exercise program plays an important role in patient outcomes as some patients may not be seen frequently in the clinic due to multiple factors (ie, client situation, insurance factors, financial factors, etc).

OTHER ASSOCIATED INJURIES

VESSELS

Brachial artery injuries associated with humeral shaft fractures can be devastating. The presence of a diaphyseal humerus fracture triples the risk of amputation when compared to an isolated brachial artery injury due to penetrating trauma.[52] Immediate debridement, vascular repair, and bony

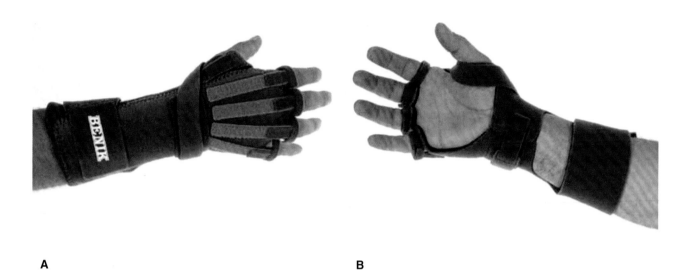

A **B**

FIGURE 13.10 Anterior (**A**) and posterior (**B**) views of a prefabricated Benik radial nerve palsy orthosis. (Reproduced with permission from Benik Corporation.)

stabilization with either external fixation or plate fixation are indicated based on the severity of soft-tissue contamination.[25] Fasciotomy should also be considered to prevent reperfusion-induced compartment syndrome.

OTHER SOFT-TISSUE INJURIES

The mechanism of injury determines the extent of muscle damage. Industrial accidents, motor vehicle accidents, and open injuries will likely cause more soft-tissue and muscle damage than a discrete blow or a single penetrating injury. It should be noted that up to 63% of patients with a humeral shaft fracture have concomitant shoulder pathology present at the time of injury. These injuries can be exacerbated by the traumatic event and should be identified and addressed during rehabilitation for optimal outcomes.[53]

SPECIAL CONSIDERATION OF THE FRACTURE

OPEN FRACTURES

The severity of soft-tissue injury and contamination will determine the most appropriate treatment in open humeral shaft fractures. The Gustilo-Anderson classification is commonly used to classify these injuries[54]:

- Type I: low-energy injury, typically an inside-out puncture wound to the skin caused by the fracture.
- Type II: higher velocity injury, and the wound is greater than 1 cm without extensive soft-tissue damage, flaps, or avulsions.
- Type III: severe injury with extensive soft-tissue damage that is further divided into three subgroups: (1) with

adequate soft tissue coverage, (2) with significant soft-tissue loss with periosteal stripping and bone exposure that will require flap coverage, and (3) with vascular injury that will require repair.

Early initiation of antibiotics is essential in all open fractures. A first-generation cephalosporin is indicated in type I and II open fractures while type III fractures should be treated with a first-generation cephalosporin and an aminoglycoside.[55] Formal operative debridement is indicated in all open fractures. The more severe the soft-tissue injury, the more appropriate the treatment with external fixation, either as a temporizing measure or definitive treatment. Low-grade open injuries can be managed with immediate plate or rodding techniques at the same time as the operative debridement.[56-58]

PATHOLOGIC FRACTURES

The humerus is the second most common long bone affected by metastatic disease and the incidence of pathologic fractures ranges from 16% to 27%.[59] Goals of surgical fixation include pain relief, immediate stabilization of the extremity for optimal function, or preventing impending fracture. Intramedullary nails and plating are both treatment options for diaphyseal lesions. Intramedullary nails provide the advantage of splinting the entire bone when used to prophylax against an impending fracture.[60,61]

MULTIPLE TRAUMA PATIENTS

Seriously consider operative stabilization of humeral shaft fractures in polytrauma patients that would otherwise be treated nonoperatively in isolation. Operative fixation allows for immediate weight bearing and facilitates rehabilitation. This can be achieved with either plate or intramedullary nail fixation with no adverse effects on outcomes.[28,30,31] It also helps avoid malunion in patients who will be lying recumbent for long periods of time due to other injuries. Not having to wear a splint allows for easier nursing care and is more comfortable for the patient.[28]

AGE

Elderly patients may be more difficult to immobilize because they are less able to tolerate treatment (eg, they are more vulnerable to axillary irritation from a coaptation splint). Elderly patients in particular need early, aggressive rehabilitation to avoid loss of joint motion. The shoulder and elbow are particularly susceptible when closed treatment is undertaken because of immobilization by the coaptation splint. A case-by-case discussion should be held with the patient and family to determine whether surgical intervention or functional bracing is desired.

CONCLUSION

In summary, humeral shaft fractures are common injuries that are encountered frequently by orthopaedic surgeons and rehabilitation specialists. The mainstay of treatment is conservative, nonoperative management with a coaptation splint followed by functional bracing. It is important to instruct patients on weight bearing limitations as well as emphasize the importance of active elbow ROM to aid in fracture healing while wearing a functional brace. However, operative treatment is indicated at times and has the advantage of allowing early weight bearing when dynamic compression plating is utilized for stable fracture patterns. Regardless of the treatment utilized, explicit communication regarding weight bearing status, ROM limitations, and brace/splint wear schedule between surgeons and therapists is imperative for optimal patient outcomes. In addition, elbow and digital ROM should only be delayed as long as absolutely necessary to prevent secondary stiffness.

HIGH YIELD POINTS

- Humeral shaft fractures are relatively common accounting for approximately 20% of all fractures.
- The treatment of choice for the majority of humeral shaft fractures is nonoperative management with acute stabilization in a coaptation splint followed by transition to a functional brace once swelling subsides.
- Functional braces allow freedom for the flexor and extensor muscles of the arm to exert a hydraulic force within their soft-tissue compartments on the fracture site, stabilizing the fracture for healing.
- Operative intervention is indicated at times and includes plate fixation, intramedullary nailing, and external fixation.

- The focus of rehabilitation following a humeral shaft fracture is on restoration of shoulder complex, elbow, wrist, and hand function.
- The ROM goals for the upper limbs should always be put in the context of individual functional demands during daily living (see **Tables 13.1** and **13.2**). At a minimum, the goal is to restore function of the involved extremity in self-care and personal hygiene.
- There is little evidence-based literature regarding optimal postoperative rehabilitation following surgical intervention, so protocols are based upon therapist experience and surgeon preference according to tissue healing and types of fixations.
- The close proximity of the radial nerve along the posterior humerus puts it at risk with humeral shaft fractures.
- When humeral shaft fractures are associated with radial nerve palsies, a custom radial nerve palsy orthosis should be fabricated to prevent contractures and optimize ADL independence until nerve function returns (referral to a certified and therapist is recommended).
- Uncomplicated humeral shaft fractures typically achieve complete union by 12 weeks and the majority of radial nerve injuries will be showing signs of recovery at this point as well.
- Explicit communication regarding weight bearing status, ROM limitations, and brace/splint wear schedule between surgeons and therapists is imperative for optimal patient outcomes.

REFERENCES

1. Rose SH, Melton LJ III, Morrey BF, Ilstrup DM, Riggs BL. Epidemiologic features of humeral fractures. *Clin Orthop.* 1982;168:24-30.
2. Ekholm R, Adami J, Tidermark J, Hansson K, Törnkvist H, Ponzer S. Fractures of the shaft of the humerus. An epidemiological study of 401 fractures. *J Bone Joint Surg Br* 2006;88:1469-1473. doi:10.1302/0301-620X.88B11.17634.
3. Bumbasirevic M, Palibrk T, Lesic A, Atkinson HDE. Radial nerve palsy. *EFORT Open Rev.* 2016;1:286-294. doi:10.1302/2058-5241.1.000028.
4. Gerwin M, Hotchkiss RN, Weiland AJ. Alternative operative exposures of the posterior aspect of the humeral diaphysis with reference to the radial nerve. *J Bone Joint Surg Am.* 1996;78:1690-1695.
5. Guse TR, Ostrum RF. The surgical anatomy of the radial nerve around the humerus. *Clin Orthop Relat Res.* 1995;320:149-153.
6. Klepps S, Auerbach J, Calhon O, Lin J, Cleeman E, Flatow E. A cadaveric study on the anatomy of the deltoid insertion and its relationship to the deltopectoral approach to the proximal humerus. *J Shoulder Elbow Surg.* 2004;13:322-327. doi:10.1016/j.jse.2003.12.014.
7. Zlotolow DA, Catalano LW, Barron OA, Glickel SZ. Surgical exposures of the humerus. *J Am Acad Orthop Surg.* 2006;14:754-765. doi:10.5435/00124635-200612000-00007.
8. Holstein A, Lewis GF. Fractures of the humerus with radial-nerve paralysis. *J Bone Joint Surg Am.* 1963;45:1382-1388.
9. Levangie PK, Norkin CC. *Joint Structure and Function: A Comprehensive Analysis.* 5th ed. Philadelphia, PA: FA Davis Company; 2011.
10. Hoppenfeld S, Murthy VL. *Treatment and Rehabilitation of Fractures.* Philadelphia, PA: Lippincott Williams & Wilkins; 2000.
11. Gates DH, Walters LS, Cowley J, Wilken JM, Resnik L. Range of motion requirements for upper-limb activities of daily living. *Am J Occup Ther.* 2016;70(1):7001350010p1-7001350010p10. doi:10.5014/ajot.2016.015487.

12. Smith J, Dahm DL, Kaufman KR, et al. Electromyographic activity in the immobilized shoulder girdle musculature during scapulothoracic exercises. *Arch Phys Med Rehabil.* 2006;87(7):923-927. doi:10.1016/j.apmr.2006.03.013.

13. Gopura RARC, Kiguchi K, Horikawa E. A study on human upper-limb muscles activities during daily upper-limb motions. *Int J Biolectromagn.* 2010;12(2):54-61.

14. Klenerman L. Fractures of the shaft of the humerus. *J Bone Joint Surg Br.* 1966;48:105-111.

15. Shields E, Sundem L, Childs S, et al. The impact of residual angulation on patient reported functional outcome scores after non-operative treatment for humeral shaft fractures. *Injury.* 2015;47:1-5. doi:10.1016/j.injury.2015.12.014.

16. Koch PP, Gross DF, Gerber C. The results of functional (Sarmiento) bracing of humeral shaft fractures. *J Shoulder Elbow Surg* 2002;11:143-150. doi:10.1067/mse.2002.121634.

17. Sarmiento A, Zagorski JB, Zych GA, Latta LL, Capps CA. Functional bracing for the treatment of fractures of the humeral diaphysis. *J Bone Joint Surg Am.* 2000;82:478-486.

18. Sarmiento A, Kinman PB, Galvin EG, Schmitt RH, Phillips JG. Functional bracing of fractures of the shaft of the humerus. *J Bone Joint Surg Am.* 1977;59:596-601.

19. Balfour GW, Mooney V, Ashby M. Diaphyseal fractures of the humerus treated with a readymade fracture brace. *J Bone Joint Surg Am.* 1982;64:11-13.

20. Shields E, Sundem L, Childs S, et al. Factors predicting patient-reported functional outcome scores after humeral shaft fractures. *Injury* 2015;46:693-698. doi:10.1016/j.injury.2015.01.027.

21. Matsunaga FT, Tamaoki MJ, Matsumoto MH, Netto NA, Faloppa F, Belloti JC. Minimally invasive osteosynthesis with a bridge plate versus a functional brace for humeral shaft fractures: a randomized controlled trial. *J Bone Joint Surg Am* 2017;99:583-592. doi:10.2106/JBJS.16.00628.

22. Ostermann PAW, Ekkernkamp A, Muhr G. Functional bracing of shaft fractures of the humerus – an analysis of 195 cases. *Orthop Trans.* 1993-1994;17:937-946.

23. Sharma VK, Jain AK, Gupta RK, Tyagi AK, Sethi PK. Non-operative treatment of fractures of the humeral shaft: a comparative study. *J Indian Med Assn.* 1991;89:157-160.

24. Zagorski JB, Latta LL, Zych GA, Finnieston AR. Diaphyseal fractures of the humerus. Treatment with prefabricated braces. *J Bone Joint Surg.* 1988;70-A:607-610.

25. Paryavi E, Pensy RA, Higgins TF, Chia B, Eglseder WA. Salvage of upper extremities with humeral fracture and associated brachial artery injury. *Injury* 2014;45:1870-1875. doi:10.1016/j.injury.2014.08.038.

26. Brien WW, Gellman H, Becker V, Garland DE, Waters RL, Wiss DA. Management of fractures of the humerus in patients who have an injury of the ipsilateral brachial plexus. *J Bone Joint Surg.* 1990;72:1208-1210.

27. Muramatsu K, Ihara K, Iwanagaa R, Taguchi T. Treatment of metastatic bone lesions in the upper extremity: indications for surgery. *Orthopedics.* 2010;33:807.

28. Bell MJ, Beauchamp CG, Kellam JK, et al. The results of plating humeral shaft fractures in patients with multiple injuries. The Sunnybrook experience. *J Bone Joint Surg Br.* 1985;67(2):293-296.

29. Korompilias AV, Lykissas MG, Kostas-Agnantis IP, Vekris MD, Soucacos PN, Beris AE. Approach to radial nerve palsy caused by humerus shaft fracture: is primary exploration necessary? *Injury.* 2013;44:323-326. doi:10.1016/j.injury.2013.01.004.

30. Tingstad EM, Wolinsky PR, Shyr Y, Johnson KD. Effect of immediate weightbearing on plated fractures of the humeral shaft. *J Trauma.* 2000;49:278-280.

31. Kosmopoulos V, Luedke C, Nana AD. Dual small fragment plating improves screw-to-screw load sharing for mid-diaphyseal humeral fracture fixation: a finite element study. *Technol Health Care.* 2015;23:83-92. doi:10.3233/THC-140875.

32. Apivatthakakul T, Phornphutkul C, Laohapoonrungsee A, et al. Less invasive plate osteosynthesis in humeral shaft fractures. *Oper Orthop Traumatol.* 2009;21(6):602-613.

33. Wali MG, Baba AN, Latoo IA, Bhat NA, Baba OK, Sharma S. Internal fixation of shaft humerus fractures by dynamic compression plate or interlocking intramedullary nail: a prospective, randomised study. *Strateg Trauma Limb Reconstr* 2014;9:133-40. doi:10.1007/s11751-014-0204-0.

34. Kurup H, Hossain M, Andrew JG. Dynamic compression plating versus locked intramedullary nailing for humeral shaft fractures in adults. *Cochrane Database Syst Rev.* 2011;6:CD005959. doi:10.1002/14651858.CD005959.pub2.

35. Ma J, Xing D, Ma X, et al. Intramedullary nail versus dynamic compression plate fixation in treating humeral shaft fractures: grading the evidence through a meta-analysis. *PLoS One* 2013;8:e82075. doi:10.1371/journal.pone.0082075.

36. Ouyang H, Xiong J, Xiang P, Cui Z, Chen L, Yu B. Plate versus intramedullary nail fixation in the treatment of humeral shaft fractures: an updated meta-analysis. *J Shoulder Elbow Surg.* 2013;22:387-953. doi:10.1016/j.jse.2012.06.007.

37. Gottschalk MB, Carpenter W, Hiza E, Reisman W, Roberson J. Humeral shaft fracture fixation: incidence rates and complications as reported by American Board of Orthopaedic Surgery Part II Candidates. *J Bone Joint Surg Am.* 2016;98:e71. doi:10.2106/JBJS.15.01049.

38. Cheng HR, Lin J. Prospective randomized comparative study of antegrade and retrograde locked nailing for middle humeral shaft fracture. *J Trauma.* 2008;65:94-102. doi:10.1097/TA.0b013e31812eed7f.

39. Scheerlinck T, Handelberg F. Functional outcome after intramedullary nailing of humeral shaft fractures: comparison between retrograde Marchetti-Vicenzi and unreamed AO antegrade nailing. *J Trauma.* 2002;52(1):60-71.

40. Liebergall M, Jaber S, Laster M, et al. Ender nailing of acute humeral shaft fractures in multiple injuries. *Injury.* 1997;28(9-10):577-580.

41. Garnavos C, Lasanianos N, Kanakaris NK, et al. A new modular nail for the diaphyseal fractures of the humerus. *Injury.* 2009;40(6):604-610.

42. Scaglione M, Fabbri L, Dell'Omo D, Goffi A, Guido G. The role of external fixation in the treatment of humeral shaft fractures: a retrospective case study review on 85 humeral fractures. *Injury* 2015;46:265-269. doi:10.1016/j.injury.2014.08.045.

43. Catagni MA, Lovisetti L, Guerreschi F, et al. The external fixation in the treatment of humeral diaphyseal fractures: outcomes of 84 cases. *Injury.* 2010;41(11):1107-1111.

44. Ruland WO. Is there a place for external fixation in humeral shaft fractures? *Injury.* 2000;31(suppl 1):27-34.

45. Spiguel AR, Steffner RJ. Humeral shaft fractures. *Curr Rev Musculoskelet Med.* 2012;5(3):177-183. doi:10.1007/s12178-012-9125-z.

46. Shao YC, Harwood P, Grotz MR, Limb D, Giannoudis PV. Radial nerve palsy associated with fractures of the shaft of the humerus: a systematic review. *J Bone Joint Surg Br.* 2005;87(12):1647-1652.

47. Sonneveld GJ, Patka P, van Mourik JC, Broere G. Treatment of fractures of the shaft of the humerus accompanied by paralysis of the radial nerve. *Injury.* 1987;18(6):404-406.

48. Foster RJ, Swiontkowski MF, Bach AW, Sack JT. Radial nerve palsy caused by open humeral shaft fractures. *J Hand Surg Am.* 1993;18(1):121-124.

49. Ring D, Chin K, Jupiter JB. Radial nerve palsy associated with high-energy humeral shaft fractures. *J Hand Surg Am.* 2004;29(1):144-147.

50. Elton SG, Rizzo M. Management of radial nerve injury associated with humeral shaft fractures: An evidence-based approach. *J Reconstr Microsurg.* 2008;24(8):569-573.

51. Noble J, Munro CA, Prasad VS, et al. Analysis of upper and lower extremity peripheral nerve injuries in a population of patients with multiple injuries. *J Trauma.* 1998;45(1):116-122.

52. Debakey ME, Simeone FA. Battle injuries of the arteries in World War II: an analysis of 2,471 cases. *Ann Surg.* 1946;123:534-557.

53. O'Donnell TM, McKenna JV, Kenny P, et al. Concomitant injuries to the ipsilateral shoulder in patients with a fracture of the diaphysis of the humerus. *J Bone Joint Surg Br.* 2008;90(1):61-65.

54. Gustilo RB, Anderson JT. Prevention of infection in the treatment of one thousand and twenty-five open fractures of long bones: Retrospective and prospective analyses. *J Bone Joint Surg Am.* 1976;58(4):453-458.

55. Gustilo RB, Mendoza RM, Williams DN. Problems in the management of type III (severe) open fractures: a new classification of type III open fractures. *J Trauma.* 1984;24(8):742-746.

56. Connolly S, McKee MD, Zdero R, et al. Immediate plate osteosynthesis of open fractures of the humeral shaft. *J Trauma.* 2010;69(3):685-690.

57. Idoine JD III, French BG, Opalek JM, et al. Plating of acute humeral diaphyseal fractures through an anterior approach in multiple trauma patients. *J Orthop Trauma.* 2012;26(1):9-18.

58. Schoots IG, Simons MP, Nork SE, et al. Antegrade locked nailing of open humeral shaft fractures. *Orthopedics.* 2007;30(1):49-54.

59. Piccioli A, Maccauro G, Rossi B, et al. Surgical treatment of pathologic fractures of humerus. *Injury*. 2010;41(11):1112-1116.

60. Damron TA, Rock MG, Choudhury SN, Grabowski JJ, An KN. A biomechanical analysis of prophylactic fixation for middle third humeral impending pathological fractures. *Clin Orthop Relat Res*. 1999;363:240-248.

61. Sarahrudi K, Wolf H, Funovics P, et al. Surgical treatment of pathological fractures of the shaft of the humerus. *J Trauma*. 2009;66(3):789-794.

14

The Elbow

Michael Suk

Lisa G. M. Friedman

Ryan Corbin Zitzke

ANATOMY AND BIOMECHANICS

The proximal portions of the radius and ulna, together with the distal humerus, form the elbow joint. Flexion and extension occur through the ulnohumeral joint, which forms a ginglymoid joint and resembles a hinge. The radiohumeral and proximal radioulnar joints allow for axial rotation and a pivoting (trochoid) type of motion.[1] The normal arc of motion about the elbow is 0° to 145°, 80°, and 85° for flexion, pronation, and supination, respectively.[2] The normal valgus orientation of the ulnohumeral articulation forms the carrying angle, which is typically 10° in males, and approaches 13° in females.[3] Although the elbow affords a large arc of motion, most activities of daily living (ADLs) are performed within an arc of 30° to 130° of flexion and 50° each of pronation and supination.[4]

The distal humerus can be thought of as being composed of a medial and lateral column (**Figure 14.1**). The lateral supracondylar ridge gives rise to the lateral epicondyle, which serves as the attachment site of the lateral collateral ligament and the supinator-extensor muscle mass. The capitellum forms the joint surface of the distal humerus that articulates with the radial head and is nearly spherical in shape. Medially, the more prominent medial epicondyle serves as the origin of the medial ulnar collateral ligament and the flexor-pronator muscle mass. Distally, the spool-like trochlea articulates with the proximal ulna.[5] On average, the articular surface of the humerus is rotated 30° anteriorly, has a valgus tilts of 5° to 7°, and, when viewed on end, is externally rotated 3° to 5°.[4]

The radial head is cylindrical in shape, of which two-thirds of the circumference are covered in hyaline cartilage. The remaining portion of its circumference is devoid of cartilage and is thus without underlying strong subchondral bone.[4] Because of these characteristics, this region of the radial head is most susceptible to fracture.[6] To allow an arc of forearm rotation approaching 180°, the radial neck makes an angle of nearly 15° with respect to the radial tuberosity. Throughout this arc of motion, the radial head maintains a specific angular relationship with the capitellum, and any variations can dramatically alter forearm rotation.[7]

The proximal ulna can be thought of as having three distinct areas: the olecranon, the greater sigmoid notch, and the coronoid process (**Figure 14.2**). The olecranon is the most proximal structure and is the attachment site for the triceps tendon. Anteriorly, the greater sigmoid notch is covered with hyaline cartilage and articulates with the trochlea. The arc of motion at this joint is approximately 185°. The coronoid process serves as the distal border for the greater sigmoid notch and is the insertion site of the brachialis and the oblique cord.[5] To complement the aforementioned anterior rotation and valgus angulation of the distal humerus, the articular surface of the ulna is oriented 30° posteriorly and is in 5° to 7° of valgus angulation. This establishes a stable articulation to perform activities with the elbow extended.[7]

REHABILITATION OF FRACTURES AT THE ELBOW

The elbow serves as a load-bearing joint and allows for hand placement in space to facilitate activities such as eating, grooming, dressing, manipulating and reaching objects, pushing, pulling, catching, throwing, and lifting. In order to perform these activities well, the joint must be pain free and have the requisite stability, range of motion (ROM), and strength.[8-11] According to Morrey et al.,[8] an elbow requires 30° of elbow extension, 130° of flexion, and 50° of supination and pronation, for the patient to return to most functional activities.

Rehabilitation of postoperative distal humeral fractures is complex as several structures surrounding this joint contribute to the static and dynamic stability of the elbow. The articular surface of the elbow joint, as well as the collateral ligaments and capsule, provides the static stability, while the elbow flexors and extensors provide the dynamic stability.[9,12,13] If there is an injury to any of these structures, the elbow has a propensity to develop stiffness and contractures, particularly in flexion.

After an injury to the joint capsule, it can thicken as much as 3 to 4 mm due to extensive collagen cross-linking and contracture. This, in turn, can block flexion and tether extension.[9,14-17]

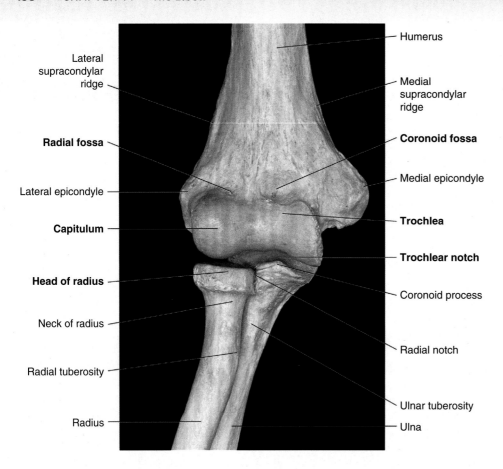

Lateral supracondylar ridge

Radial fossa

Lateral epicondyle

Capitulum

Head of radius

Neck of radius

Radial tuberosity

Radius

Humerus

Medial supracondylar ridge

Coronoid fossa

Medial epicondyle

Trochlea

Trochlear notch

Coronoid process

Radial notch

Ulnar tuberosity

Ulna

FIGURE 14.1 Anterior view of the osteology of the distal humerus. (Reproduced from Moses KP, Banks JC, Nava PB, Petersen DK. *Atlas of Clinical Gross Anatomy.* 2nd ed. Elsevier; 2013:232-247.)

The brachialis muscle, which is in contact with the capsule, can often scar down due to posttraumatic hematoma formation, further limiting ROM.[9,15,18] The patient also has a natural tendency of positioning the injured elbow in flexion, which when held between 70° and 100° of flexion, the collateral ligaments are on slack, which further encourages flexion contractures.[10,19] Additionally, scar tissue adherence of the triceps, as well as adaptive shortening of the biceps and forearm muscles, can also play a factor in loss of ROM at the elbow. Other reported reasons for loss of motion include severity of trauma, intra-articular trauma, heterotopic ossificans, and prolonged immobilization.[10,15]

The treating therapist must be able to identify and effectively treat any structures that may be contributing to loss of motion. See **Table 14.1** for other factors the treating therapist should consider when evaluating for loss of motion. The goal of rehabilitation is to protect healing structures and

Humerus

Lateral epicondyle

Capitulum of humerus

Medial epicondyle

Trochlea of humerus

Trochlear notch

Coronoid process

Head of radius

Radial notch

Neck

Tuberosity of ulna

Radial tuberosity

Radius

Ulna

FIGURE 14.2 Anterior view of the proximal radioulnar joint. (Reproduced from Hombach-Klonisch S, Klonisch T, Peeler J. *Sobotta Clinical Atlas of Human Anatomy*, one voume, Engish. 2019:83-151.)

TABLE 14.1 Postoperative Factors Physical and Occupational Therapists Should Consider in Evaluating for Loss of Elbow Range of Motion

- Adherent scar formation/incisional scars
- Postoperative edema
- Pain
- Muscle spasms
- Nerve compressions or neuropraxias
- Muscle weakness
- Cognitive/psychosocial factors that may inhibit patient education
- Status of wound

restore motion, strength, and stability, while remaining cognizant of the current stage of wound healing. Early, appropriate management is paramount to prevent fixed elbow contractures, poor functional outcomes, and decreased patient satisfaction.[9,11,16,17,20-24]

The following guidelines are for the postoperative rehabilitation of stable fixation of fractures of the distal humerus, proximal ulna, and radial head without associated ligament reconstruction or nerve injuries. Please see the "Special Considerations" section for further guidance if these structures need to be addressed.

Week 0 to 2 Post-Op: Inflammatory Stage

Rehabilitation Goals

The goals during this period are to minimize edema and scar adhesions; manage pain; protect the repair; and initiate active range of motion (AROM) exercises, patient education on therapy program and precautions, and a home exercise program (HEP).

During the first week of fracture healing (inflammatory stage), a fracture hematoma is developing, predominantly by inflammatory cells. No callous formation is yet noted. The stability of the fracture is afforded by the internal fixation only.

Therapy is initiated within 1 week of surgery. During the first few visits, therapy consists of teaching precautions regarding weight-bearing and lifting, instructions about the HEP consisting of ROM to uninvolved joints, and the management of pain and edema. ADLs modifications and adaptive aids need to be addressed so that the patient can continue modified independence with all self-care activities.

Week 2 to 4 Post-Op: Fibroblastic Stage

Rehabilitation Goals

The rehabilitation goals during this phase are the same as during the inflammatory stage. ROM is progressed.

Osteoblasts are evident, which is important in laying down woven bone. It is during this stage that early callous formation is hopefully evident on x-ray films. The therapist still has to take great care with the amount of stress that is placed on the fracture site during this stage, as the callous formation strength is much lower than that of normal bone, and the therapist is still relying on the strength of the fixation. Communication with the surgeon needs to be ongoing during this stage regarding the strength of the fixation as well as the status of bridging callous seen on x-ray films during follow-up visits.

AROM and active-assisted range of motion (AAROM) exercises to the elbow in flexion and extension are initiated, via gravity-assist or gravity-eliminated planes. The patient is initially placed in supine to control compensatory movements from the shoulder during AROM exercises. This position also provides patients with proprioceptive feedback needed to minimize shoulder compensation, especially during elbow extension. Forearm rotation AROM exercises

with the elbow at 90° of flexion are initiated within a pain-free ROM. AROM should be ongoing to all unaffected joints and emphasized in a HEP to prevent joint stiffness (see patient handout exercises). Composite stretching to the forearm flexor and extensor compartments, initially with the elbow in slight flexion, will prevent future muscle-tendon shortening. Light putty exercises are provided to maintain grip and pinch strengths. Gentle isometric exercises to the wrist, biceps, and triceps can be initiated only if compressive forces are not contraindicated, as dictated by the strength of the surgical fixation and the rehabilitative needs of any associated injuries, during this phase.

Edema is managed via elevation, ice, retrograde massage, and AROM exercises. For severe edema, compression garments assist greatly in reducing edema. If distal edema is present, compression sleeves to the hand and digits also should be provided to assist in lymphatic drainage (**Figure 14.3**).

Modalities used during this stage, such as ice packs, traditional or premodulated interferential current stimulation, transcutaneous electric nerve stimulation, and high-voltage galvanic stimulation, can assist with pain management as well as edema control. Neuromuscular electric stimulation (NMES) can be initiated by week 3 and can help regain volitional movements of the weakened triceps and/or biceps/brachioradialis. However, if any soft tissue structures were repaired at the time of the fixation, NMES should be avoided for up to 6 weeks postoperatively to allow appropriate healing time of the repaired tissue.

Serial static elbow extension splinting for night use can be utilized for the patient if progressive loss of elbow extension is noted within the first 3 weeks (**Figure 14.4**). See "Special Considerations" section for any distal splinting needs, if any associated nerve injuries are present, or if any ligaments were repaired and need to be protected. A cuff and collar sling can be provided for patients during the day to use for comfort between exercises (**Figure 14.5**).

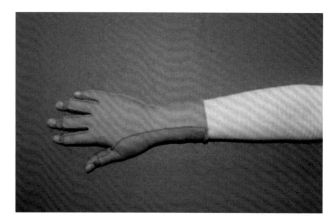

FIGURE 14.3 A compression glove can be used for edema control. (Reproduced with permission from Williams T, Berenz T. Postburn upper extremity occupational therapy. *Hand Clin.* 2017;33(2):293-304.)

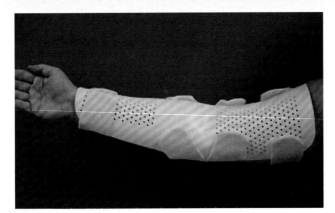

FIGURE 14.4 Serial nighttime extension splitting can be used to prevent loss of extension.

Scar mobilization is initiated once sutures are removed, typically 2 weeks postoperatively. Scar pads are provided to promote a soft, pliable scar with minimal adhesions to underlying tissues, which also improves the excursion needs of the muscle-tendon units.

During this stage of healing, the treating therapist should also identify any soft tissue structures that have become adaptively shortened or tight due to immobilization, which could also be contributing to limitations in elbow ROM, such as in the triceps, biceps, brachioradialis, forearm extensors/flexors, supinator, or pronator. Capsular adhesions, muscle inhibition, muscle cocontraction, and guarding also must be considered and be treated effectively as tissue healing continues to allow for motion to be regained.

Week 4 to 8 Post-Op: Fibroblastic Stage Continued
Rehabilitation Goals
The goals of this stage are to continue to progress ROM and strength, minimize pain and edema, and progress toward light use of the extremity during ADLs.

The organization of callus and lamellar bone deposition begins during this stage and the stability of the fracture is now afforded not only by the fixation but also by the bridging callus. This needs to be monitored by x-ray films during ongoing postoperative clinical visits. Communication between the surgeon and the therapist on the amount of stress that can be placed on the bone needs to be clarified in order to safely progress patients through the rehabilitation program.

AROM/AAROM to the elbow, wrist, and hand are continued. Patients can progress to AAROM exercises to the elbow in an upright position using a cane to achieve end ROM and blocking the shoulder from compensatory motion. These exercises should be added to their HEP. Upper body ergometer for 8 to 10 minutes on zero resistance is effective in warming the elbow joint at the beginning of the session.

Gentle passive range of motion (PROM) to the elbow and forearm can be initiated by week 6 as fracture healing and surgeon discretion allows. As PROM is cleared by the surgeon, static progressive splinting (**Figure 14.6**) and joint mobilizations to the elbow can be utilized by week 6 to assist in regaining motion that continue to be restricted by capsular or soft tissue contractures.

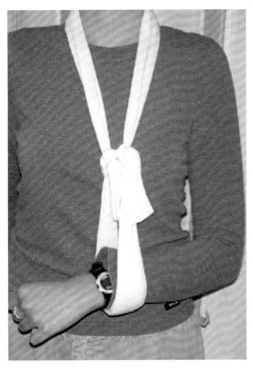

FIGURE 14.5 A cuff and collar sling can be used during the day for comfort between exercises. (Reproduced with permission from King GJW. Fractures of the radial head. In: Wolfe SW, Hotchkiss RN, Pederson WC, Kozin SH, Cohen MS, eds. *Green's Operative Hand Surgery.* Elsevier; 2016:734-769:Figure 19.11c. © 2017.)

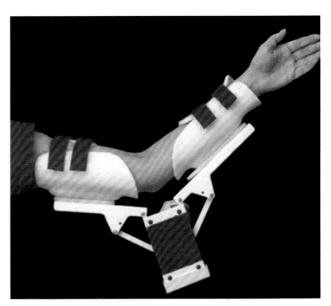

FIGURE 14.6 A static progressive splinting system can be utilized to help regain range of motion. (Reproduced with permission from Ulrich SD, Bonutt PM, Seyler TM, Marker DR, Morrey BF, Mont MA. Restoring range of motion via stress relaxation and static progressive stretch in posttraumatic elbow contractures. *J Shoulder Elbow Surg.* 2010;19(2):196-201.)

Gentle stretching to any restricted tissues is performed during this stage to maximize tissue excursion (N.B. see patient handout on forearm extensor/flexor stretches, triceps/biceps stretches).

Isotonic exercises to biceps, triceps, wrist flexors/extensors, and forearm supinators/pronators with low resistance can be added to the rehabilitation program.

Myofascial soft tissue mobilization, proprioceptive neuromuscular facilitation (PNF) hold-relax and contract-relax techniques to inhibit cocontraction of muscles, and muscle energy techniques are also all effective in regaining motion.

Modalities such as hot packs, fluidotherapy, and ultrasound are effective in providing therapeutic heat to increase tissue extensibility and to mobilize any surgical scar adhesion. Note all modalities are to be used with precaution and attention to contraindications.

Patient education on the light use of the operative extremity during self-care tasks can be started as early as postoperative week 6. However, patients, still need to adhere to lifting and weight-bearing restrictions.

Week 8 to 12 Post-Op: Remodeling Stage

Rehabilitation Goals

In this stage, the goals are to maximize end range active motion of the elbow, regain strength of the entire upper extremity, and maximize the return to independent ADL status.

Fracture healing is characterized by remodeling during this stage. Lamellar bone is replacing callus bridging and continues to do so for up to 9 months. The fracture is fairly stable to withstand the more aggressive therapy needed to regain motion and strength.

More aggressive PROM and joint mobilizations to the elbow can safely be utilized by the therapist if capsular adhesions continue to be present in order to regain normal arthrokinematics. Progressive resistive exercises utilizing isotonic, concentric, and eccentric contraction to elbow flexors and extensors, forearm supinator, pronators, wrist extensors, and flexors are added to the rehabilitation program to regain functional strength. Rotator cuff and periscapular strengthening also need to be included for proximal stabilization.

The use of muscle energy, myofascial techniques, PNF, and hold-relax and contract-relax techniques may continue to be beneficial in regaining strength and endurance.

Modalities such as fluidotherapy, heat with stretching, and ultrasound with stretching may also continue to be effective in improving tissue extensibility and excursion.

The rehabilitation program during this phase should progress patients with the goals to assist patients to return to work-related and sport-related activities.

DISTAL HUMERAL FRACTURES

By definition, fractures of the distal humerus involve the metaphyseal region of the distal humerus. They may have intra-articular extension or remain extra-articular. Injuries most commonly result from compressive forces across the elbow in varying degrees of flexion, with varus or valgus angulation. The incidence of distal humerus fractures in the United States has been estimated at 287 per 100,000 person-years.[25] Distal humerus fractures occur in a bimodal distribution with low-energy fractures occurring in the elderly and higher energy fractures in younger patients. The principles of treatment, as in all articular fractures, are anatomical reduction, stable fixation, and early mobilization.

CLASSIFICATION

There are many classification systems available for distal humerus fractures. For the sake of simplicity, the Arbeitsgemeinschaft fur Osteosynthesegragen/Orthopaedic Trauma Association (AO/OTA) classification will be utilized here (**Figure 14.7**).

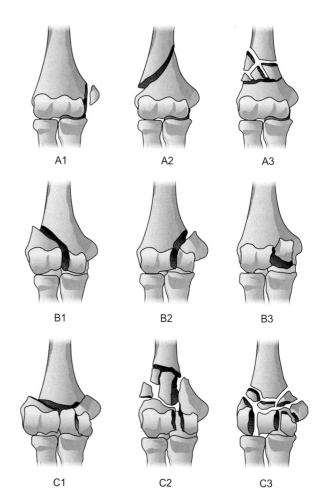

FIGURE 14.7 The OTA/AO classification for distal humerus fractures. Type 13 A: Extra-articular fracture—A1, apophyseal avulsion; A2, metaphyseal simple; A3, metaphyseal multifragmentary. Type 13 B: Partial articular fracture—B1, sagittal lateral condyle; B2, sagittal medial condyle; B3, frontal. Type 13 C: Complete articular fractures—C1, articular simple, metaphyseal simple; C2, articular simple, metaphyseal multifragmentary; C3, articular, multifragmentary.

DIAGNOSIS

History and Physical Examination

Distal humeral fractures that occur in young patients tend to be the result of high-energy trauma: motor vehicle collisions or falls from height. Fractures occurring in the elderly are typically secondary to a fall from a standing height onto an outstretched hand or secondary to a direct blow mechanism. A painful swollen elbow with limited ROM is common, as well as a sense of instability about the elbow. A ligamentous examination aids in ruling out concomitant ligament injury, but is not always tolerated by patients in the setting of acute trauma.

TREATMENT

Nonoperative

Nondisplaced fractures, displaced fractures with adequate reduction, and extra-articular distal humerus fractures can be managed nonoperatively with close radiographic follow-up. This can be accomplished with a variety of splints, braces, and casts. A comparative study of nonoperative treatments utilizing anterior and posterior U-shape plaster with the elbow in extension compared to conventional single posterior plaster slab showed the former led to a statistically significant reduction in cubitus varus deformity. This method also had a significantly lower risk of displacement following reduction and secondary redisplacement.[26]

Operative

For fractures that have significant displacement and intra-articular extension, open reduction and internal fixation is the most common operative choice. The benefits include early functional return following treatment and reduced risk of degenerate joint disease. Operative fixation can be achieved with various techniques, including 90-90 plating with precontoured plates and locked plates (**Figure 14.8**). The goal of any intra-articular fracture treated operatively is anatomical reduction, stable fixation, and early mobilization of the joint.

POSTOPERATIVE REHABILITATION

The importance of physical therapy was highlighted in a randomized comparative study comparing formal physical therapy with no formal therapy after the treatment of distal humerus fractures.[27] Physical therapy resulted in statistically significant better ROM in the first 19 weeks following reduction compared with no formal physical therapy.

With stable fixation, active exercises involving the elbow should be initiated within a few days postoperatively as the elbow is prone to stiffness. A splint may be used postoperatively, but its use should be discouraged after 48 to 72 hours.

Active-assisted elbow motion exercises are performed by having the patient bend the elbow as much as possible using their own strength while simultaneously using their opposite well-arm to push the arm gently into further flexion. By using AROM, reflexive relaxation of opposing muscle groups is minimized, and the risk of loss of fixation significantly decreases.

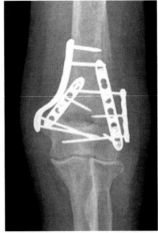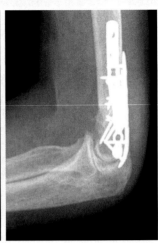

FIGURE 14.8 Bicondylar 90-90 plating technique for fixation of distal humerus fracture. (Reproduced with permission from Leigey DF, Farrell DJ, Siska PA, Tarkin IS. Bicolumnar 90-90 plating of low-energy distal humeral fractures in the elderly patient. *Geriatr Orthop Surg Rehabil.* 2014;5(3):122-126. doi:10.1177/2151458514526882.)

Passive motion, on the other hand, may result in unintended resistance, due to pain, and greater loads on the fixation construct, leading to early failure. Patients should remain non–weight-bearing for a minimum of 6 to 8 weeks, and follow-up radiographs should be obtained every 2 weeks to assess for bony union. After 6 to 8 weeks, resistive strengthening is initiated and gentle passive stretching by a qualified therapist can be started to increase the flexion/extension arc.

OLECRANON FRACTURES

The olecranon is the most proximal portion of the ulna and articulates with the trochlea of the distal humerus (**Figure 14.9A and B**). This articulation provides the flexion-extension movement of the elbow. The triceps attaches on the proximal tip of the olecranon, and the integrity of this attachment is integral in treatment decisions regarding olecranon fractures. While olecranon fractures commonly occur in the elderly secondary to indirect trauma, they more frequently occur in the younger population secondary to direct trauma. By definition, all olecranon fractures are intra-articular and should be treated as such.

CLASSIFICATION

Many attempts have been made to classify olecranon fractures, but none are consistently used throughout the orthopaedic literature. The most important considerations are the amount of fracture displacement and the integrity of the triceps, which is the extensor mechanism of the elbow.

DIAGNOSIS

History and Physical Examination

The typical history in an elderly patient is a fall onto an outstretched hand with the elbow in flexion, leading to

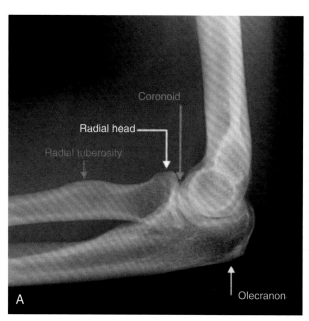

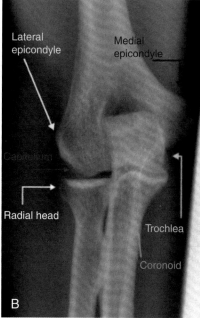

FIGURE 14.9 A, A normal lateral radiograph of the elbow indicating osteological landmarks. **B**, A normal anteroposterior (AP) radiograph of the elbow indicating osteological landmarks.

contraction of the triceps. Because of its subcutaneous location, olecranon fractures can also be a result of direct trauma. Patients will commonly have pain, swelling, ecchymosis, and an inability to extend the elbow. Other injuries about the elbow, such as a concomitant radial head fracture, should be evaluated during examination and on radiographs. A thorough neurovascular examination is necessary as the ulnar nerve is at risk in higher energy trauma.

TREATMENT

The goals of treatment of olecranon fractures include articular restoration, preservation of motor power of extension, stability, the avoidance of stiffness, and limiting the possible associated complications.[26]

Nonoperative

Nondisplaced fractures and stable fractures displaced less than 2 mm can successfully be treated by closed means utilizing a long arm posterior splint or a long arm cast. The elbow should be held in 60° to 90° of flexion for 1 to 2 weeks with gradual resumption of ROM thereafter. In addition, some elderly, frail patients with displaced fracture but retained ability to extend the elbow may be considered for nonoperative treatment with extension splinting or casting for 6 weeks.

Operative (Figures 14.10 and 14.11)

Fractures with >2 mm of displacement and those that are unstable are best treated with surgery. The best method of fixation is dependent on the characteristics of the fracture. For example, transverse fractures can be treated with Kirschner wires (K-wires) utilizing a tension band technique. This is inappropriate in comminuted or oblique fractures, which are best treated with a plate and screw construct. In a study

comparing plate fixation to tension band wiring, plate fixation resulted in a higher percentage of "good" clinical and x-ray results. In addition, the reported complications with tension band wiring were significantly higher at 74% compared to 5% with plate fixation.[25]

RADIAL HEAD FRACTURES

The proximal portion of the radius, the cylindrically shaped radial head, articulates with the capitellum of the distal humerus. It is mostly covered with cartilage, except on the lateral aspect, and is recognized as an important secondary stabilizer against valgus stress. It also functions to prevent proximal migration of the radius and shares ~50% of the axial load at the elbow. Injury to the radial head occurs in ~20% of acute elbow injuries and typically occurs secondarily to a fall on an outstretched hand. Varying degrees of associated injuries can occur simultaneously depending on the amount of varus or valgus load at the time of injury and must be evaluated with a thorough physical examination.

CLASSIFICATION

Over the years, many different schemes have been devised to classify these injuries. The Mason classification, which was further modified by Johnston, is most commonly utilized (**Figure 14.12**).

DIAGNOSIS

History and Physical Examination

A fall onto an outstretched hand is the typical history given by a patient with a radial head fracture. On physical examination,

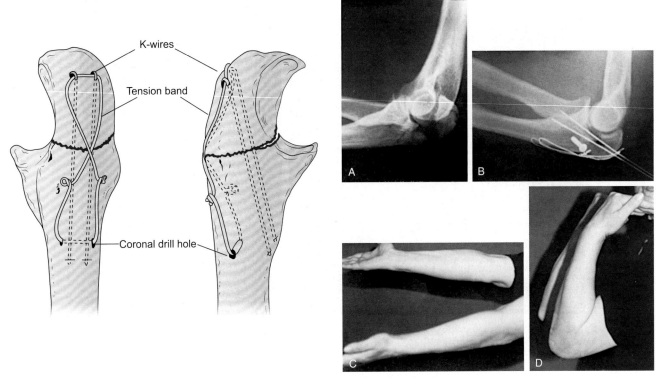

FIGURE 14.10 Left: Cartoon image of tension-band technique utilizing Kirschner wires (K-wires) for the fixation of olecranon fracture. Right: **A**, A simple transverse olecranon fracture. **B**, Olecranon fracture treated with a tension-band technique. **C**, Postoperative extension. **D**, Postoperative flexion. (Reproduced with permission from Chan W, Donnelly KJ. Does K-wire position in tension band wiring of olecranon fractures affect its complications and removal of metal rate? *J Orthop.* 2014;12(2):111-117.)

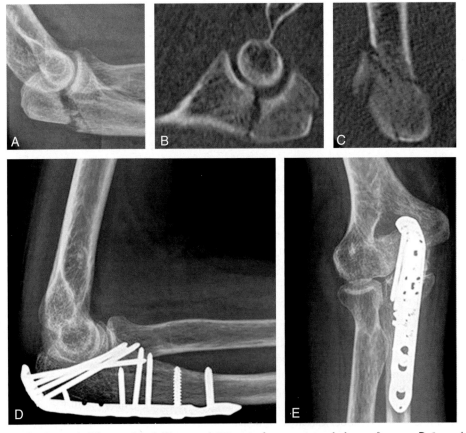

FIGURE 14.11 A, Lateral radiograph (**B**) sagittal and (**C**) coronal CT scan of a comminuted olecran fracture. **D**, Lateral and (**E**) anteroposterior postoperative radiograph following open reduction internal fixation of the olecranon fracture with a plate. (Reprinted from Midtgaard KS, Ruzbarsky JJ, Hackett TR, Viola RW. Elbow fractures. *Clin Sports Med.* 2020;39(3):623-636.)

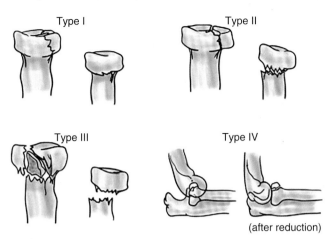

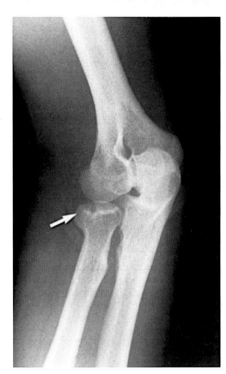

(after reduction)

FIGURE 14.12 The Mason classification of radial head fractures. Type I—minimally displaced fractures (<2mm) without angulation. Type II—partial articular fractures with >2mm of displacement. Type III—complete articular fractures with severe comminution. Type IV—radial head fracture associated with an elbow dislocation. (Reproduced with permission from Morrey BF. *The Elbow and its Disorders*. Philadelphia: W.B. Saunders Company; 1993.)

FIGURE 14.13 Oblique x-ray of the elbow demonstrating a radial head fracture (arrow).

there is often an effusion present as well as a limited ROM. It is important to ascertain if the decrease in ROM is secondary to patient discomfort or if a mechanical block is present. This can be done by aspirating any present effusion to relieve discomfort and injecting local anesthetic into the joint, followed by reexamination of ROM. A randomized controlled trial found that for patients with radial head fractures, 92% of the patients who received aspiration reported immediate and lasting relief from pain compared to those who were not aspirated.[28]

TREATMENT

Nonoperative

For type I fractures, treatment consists of symptomatic management with analgesics, sling for comfort, and early ROM, typically within a week of injury (**Figure 14.13**). When cast immobilization was compared to immediate mobilization, no differences were found in terms of pain or loss of motion.[29] Weight-bearing is protected for 6 weeks.

Identifying if a mechanical block is present is paramount in treating type II fractures. If there is no mechanical block, treatment follows the same course as in type I fractures.

In rare occasions, type III fractures without a mechanical block, any associated fractures, or instability can be considered for nonoperative treatment, similar to type I fractures.

Operative

The indications for operative treatment of type II fractures are the presence of a mechanical block to motion and fracture displacement of >2 mm with associated elbow instability. The treatment consists of open reduction and internal fixation of the fracture or excision of the radial head fragment if it is not amendable to fixation (**Figure 14.14**).

Type III fractures with a mechanical block necessitate open treatment to remove impinging structures and to reconstruct the radial head, when feasible. In cases in which the radial head is not reconstructible, a strong consideration for arthroplasty must be given. Excision of the radial head is a viable option, but is not without complications, particularly in cases with an associated ligamentous injury.

AFTER TREATMENT

A splint may be utilized postoperatively but should be discontinued within a few days to prevent soft tissue contracture. AROM and AAROM is encouraged immediately, while loading of the elbow is avoided for 6 to 8 weeks (**Figure 14.15A and B**).

THERAPEUTIC INTERVENTIONS

STABLE FRACTURES

There are general guidelines that can help direct the rehabilitation progression of stable fractures (**Table 14.2**). The time spent in each fracture healing stage may vary with each patient. Communication between the surgeon and the therapist is vital to safely advance the stress placed on healing tissue.

SPECIAL CONSIDERATIONS WITH REHABILITATION

FRACTURES COMBINED WITH SOFT TISSUE AND/OR NERVE INJURY/REPAIR

The previous section on rehabilitation guidelines of fractures around the elbow addressed stable fractures. If there are

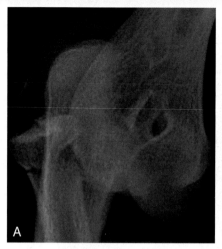
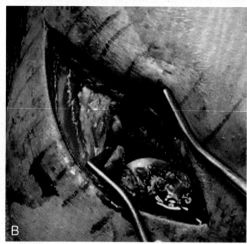
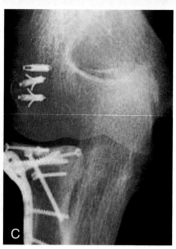

FIGURE 14.14 A, Oblique radiograph demonstrating an elbow dislocation and a comminuted radial head fracture. **B**, Intraoperative photograph demonstrating comminution and bone loss. **C**, Postoperative anterioposterior radiograph after open reduction internal fixation of the radial head fracture. (Reprinted from Midtgaard KS, Ruzbarsky JJ, Hackett TR, Viola RW. Elbow fractures. *Clin Sports Med.* 2020;39(3):623-636.)

accompanying injuries to the fracture, there must be good communication between the surgeon and the therapist to appropriately rehabilitate the patient and functionally optimize outcomes. Information from the surgeon on the rigidity of the fixation, ligamentous stability, and the status of nerves and soft tissues will guide the treatment plan. As previously stated, elbow contracture can be a common complication of elbow fractures if not treated appropriately and in a timely manner. Schippinger et al. demonstrated that immobilization over 3 weeks after a simple elbow dislocation may result in inferior function versus those that were immobilized for only 2 weeks.[30]

In order to prevent these adverse effects, the treating therapist must have a good understanding of how to perform prescribed ROM exercises in the early phases of healing to optimize motion, while maintaining stability. There have been numerous biomechanical studies that have examined elbow stability and ligamentous stress through elbow ROM with different forearm positions.[31-39] When nerve injury also occurs along with the elbow fracture, the therapist must be knowledgeable on splinting and rehabilitation considerations in order to avoid overstressing the repair and prevent further injury and joint contractures. It is beyond the scope of this chapter to discuss the rehabilitative approach these injuries, but they will be summarized in the following section and outlined in the table.

LIGAMENT REPAIRS

Along with fractures around the elbow, there may be instability requiring repair of the ligaments. It is vital for the therapist to understand, either through reviewing the documentation

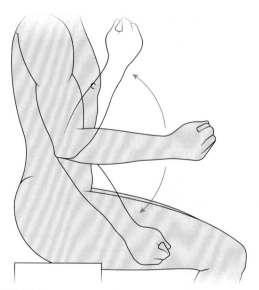
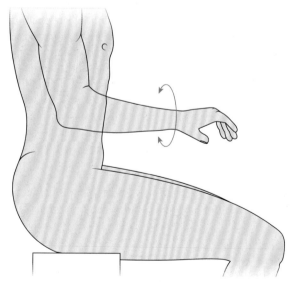

FIGURE 14.15 A and **B**, Postoperatively, patients work on active range of motion in (**A**) flexion and extension and (**B**) pronation and supination.

TABLE 14.2 General Guidelines for the Progression of Rehabilitation for the Operative Fixation of Stable Elbow Fractures

	0-4 wk	4-8 wk	8-12 wk
Precautions			
Weight-bearing	NWB	Progress to WBAT per MD clearance	Progress to FWB per MD clearance
Lifting	No lifting, pushing/pulling	Progress per MD	Progress per MD
Modalities	• Ice packs for edema • IFC or premod for pain/edema • NMES by week 3 for neuromuscular reeducation • Compression sleeves to digits and UE for edema • HGVS for edema • TENS	• Fluidotherapy • Hot pack w/ stretch • Ultrasound to heat tissue for stretch if fracture healed • NMES for neuromuscular reeducation	• Hot packs w/ stretch • Ultrasound • Fluidotherapy
Splinting	• Serial static elbow extension splint for night use if progressive loss of elbow extension noted • Cuff and collar for comfort between exercises	• Static progressive elbow brace by week 6 per MD clearance	• Static progressive elbow brace as indicated
ROM/exercises	• No PROM to elbow • AROM/AAROM elbow flexion/extension supine and gravity-eliminated positions • AAROM elbow using cane • AROM/PROM to unaffected joints of wrist and digits • AROM to shoulder all planes • Gentle isometrics to shoulder, wrist and elbow by week 2-3 • Light putty exercises by week 2-3 • Scar mobilization and use of scar pad by week 2 post suture removal	• A/AAROM elbow using cane • Gentle PROM to elbow by week 6 per fracture healing • UBE • PNF contract relax/hold relax • Low-resistance isotonic exercises • Stretching to restricted tissues • Myofascial release techniques • Muscle energy techniques • Joint mobilization if cleared by week 6	• PROM/AROM elbow and FA • UBE with increased resistance • PREs to wrist/FA/elbow • RTC and periscapular strengthening • Joint mobilizations by week 8 • ADL simulation tasks • Job-specific/sport-specific exercises • Closed chain/open chain exercises • T-Band exercises utilizing concentric/eccentric control of isolated muscle groups
Patient education	• HEP on all exercises • Patient education handout • ADL retraining/adaptive equipment needs	• Light use of UE for self care • Update HEP	• Update HEP

AAROM, active-assisted range of motion; ADL, activities of daily living; AROM, active range of motion; FWB, full weight bearing; HEP, home exercise program; HGVS, high voltage galvanic stimulator; IFC, interferential current therapy; NMES, neuromuscular electrical stimulation; NWB, non–weight-bearing; PNF, proprioceptive neuromuscular facilitation; PRE, passive resistance exercises; PROM, passive range of motion; ROM, range of motion ; RTC, rotator cuff; TENS, transcutaneous electrical nerve stimulation; UBE, upper body ergometer; WBAT, weight bearing as tolerated.

or speaking to the surgeon, what the safe ROM is to prevent recurrent instability in the early phases of healing. This information is crucial in guiding the early therapy treatment plan. For example, the elbow may be limited to within the stable arc of motion for the first 3 weeks and then can be progressed by 10° to 15° with each following week.

LATERAL LIGAMENT INJURIES

The lateral ulnar collateral ligament is the primary stabilizer against posterolateral rotatory instability and varus

instability.[33,34] It is uniformly taut during elbow motion.[35,36] Cadaveric studies have demonstrated that forearm pronation increases posterolateral rotatory stability in cases in which the lateral ligamentous complex is disrupted.[37] Therapists must also be cautious of abduction of the shoulder due to the resultant varus stress across to the elbow.

MEDIAL LIGAMENT INJURIES

The anterior bundle of the medial collateral ligament is considered the primary restraint to valgus torque between 20° and

120° of motion. From 0° to 80° of flexion, the anterior band plays the primary role, and from 80° to 120°, the posterior band plays a primary role.[38] Overlap is noted between the anterior and posterior band in the the deep middle fibers, which remain isometric throughout the arc of motion. Eccentric forces concentrate in this portion of the ligament. Dynamic stabilizers to the medial elbow primarily are the flexor carpi ulnaris and the flexor digitorum superficialis. The flexor carpi ulnaris is the primary stabilizer to valgus loads at 45° and 90° of elbow flexion.[39] Strengthening of these muscles should be incorporated to a rehabilitation program to increase stability. Several studies have demonstrated that AROM with the forearm supinated stabilizes the medial elbow more than with the forearm in pronation.[38]

If both medial and lateral ligaments are disrupted, the forearm should be kept in a neutral position during ROM exercises. When performing forearm ROM exercises, the elbow should be flexed to 90°.

ESSEX-LOPRESTI INJURY

This injury occurs with radial head fractures plus dislocation of the distal radial ulnar joint (DRUJ) and interosseous membrane. Patients will complain of ulnar-sided wrist pain. If this injury is suspected by the therapist, a referral back to the physician should be made to stabilize the DRUJ.

NERVE INJURIES AROUND THE ELBOW

If a nerve is injured or repaired around the elbow, the therapist must educate the patient on sensory precautions to avoid further injury. It is also important to provide encouragement to the patient because of the length of time it takes for a nerve to regenerate when injured at the level of the elbow. Any joint contractures must be prevented or addressed with splinting. Splinting can also be implemented to compensate for muscle imbalances and to increase the patient's functional use of the extremity. The appropriate sensory tests and manual muscle testing should also be performed monthly to determine clinical progress and neurological recovery.

If a nerve conduit was performed with the nerve repair, there exist rehabilitation precautions. It is recommended that no scar massage be performed for 4 weeks postoperatively and ultrasound should never be performed to avoid degrading the conduit.[40]

Fractures combined with soft tissue and/or nerve injury/repair (Table 14.3)

MD prescription (0-4/6 weeks after injury) for elbow fracture (Figure 14.16)

MD prescription (weeks 6-12) for elbow fracture (Figure 14.17)

MD prescription (0-4/6 weeks after injury) for elbow fracture with associated injuries (Figure 14.18)

PATIENT EDUCATION ON FRACTURE HEALING AND LIMITATIONS

You have broken (fractured) a bone in your elbow. It is important to understand what to do and not do throughout

TABLE 14.3 Postoperative Occupational Therapy Protocols for Various Elbow Surgical Repairs

Structure Involved	Rehabilitation Implications
Lateral collateral ligament repair	Perform ROM with the forearm pronated for 6 wk and avoid varus stress Avoid shoulder abduction to avoid varus stress to elbow
Medial ulnar collateral ligament repair	Perform ROM with the forearm in supination for 6 wk and avoid valgus stress Avoid shoulder external rotation to avoid valgus stress to elbow
Medial and lateral collateral ligament repairs	Perform ROM with forearm neutral position for 6 wk
Ulnar nerve injury/repair	Teach patient sensory precautions to avoid further injury Anticlaw splint to avoid hyperextension of MP joints of ring and small finger and to prevent PIP contractures while increasing functional use of hand
Median nerve injury/repair	Teach patient sensory precautions to avoid further injury Patient may need thumb web spacer splint Short opponens splint to increase ability to grasp objects Patient may need splints to keep IF DIP and thumb IP flexed to increase fine motor coordination skills
Radial nerve injury/repair	Teach patient sensory precautions to avoid further injury Patient will need dynamic forearm- or wrist-based splint to extend digit MPs and wrist

DIP, distal interphalangeal; IF, index finger; IP, interphalangeal; MP, metacarpophalangeal; PIP, proximal interphalangeal; ROM, range of motion.

Patient name:_____Date_____

Date of birth:_____

Diagnosis:_____

Date of injury/surgery_____

_____PT/OT evaluate and treat

Frequency and duration: 2-3 x a week for 10-12 weeks

***No weightbearing/lifting with upper extremity > than 2 pounds**

RX:

-A/AAROM to elbow and forearm until next x ray

-A/AROM/PROM to shoulder, wrist, forearm, and hand

-Modalities as needed

___**MHP/CP**

___**Electrical stimulation for pain and edema**

___**Fluidotherapy**

_____Date_____

Physician signature-this indicates medically necessary

FIGURE 14.16 Therapy prescription for postoperative elbow fracture 0 to 4/6 weeks after injury.

Patient name:_____Date_____

Date of birth:_____

Diagnosis:_____

Date of injury/surgery_____

_____PT/OT evaluate and treat

Frequency and duration: 2-3 x a week for 6 weeks

*Weightbearing as tolerated

RX:

-A/AA/PROM to elbow and FA

-Static progressive splinting as needed

-Progressive strengthening throughout entire UE

-Continue modalities as needed

__**MHP/CP**

__**Ultrasound**

__**Electrical stimulation**

__**Fluidotherapy**

_____Date_____

Physician signature-indicates medically necessary

FIGURE 14.17 Therapy prescription for postoperative elbow fracture 6 to 12 weeks after injury.

your healing process to help the bone heal. When a bone breaks, it heals in three stages. You will also go through three stages of rehabilitation. You will see your doctor at the following times after your injury: 2 weeks (if you had surgery for suture removal), 6 weeks, and 12 weeks. Your doctor will recommend you start therapy within the first week of your surgery because the elbow gets very stiff if early motion is not performed. It is important for you to participate in therapy to improve the use of your arm while the fracture heals. If therapy and the appropriate exercises are not performed after elbow fractures, stiffness, loss of strength, prolonged pain, and inability to use the arm may result.

The first stage of therapy is started before you see your doctor at 6 weeks. At this time, the bone is not strong enough to lift, push, pull, or bear weight. Some examples of things you should avoid during this time are:

- Getting the operative elbow wet before the stitches are taken out.
- Pushing off a surface with your injured arm.
- Carrying anything with that injured arm.
- Pushing or pulling open a door with the injured arm.
- Use your injured arm only as tolerated for doing everyday basic self-care activities such as bathing, dressing, and grooming. At this time, you will probably be relying on your other arm for most daily tasks. Tasks will get easier as you gain more motion and your pain decreases.

Patient name:_____Date_____

Date of birth:_____

Diagnosis:_____

Date of injury/surgery_____

_____PT/OT evaluate and treat

Frequency and duration: 2-3 X a week for 10-12 weeks

*No weightbearing/lifting with upper extremity until next MD

Appointment

*Degree of elbow stability in OR:

1. Stable from_____deg ext to _____ deg flex(perform in this range X3 weeks then progress 10-

15 degrees every week after)

2.___Elbow stable through full ROM-perform A/AAROM to patient tolerance

*Other structures involved:

_____**Repair of LCL (therapist to perform ROM with FA pronated for 6 weeks and avoid**

varus stress.)

_____**Repair of MCL (therapist to perform ROM with FA supinated for 6 weeks and avoid**

valgus stress)

_____**Repair of LCL and MCL (therapist to perform ROM with FA neutral X 6 weeks and**

avoid valgus and varus stress)

_____**Nerve injury** _____**Median** _____**Ulnar** _____**Radial**

(Teach sensory precautions to avoid injury)

_____**Nerve repair** _____**Median** _____**Ulnar** _____**Radial** ____**Nerve conduit**

(No scar massage X 4 weeks, no ultrasound)

_____**Other:**_____

_____   Date_____

Physician signature-indicates medically necessary

FIGURE 14.18 Therapy prescription for postoperative elbow fracture 0 to 4/6 weeks after injury with concomitant injuries.

Your therapist will be giving you exercises to perform that are safe during phase time. It is vital to your outcome that you perform these exercises every 2 to 3 hours every day when awake because, once the elbow gets stiff, it is very hard to gain the motion back as time passes.

The second stage of rehabilitation begins with the 6-week visit to your doctor. X-rays should show more healing. At this time, you will be able to do more with your arm. You will be able to lift up to 10 pounds. You still will not have enough strength to push yourself up with the arm or push or pull heavy objects. At this stage, therapy will be more aggressive with regaining motion and you will start light strengthening, granted the bone is healing as expected. You will find it easier to perform your daily activities, and your pain should be less, allowing more use of your arm.

The final stage of rehabilitation emphasizes increasing your strength and maintaining your motion. Your doctor will see you around 12 weeks after your fracture for another x-ray to make sure the bone is completely healed and you will be released to unrestricted activity. Just remember that strength increases over time and to gradually increase your activities. Be sure to continue the exercises prescribed by your therapist.

At any point in your rehabilitation if you are concerned about doing an activity that was not specified, please contact your doctor or therapist. Especially in the early stages of healing, you do not want to have any setbacks that will lead to more swelling and pain. These things can prolong your rehabilitation and your return to the things that you enjoy doing.

REFERENCES

1. Morrey BF. Radial head fracture. In: Morrey BF, ed. *The Elbow and Its Disorders*. 3rd ed. WB Saunders; 2000.
2. Boone DC, Azen SP. Normal range of motion of joints in male subjects. *J Bone Joint Surg Am*. 1979;61:756.
3. Beals RK. The normal carrying angle of the elbow. *Clin Orthop*. 1976;119:194.
4. Morrey BF, Askew LJ, An KN, Chao EY. A biomechanical study of functional elbow motion. *J Bone Joint Surg Am*. 1981;63:872-877.
5. Alcid JG. Elbow anatomy and structural biomechanics. *Clin Sports Med*. 2004;23:503-517.
6. Thomas TT. A contribution to the mechanism of fractures and dislocations and dislocations in the elbow region. 1929;89:108-121.
7. Morrey BF. Elbow and forearm. In: Delee J, ed. *Delee & Drez's Orthopaedic Sports Medicine*. 3rd ed. WB Saunders; 2009.
8. Morrey BF, Askew LJ, An K-N. A biomechanical study of normal functional elbow motion. *J Bone Joint Surg Am*. 1981;63A:872-877.
9. Davila SA. Therapists management of fractures and dislocations of the elbow. In: Mackin EJ, Callahan AD, eds. *Rehabilitation of the Hand and Upper Extremity*. Vol. 2. 5th ed. Mosby; 2002:1230-1244.
10. Davila S, Jones KJ. Managing the stiff elbow: operative ,nonoperative, and postoperative techniques. *J Hand Ther*. 2006;19(2):268-281.
11. Hotchkiss RN, Davila S. Rehabilitation of the elbow. In: Nickel E, Botte MJ, eds. *Orthopedic Rehabilitation*. 2nd ed. Churchill Livingstone; 1992.
12. Stroyan M, Wilk KE. The functional anatomy of the elbow complex. *J Ortho Sports Phys Ther*. 1993;17:279-288.
13. Werner FW, An K-N. Biomechanics of the elbow and forearm. *Hand Clin*. 1994;10:439.
14. Hotchkiss RN. Elbow contracture. In: Green DP, Hotchkiss RN, Peterson WC, Wolfe SW, eds. *Greens Operative Hand Surgery*. 5th ed. Churchill-Livingstone; 2005:667-682.
15. Modabber MR, Jupiter JB. Reconstruction for post-traumatic conditions of the elbow joint: current concepts review. *J Hand Surg*. 1995;77A:1431.
16. Morrey BF. Splints and bracing at the elbow. In: Morrey BF, ed. *The Elbow and Its Disorders*. 3rd ed. Saunders; 2000:150-154.
17. Nirschl RP, Morrey BF. Rehabilitation. In: Morrey BF, ed. *The Elbow and Its Disorders*. 3rd ed. Saunders; 2000:141-146.
18. Page C, Backus SI, Lenhoff MW. Electromyographic activity in stiff and normal elbows during flexion and extension. *J Hand Ther*. 2003;16:5-11.
19. Tucker K. Some aspects of post-traumatic elbow stiffness. *Injury*. 1978;9:216-220.
20. Weiss AP, Sachar K. Soft tissue contracture about the elbow. *Hand Clin*. 1994;10:439.
21. Kuntz D, Baratz M. Fractures of the elbow, *Orthop Clin North Am*. 1999;30:37.
22. Broberg MA, Morrey BF. Results of treatment of fracture-dislocations of the elbow. *Clin Orthop*. 1987;216:109.
23. Cohen M, Hastings H. Acute elbow dislocation:evaluation and management. *J Am Acad Orthop Surg*. 1998;6:15.
24. Hildebrand KA, Patterson SD, King GJW. Acute elbow dislocation: simple and complex. *Orthop Clin North Am*. 1999;30:63.
25. Hume MC, Wiss DA. Olecranon fractures. A clinical and radiographic comparison of tension band wiring and plate fixation. *Clin Orthop Relat Res*. 1992;285:229-235.
26. Cabanela M. Olecranon fractures. In: Morrey BF, ed. *The Elbow and Its Disorders*. W.B. Saunders; 1987.
27. Hoppenfeld S. *Treatment & Rehabilitation of Fractures*. Lippincott Williams & Wilkins; 2000.
28. Holdsworth BJ, Clement DA, Rothwell PN. Fractures of the radial head--the benefit of aspiration: a prospective controlled trial. *Injury*. 1987;18:44-47.
29. Unsworth-White J, Koka R, Churchill M, et al. The non-operative management of radial head fractures: a randomized trial of three treatments. *Injury*. 1994;25:165-167.
30. Schippinger G, Seibert FJ, Kucharcrzk M. Management of simple elbow dislocations. Does the period of immobilization affect the eventual results? *Langerbecks Arch Surg*. 1999;384:294-297.
31. Morrey BF. Current concepts in the treatment of fractures of the radial head, the olecranon,and the coronoid. *J Bone Joint Surg*. 1995;77:316-327.
32. Szekerez M, Chinchalkar S, King G. Optimizing elbow rehabilitation after instability. *Hand Clin*. 2008;24:27-38.
33. O'Driscoll SW, Morrey BF, Korinek S, et al. Elbow subluxation and dislocation. A spectrum of instability. *Clin Orthop Relat Res*. 1992;(280):186-197.
34. An KN, Morrey BF. Biomechanics of the elbow. In: Morrey BF, ed. *The Elbow and Its Disorders*. 3rd ed. WB Saunders; 2000:43-60.
35. Olsen BS, Vaesel MT. Sojbjerg JO, et al. Lateral collateral ligament of the elbow joint: anatomy and kinematics. *J Shoulder Elbow Surg*. 1996;5:103-112.
36. Olsen BS, Sojberg JO, Dalstra M, et al. Kinematics of the lateral ligamentous constraints of the elbow joint. *J Shoulder Elbow Surg*. 1996;5(5):333-341.
37. Cohen MS, Hastings H II. Rotatary instability of the elbow. The anatomy and role of the lateral stabilizers. *J Bone Joint Surg Am*. 1997;79(2):225-233.
38. Armstrong AD, Dunning CE, Faber KJ, et al. Rehabilitation of the medial collateral ligament-deficient elbow: an in vitro biomechanical study. *J Hand Surg Am*. 2000;25(6):1051-1057.
39. Park MC, Ahmad CS. Dynamic contributions of the flexor-pronator mass to elbow valgus stability. *J Bone Joint Surg Am*. 2004;86-A(10):2268-2274.
40. Taras JS, Nanavat V, Steelman P. Nerve Conduits. *J Hand Ther*. 2005;18:191-197.

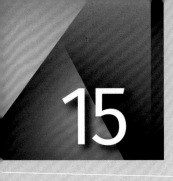

15

Forearm Fractures

Maureen A. O'Shaughnessy
Amy L. Ladd

ANATOMY AND BIOMECHANICS

The radius and the ulna comprise the bony architecture of the forearm. They are constrained proximally at the proximal radioulnar joint (PRUJ), distally at the distal radioulnar joint (DRUJ), and longitudinally by the interosseous membrane (IOM). Load is transmitted from the wrist to the elbow through the intricate balance of the bony, ligamentous, and musculotendinous anatomy of the forearm.

The DRUJ consists of the sigmoid notch on the radius in which the round articular surface of the ulnar head articulates. Little inherent bony stability exists between the distal radius and ulna; thus, the soft tissues about the joint play a crucial role. The main stabilizers of the DRUJ are the distal radioulnar ligaments (volar and dorsal radioulnar ligaments) and the triangular fibrocartilage complex (TFCC). The TFCC is a soft-tissue confluence made up of several structures which provide additional stability. The TFCC complex consists of the triangulofibrocartilage, extensor carpi ulnaris subsheath, and the ulnar extrinsic ligaments. Hotchkiss and colleagues noted that the TFCC contributes 8% to the forearm's overall mechanical stiffness.[1]

The PRUJ consists of the bony articulation between the radial head and the proximal ulna. The radial head articulates in the lesser sigmoid notch of the proximal ulna. The annular ligament links the radius and ulna proximally; it is a stout, circumferential band that arises and inserts on the lesser sigmoid notch and wraps circumferentially around the radial head and neck, forming a strong but flexible sling. Several studies have shown that the radial head is not round but rather an oval shape; thus, the contact area of the articular surface within the lesser sigmoid notch and radiocapitellar joints changes based on the position of the forearm.[2,3] The radial head serves an important role as the primary constraint to longitudinal stability of the forearm. Whereas elbow flexion and extension occurs at the radiocapitellar and ulnohumeral joints at the elbow, forearm rotation at the elbow occurs through pronosupination at the PRUJ.

The IOM consists of stout oblique fibrous tissue running from the radius to the ulna. The fibers serve to link the bones as well as the important job of transferring load from the radius to the ulna. Load sharing in the upper extremity changes from primarily at the radiocarpal joint distally to primarily at the ulno-humeral joint proximally. This load transfer is achieved through an intact IOM. The major component of the IOM is the central band, also called the interosseous ligament of the forearm.[4] The central band consists of collagenous tissue which is approximately twice the thickness of the rest of the IOM.[4] The band is found about 60% of the distance from the radial styloid and accounts for 71% of the IOM's total stiffness.[4] It runs at approximately a 20° angle from proximal-radial to distal-ulnar direction.[5] It is the primary stabilizer of longitudinal stability when the radial head is fractured or resected.[4] The IOM also serves as a site of origin for musculature in the forearm.

Five discrete components of the IOM have been identified: the **central band**, the **distal oblique bundle**, an **accessory band**, a **dorsal oblique accessory cord**, and a **proximal oblique accessory cord**[5]. The distal oblique bundle has been found to be involved in the stability of the DRUJ in all forearm positions.[5] Because the IOM has no attachment to the distal third of the radius, fractures in this location may have a higher incidence of shortening.

The radius rotates around a fixed ulna to allow forearm rotation, although this relationship is often mistaken—a common misconception that the ulnar head rotates distally. An intact radius reveals a gentle curvature or "bowing" of the radius. This diaphyseal bowing of the radius is critical to allow full pronation and supination of the forearm as the radius rotates around the fixed ulna. Disorders of the shape of the radius, either congenital or acquired, will lead to limitations in the pronosupination of the forearm.

The position of the apparent length of the ulnar head (termed ulnar variance radiographically) changes based on the position of the forearm. In neutral, the ulnar head is roughly equivalent length of the distal radius. The ulna appears longest (ulnar positive) in full pronation and shortest (ulnar negative) in full supination.

In an ulnar-neutral wrist, 80% of the axial load is transmitted across the radiocarpal joint and 20% through the ulnocarpal joint. At the elbow the load is equilibrated via load transmission across the IOM from the radius to the ulna. Forces borne at the elbow are 60% radiocapitellar and 40% ulnohumeral.[6-8]

Positive ulnar variance increases the load transmitted through the distal ulnocarpal joint. Studies have shown that positive ulnar variance of 2 mm will increase the load transmission of the distal ulna from a normal 20% to 40% which may ultimately lead to ulnocarpal impaction and wrist pain.[9] Patients with proximal radial translation >1 cm typically experience pain and loss of motion while those with <1 cm report pain but preserved motion.[10]

The forearm is linked carefully between the five components—the PRUJ, DRUJ, IOM, radial shaft, and ulnar shaft. A break in any one of these five components can lead to instability or pathology in the remaining link. An understanding of this crucial fundamental anatomy will help the reader understand the complex pathology of the forearm.

DEFINITION AND CLASSIFICATION

Forearm fractures include fractures of the shaft of the radius, ulna, or combined fracture to the radius and ulna, typically called a "both-bone" fracture.

Forearm fractures are classified according to the location (proximal third, middle third, or distal third), fracture pattern (transverse, oblique, spiral, comminuted, or segmental), displacement (displaced or nondisplaced), and finally angulation (volar or dorsal and radial or ulnar) (**Figures 15.1-15.6**). Angulation references the direction the distal segment moves in comparison to the proximal segment.

A **nightstick** fracture is an isolated midshaft ulnar fracture. Mechanism of injury is typically a direct blow to the ulnar shaft, often while the patient is protecting the face or body from injury using the forearm. The term comes from the historical "nightstick" club carried as a compliance tool or defensive weapon by police or military personnel and associated injury caused by this device.

The muscular forces acting on the proximal and distal fragments determine displacement according to the location of the fracture. A proximal third radius fracture, between the insertion of the supinator and pronator teres muscles, leads to supination of the proximal fragment by the action of the supinator muscle and pronation of the distal fragment

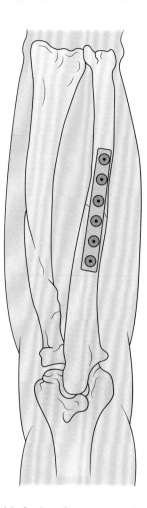

FIGURE 15.2 Midshaft ulnar fracture treated with compression plate fixation. This fixation restores anatomic alignment of the shaft of the ulna and allows early range of motion of the elbow, forearm, and wrist. (Reprinted with permission from Hoppenfeld S, Murthy VL. *Treatment and Rehabilitation of Fractures*. Philadelphia: Lippincott Williams & Wilkins; 2000.)

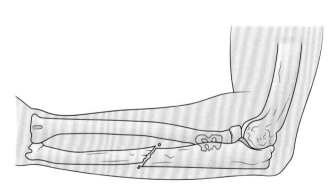

FIGURE 15.1 Minimally displaced oblique fracture of the middle third of the ulna. (Reprinted with permission from Hoppenfeld S, Murthy VL. *Treatment and Rehabilitation of Fractures*. Philadelphia: Lippincott Williams & Wilkins; 2000.)

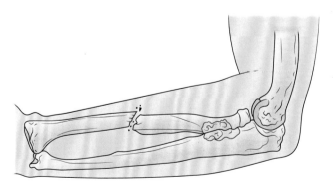

FIGURE 15.3 Displaced oblique fracture of the midshaft of the radius. This fracture generally requires internal fixation to anatomically align the radius and restore radial. (Reprinted with permission from Hoppenfeld S, Murthy VL. *Treatment and Rehabilitation of Fractures*. Philadelphia: Lippincott Williams & Wilkins; 2000.)

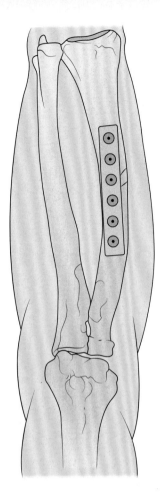

FIGURE 15.4 Midshaft radius fracture treated with compression plate fixation. This fixation restores the anatomic alignment of the radius and the radial blow and allows for early range of motion of the elbow, forearm, and wrist. (Reprinted with permission from Hoppenfeld S, Murthy VL. *Treatment and Rehabilitation of Fractures.* Philadelphia: Lippincott Williams & Wilkins; 2000.)

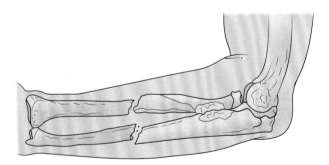

FIGURE 15.5 Oblique displaced midshaft fractures of the radius and ulna both-bone forearm fracture. These fractures require open reduction and internal fixation with a compression plate in order to restore the anatomic alignment of the radius and ulna and allow early range of motion. (Reprinted with permission from Hoppenfeld S, Murthy VL. *Treatment and Rehabilitation of Fractures.* Philadelphia: Lippincott Williams & Wilkins; 2000.)

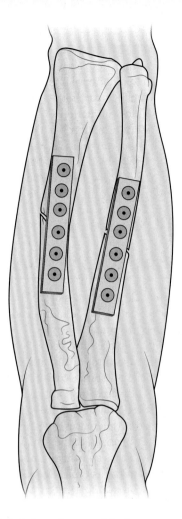

FIGURE 15.6 Both-bone fracture of the forearm treated with compression plate fixation of both the radius and the ulna. This fixation restores anatomic alignment of the shaft of the ulna and allows early range of motion of the elbow, forearm, and wrist. (Reprinted with permission from Hoppenfeld S, Murthy VL. *Treatment and Rehabilitation of Fractures.* Philadelphia: Lippincott Williams & Wilkins; 2000.)

caused by the action of the pronator teres and pronator quadratus muscles. A distal third radius fracture leads to a proximal fragment held in neutral by the counteracting forces of the supinator and pronator teres. The distal fragment will pronate due to the pull of the pronator quadratus muscle.

Associated injuries include fractures of the shaft with an associated dislocation. In the forearm, associated injuries include the Monteggia fracture (radial head dislocation with fracture of the ulna), Galeazzi fracture (DRUJ dislocation with fracture of the radius), and Essex-Lopresti fracture (fracture of the proximal radius with complete disruption of the IOM and DRUJ dislocation). An Essex-Lopresti equivalent is injury to the IOM leading to radial longitudinal instability without associated fracture or dislocation. See section titled "Associated Injuries" for more details of these variants.

Fractures of the ulna and radius require evaluation of the elbow and wrist, respectively. Satisfactory anteroposterior and lateral radiographs of both joints should be obtained for all forearm fractures. Careful examination of the ulnar styloid and DRUJ should be performed. Ulnar styloid fractures and widening of the DRUJ are suggestive of DRUJ injury and help in diagnosing Galeazzi fractures. Distal radial shortening of greater than 5 mm is also associated with Galeazzi fractures. Prominence of the radial head, pain on radial head palpation, and ulnar shortening without a radius fracture are all associated with radial head subluxation or dislocation and indicate a Monteggia fracture. Galeazzi and Monteggia fractures must be identified because the joint injury needs to be addressed. There is an increased risk of complications including loss of motion, malunion, nonunion, and neurovascular compromise of the posterior interosseous nerve associated with these injuries.

MANAGEMENT

Diagnosis, History, and Physical Examination

Most forearm fractures are a result of a fall onto an outstretched hand or a direct blow sustained in motor vehicle accident or altercation. Unlike the typical distal radius or distal humerus fracture which may occur in osteoporotic bone as a result of a ground level fall, forearm fractures tend to occur as a result of a high-energy mechanism.

TREATMENT

Nonoperative

Nightstick fractures, nondisplaced fractures, or displaced fractures with adequate reduction can usually be managed nonoperatively with close radiographic and clinical surveillance. This can be accomplished using splinting, bracing, or casting. Pediatric forearm fractures have a distinct treatment protocol given the unique anatomy of the skeletally immature patient, discussion of which is beyond the scope of this chapter.

Immobilization consists of splinting, casting, or functional bracing (removable plastic brace). The question of long-arm, above-elbow immobilization versus short-arm, below-elbow immobilization is an ongoing debate. Proponents of above-elbow casting claim that greater control is given when the elbow is not allowed to articulate to prevent pronation and supination. However, an above-elbow cast is poorly tolerated by patients, and some argue that below-elbow immobilization is sufficient. Prospective randomized studies of distal radius fracture nonoperative treatment show equivalent maintenance of reduction in a short versus long arm cast[11].

A recent systematic review of ulnar nightstick fractures shows a trend toward adequate rates of healing with immobilization in a below elbow cast or removable orthoses and early motion[12]. No definitive studies have demonstrated the amount of stability and immobilization required for forearm, DRUJ, or PRUJ injuries. The decision remains with the treating surgeon.

Fractures are typically immobilized for a period of 6 to 12 weeks based on clinical and radiographic progress. At the 4- to 6-week return visit, radiographs out of cast are obtained. Casting may be discontinued when there is abundant callus on radiographs, no motion at the fracture site

on examination, and fracture site is nontender to palpation. This typically occurs between the 6- to 8-week period but may vary by patient and fracture pattern. In cases of slow healing, casting may be extended. If after 3 to 4 months no change in fracture union has taken place, a fracture nonunion has occurred and consideration for open reduction with or without bone grafting should be taken.

Either a short or long arm cast is applied based on surgeon preference. Cast is trimmed at the metacarpophalangeal (MCP) joints to allow full digit range of motion (ROM). During the healing period, active motion of the digits and shoulder is encouraged; gentle motion at the elbow is encouraged if short arm cast is used. Dependent edema is treated with elevation and/or compression. Once immobilization is discontinued, an accelerated rehabilitation protocol can be used to regain motion and strength lost during immobilization.

Operative

Most forearm fractures will require surgical stabilization with open reduction and internal fixation being the most common operative technique. By necessity, an adult both-bone forearm fracture requires operative stabilization and is called a "fracture of necessity." This is due to the divergent pull of the forearm musculature which makes maintaining a closed reduction almost impossible.

Polytrauma patients who require use of the arm for weight bearing to offload weight from an injured lower extremity who have forearm fractures which may otherwise be treated nonoperatively may be treated operatively to allow immediate weight bearing. Intra-articular fracture of the radius and ulna have their own management protocols and are covered separately in their respective chapters.

Goals of surgery include reduction of overall alignment and restoration of radial bow. Although precise anatomic reduction is admirable, fractures of the shaft do not require the same precise reduction as fractures of the joint given that the diaphysis is not an articulating surface. Diaphyseal fractures may be highly comminuted and displaced, and in the case of open fractures, bone segments may be missing which preclude an anatomic reduction. Therefore, treatment of diaphyseal fractures focuses on restoring the overall alignment of the bone. Accurate restoration of alignment is key to maintain pronation, supination, and grip strength. The radial bow and interosseous space should be preserved. The exception to this rule is isolated ulnar fractures in which up to 50% displacement is tolerated without significant dysfunction.

Surgical intervention should aim to provide stable, durable internal fixation. Forearm shaft fractures often occur in the polytrauma patient who would benefit from immediate weight bearing of the upper extremity to offload a severe lower extremity injury. These factors should be considered in operative planning.

Synostosis, or bony growth/fusion between the radius and ulna, is a complication that may occur in relation to forearm fractures. Disruption of the periosteum about the radius or ulna can lead to bony growth. When bone grows between the two bones, the bones become linked and lead to a reduction or even loss of pronosupination of the forearm. Increased risk is associated with injuries at the same level. Operative fixation through a single incision and the use of bone graft may also increase the risk and therefore are avoided whenever possible.

INITIAL POST-OP TREATMENT

A splint may be used postoperatively to protect the incision but should be discontinued within a few days. Moss and Bynum report use of a splint for 5 to 7 days followed by early motion.[13] Active assisted motion is started early to prevent soft-tissue contracture. In certain cases, immediate full weight bearing of the operative arm is allowed, particularly in the polytrauma patient. Communication with the treating surgeon is required prior to allowing this.

ASSOCIATED INJURIES

MONTEGGIA FRACTURES

Diagnosis, History, and Physical Examination

Monteggia fracture/dislocation is a proximal or middle third ulnar fracture with dislocation of the radial head. The radial head may dislocate anteriorly, posteriorly, or laterally. In some instances, both the radius and the ulna may be fractured. Injury is usually a result of fall onto an outstretched hand or a direct blow sustained in motor vehicle accident or altercation. The radial head injury, particularly an isolated dislocation without fracture, can be missed if the examiner is not attuned to this associated injury. Often the radial head may self-reduce and the treating provider may believe the injury to be an isolated ulnar fracture. One has to have a high index of suspicion for a Monteggia fracture when isolated ulnar fractures are seen, as they represent a higher degree of injury and may require prolonged recovery and rehabilitation.

Monteggia fractures are classified based on the Bado classification system.[14] In this system, the direction of the radial head dislocation is the descriptor. Type I is anterior dislocation of the radial head, type II is posterior dislocation of the radial head, and type III is lateral dislocation of the radial head. Type I-III are associated with proximal or middle third ulnar fractures. A Bado type IV is proximal or middle third of both the ulna and radius with dislocation of the radial head in any direction.

The posterior interosseous nerve (PIN) lies in close proximity to the radial head, crossing the radial head on average between 3 and 5 cm from the radiocapitellar joint based on the pronosupination of the arm.[15] With radial head dislocation, the PIN may be injured from pull of the bone on the nerve. This leads to a neuropraxia (nerve contusion without disruption) that typically resolves in 6 to 8 weeks. If no recovery is noted clinically or an electrodiagnostic examination by 4 to 6 months, exploration of the nerve could be considered. Operative treatment for associated radial head fractures may similarly put the PIN at risk for injury and should be closely protected.

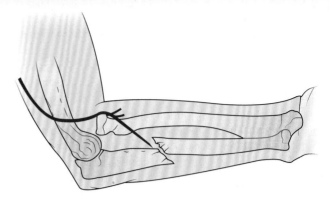

FIGURE 15.7 Fracture of the diaphysis of the ulna with a dislocated radial head. An anterior dislocation of the radial head is a Monteggia fracture type I, as seen here, requiring reduction of the radial head and internal fixation of the ulnar fracture. (Reprinted with permission from Hoppenfeld S, Murthy VL. *Treatment and Rehabilitation of Fractures.* Philadelphia: Lippincott Williams & Wilkins; 2000.)

TREATMENT AND AFTERCARE

In adults, Monteggia fractures are fractures of necessity and should be treated surgically. For Monteggia fractures, the key steps are plating of the ulnar fracture and closed reduction of the head. Simultaneous reduction of the radial head typically occurs as the ulnar shaft is anatomically reduced and fixed (**Figures 15.7** and **15.8**).

Postoperative immobilization varies depending on the stability of the radial head after reduction and the stability of the ulnar fracture fixation. Traditionally Monteggia fractures were treated in long arm cast for 6 weeks. Newer operative techniques and understanding of functional rehabilitation likely will allow treating surgeons to move these patients sooner. The arm is supported in a protective splint initially to protect the incisions and repairs, but active motion is encouraged within the first 2 weeks to prevent elbow and forearm stiffness. Some authors start active motion with gravity assistance for both flexion and extension in the first week.[16] The treating therapist should check with the referring surgeon for restrictions.

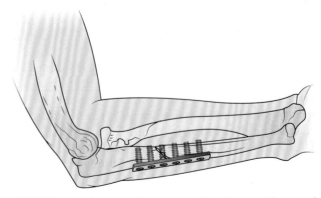

FIGURE 15.8 Reduction of the radial head and internal fixation of the ulnar fracture with compression plating. (Reprinted with permission from Hoppenfeld S, Murthy VL. *Treatment and Rehabilitation of Fractures.* Philadelphia: Lippincott Williams & Wilkins; 2000.)

GALLEAZZI FRACTURE

Diagnosis, History, and Physical Examination

A Galeazzi fracture/dislocation is a radius fracture with disruption of the DRUJ. Fracture is typically in the middle to distal one-third of the radius as this location is more likely to cause disruption to the DRUJ. Injury is typically a result of axial load with a torsional force. In order for DRUJ dislocation to occur, severe disruption of the TFCC is required. If the TFCC injury and DRUJ instability are not recognized and treated appropriately, poor outcome is common.

The Galeazzi is called a "fracture of necessity" because in this injury it is necessary to provide surgical intervention because of loss of correction and loss of bowing of the radius. Misdiagnosis or inadequate management can lead to disabling complications including DRUJ instability, malunion, limited forearm ROM, chronic wrist pain, and post-traumatic arthritis.[17] Nonoperative management of Galeazzi fractures are uniformly unsatisfactory.[18,19]

Several muscles exert deforming forces on the Galeazzi fracture. The pronator quadratus attaching distally on the radius will cause rotational deformation. Several muscles pull the distal radius proximally, in effect shortening the radius. These include the brachioradialis inserting at the radial styloid and the abductor pollicis longus and extensor pollicis brevis.

Treatment

For Galeazzi fractures, the radius is anatomically reduced and fixed with a plate. This restores the position of the radioulnar joint. Care needs to be paid to anatomically restoring the sagittal radial bow of the radius (**Figures 15.9-15.11**).

After radius fixation, the DRUJ is examined. If the DRUJ is stable, a protective splint with early motion is appropriate aftercare.[20-22]

If the DRUJ is not reduced or the reduction is unstable, attempt is made to close reduce the joint. If successful, the joint is pinned using two Kirschner wires (K-wires) to hold the reduction. Alternatively, the patient may be casted in supination if the DRUJ reduction remains stable in this position.

If reduction is unsuccessfully closed, open reduction is required. If there is a large ulnar styloid fragment, this is treated with open reduction internal fixation. The TFCC should be explored and repaired using bone tunnels or suture anchors. If the joint remains irreducible, the DRUJ should be

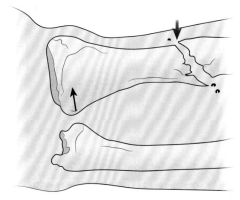

FIGURE 15.10 Galeazzi fracture/dislocation, illustrating a distal radioulnar joint disruption. The arrows represent the direction of force at time of injury. (Reprinted with permission from Hoppenfeld S, Murthy VL. *Treatment and Rehabilitation of Fractures.* Philadelphia: Lippincott Williams & Wilkins; 2000.)

opened and any interposed tissue removed. The most common interposed tissue is the extensor carpi ulnaris tendon. Depending on joint stability after these steps have been taken, K-wire fixation of the ulna to the radius may be required.

Aftercare

Typically, the arm is immobilized in supination after treatment. The DRUJ is most stable in supination; thus, immobilization in this position helps the joint, and the injured soft tissues heal in the most inherently stable position. Postoperative protocol varies by stability of the DRUJ.

As noted above, if the DRUJ is stable after radius fixation, a protective splint is used for the first days to weeks followed by early motion. However, if the DRUJ required K-wire fixation, TFCC repair, ulnar styloid fixation, or splinting in supination, then greater immobilization is required. This is typically immobilization in supination with either a long arm splint or cast for 4 to 6 weeks. K-wires are typically removed at 4 to 6 weeks once the tissues have had a chance to heal.

ESSEX-LOPRESTI INJURY/RADIOLONGITUDINAL INSTABILITY

History, Diagnosis, and Physical Examination

An Essex-Lopresti injury (ELI) is characterized by fracture of the proximal radius, usually the radial head, with

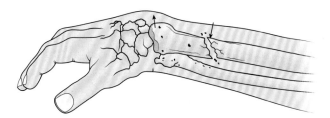

FIGURE 15.9 Fracture of the distal radius with distal radial/ulnar joint disruption (Galeazzi fracture/dislocation). The arrows represent the direction of force at time of injury. (Reprinted with permission from Hoppenfeld S, Murthy VL. *Treatment and Rehabilitation of Fractures.* Philadelphia: Lippincott Williams & Wilkins; 2000.)

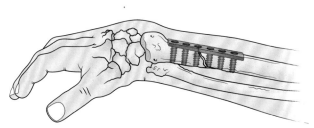

FIGURE 15.11 Reduction of a Galeazzi fracture/dislocation with compression plate fixation of the distal radioulnar joint. (Reprinted with permission from Hoppenfeld S, Murthy VL. *Treatment and Rehabilitation of Fractures.* Philadelphia: Lippincott Williams & Wilkins; 2000.)

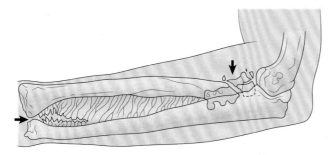

FIGURE 15.12 Fracture of the proximal radius with disruption of the interosseous membrane between the radius and ulna (Essex-Lopresti fracture). This injury is associated with proximal migration of the radius and instability of the distal radioulnar joint. The arrows represent the direction of force at time of injury. (Reprinted with permission from Hoppenfeld S, Murthy VL. *Treatment and Rehabilitation of Fractures.* Philadelphia: Lippincott Williams & Wilkins; 2000.)

disruption of the IOM and dislocation or disruption of the DRUJ (**Figure 15.12**). It is caused by a violent load transmitted from the wrist to the elbow. This is a devastating but rare injury which results from forceful axial and torsional load of the forearm. The injury is commonly missed and presents in a delayed fashion. The injury leads to axial and longitudinal instability of the forearm.

Aftercare

Postoperative protocols vary by acuity of injury. Traditionally in the acute setting, the arm should be immobilized in an above-elbow cast with the forearm in supination for 4 to 6 weeks. Grassmann et al report that early flexion and extension of the elbow is encouraged while avoiding forearm rotation for the first 6 weeks. This is done by placing the elbow in a Muenster orthosis which allows 0° to 90° of elbow flexion-extension with the forearm maintained in supination to protect the DRUJ and the IOM.[23]

Matson and Ruch report that following reconstructive surgery for the chronic injury, patients are immobilized in a sugar-tong splint for 2 weeks until suture removal.[24] They are then transitioned to a Muenster splint to immobilize forearm rotation but gentle elbow ROM is begun. At 6 weeks, the Muenster is discontinued and active ROM of the wrist is started.[24]

Adams et al treat a chronic reconstruction with 1 to 2 weeks of above-elbow immobilization in neutral, followed by a short arm cast or removable splint that is worn for 4 to 6 weeks. They do not limit forearm rotation other than the first 1 to 2 weeks.[25]

REHABILITATION OF FOREARM FRACTURES

According to Matthias and Wright, the forearm is uniquely designed to bear significant load while rotating nearly 180°.[6] The complement of shoulder circumduction and forearm rotation allows placement of the human hand in virtually all spatial directions. In order to achieve this remarkable feat, the radius and ulna must maintain an appropriate length, alignment, and congruent articulations at both the DRUJ and PRUJ. Supporting this construct is the IOM with the central band being the most crucial component. A disruption of any of these components will lead to dysfunction of the forearm resulting in loss of pronosupination and/or flexion-extension.

The goals of rehabilitation of forearm fractures are improvement in swelling, pain, ROM, strength, and, ultimately, return to preinjury function. Studies have shown that most functional activities require 30° of elbow extension, 130° of elbow flexion, and 50° of supination and pronation.[26]

The therapist aims to guide the patient through the stages of healing from early protection of wound healing, later to protect healing structures to maintain stability, and finally to restore motion and strength.

The following rehabilitation guidelines are for stable fixation of fractures of the shaft of the radius and/or ulna. Please see the following "Special Considerations" section for further guidelines for treating patients with an associated injury (i.e., Galeazzi, Monteggia, Essex-Lopresti).

SPECIAL CONSIDERATIONS

The associated fractures including Monteggia, Galeazzi, and Essex-Lopresti require special consideration. The main difference is to limit forearm rotation during the healing period. The most stable position for associated injuries of the forearm is with the forearm in supination.

The Monteggia fracture is classically immobilized in a long arm cast for 6 weeks. Newer protocols are treating with 1 to 2 weeks in a protective splint while the wounds heal followed by active early flexion-extension of the arm at 2 weeks. No forearm rotation is done until typically the 4 to 6 week mark.

The Galeazzi injury and ELI are similar. Classically, these injuries are immobilized in an above-elbow cast with the forearm in supination for 6 weeks. More recent protocols have shown that an injury in which the DRUJ is stable after fixation of the radius, it is reasonable to be more aggressive with motion. The surgeon will typically use a protective splint for the first 1 to 2 weeks while wounds are healing and then start early motion including flexion/extension and pronosupination at 1 to 2 weeks postoperatively.

However, if the DRUJ was unstable, especially if K-wires were placed to immobilize the DRUJ, the arm is immobilized with above-elbow cast in supination for 4 to 6 weeks. More recent protocols have shown that in this scenario, it is safe to use a protective splint for the first 1 to 2 weeks and then begin active flexion-extension with the arm in supination at week 1 to 2. This is achieved by a Muenster orthosis which allows elbow flexion-extension but no forearm rotation.

The chronic ELI can be treated similarly with 1 to 2 weeks of protection followed by early flexion-extension of the elbow while limiting forearm rotation.

PROTOCOLS AND REHABILITATION GOALS OF FOREARM FRACTURES

OPERATIVE

Week 0 to 2 rehabilitation goals: Rest surgical wound and repair site. Edema control and pain relief. Full digit and shoulder motion (active range of motion/active-assist range of motion/passive range of motion [AROM/AAROM/PROM]). Very gentle motion of forearm and elbow (AAROM only).

Week 2 to 4 rehabilitation goals: Edema control, scar mobilization by 2 weeks post suture removal. Light putty exercises by week 2 to 3. Full digit and shoulder motion (AROM/AAROM/PROM). Progress gentle motion of forearm and elbow, gentle isometrics by week 2 to 3.

Week 4 to 8 rehabilitation goals: Edema control, scar desensitization. Light use of operative arm for activities of daily living (ADLs). Full digit and shoulder motion (AROM/AAROM/PROM). Progress gentle motion of forearm and elbow focusing on pronosupination, elbow and wrist flexion/extension, and advancing gentle isometrics.

Week 8 to 12 rehabilitation goals: Full active and passive ROM exercises to all joints of the extremity while focusing on pronation and supination of the forearm. Putty and ball-squeezing exercises improve grip strength. Introduce gentle resistive exercises using weights in gradation.

NONOPERATIVE/TENUOUS OPERATIVE FIXATION

Week 0 to 2 rehabilitation goals: Immobilized in cast/splint. Edema control of digits. Full digit and shoulder motion in all planes (AROM/AAROM/PROM). Very gentle motion of elbow if short arm cast flexion/extension only.

Week 2 to 4 rehabilitation goals: Immobilized in cast/splint. Edema control of digits. Full digit and shoulder motion in all planes (AROM/AAROM/PROM). Very gentle motion of elbow if short arm cast flexion/extension only. Progress gentle motion of elbow and flexion/extension only.

Week 4 to 8 rehabilitation goals: Edema control. Once cast removed, desensitization. Light use of operative arm for ADLs. Full digit and shoulder motion (AROM/AAROM/PROM). Progress gentle motion of forearm and elbow focusing on pronosupination, elbow and wrist flexion/extension, and advancing gentle isometrics. Light putty and ball-squeezing exercises.

Week 8 to 12 rehabilitation goals: Edema control. Full active and passive ROM exercises to all joints of the extremity while focusing on pronation and supination of the forearm. Putty and ball-squeezing exercises improve grip strength. Introduce gentle resistive exercises using weights in gradation.

REFERENCES

1. Hotchkiss RN, An KN, Sowa DT, Basta S, Weiland AJ. An Anatomic and mechanical study of the interosseous membrane of the forearm: pathomechanics of proximal migration of the radius. *J Hand Surg Am.* 1989;14(2 pt 1):256-261.

2. van Riet RP, Van Glabbeek F, Baumfeld JA, et al. The effect of the orientation of the radial head on the kinematics of the ulnohumeral joint and force transmission through the radiocapitellar joint. *Clin Biomech (Bristol, Avon).* 2006;21:554-559.

3. van Riet RP, Van Glabbeek F, Baumfeld JA, et al. The effect of the orientation of the noncircular radial head on elbow kinematics. *Clin Biomech (Bristol, Avon).* 2004;19:595-599.

4. Rozental TD, Beredjiklian PK, Bozentka DJ. Longitudinal radioulnar dissociation. *J Am Acad Orthop Surg.* 2003;11:68-73.

5. Adams JE. Forearm instability: anatomy, biomechanics, and treatment options. *J Hand Surg.* 2017;42(1):47-52.

6. Matthias R, Wright TW. Interosseous membrane of the forearm. *J Wrist Surg.* 2016;5:188-193.

7. Birkbeck DP, Failla JM, Hoshaw SJ, Fyhrie DP, Schaffler M. The interosseous membrane affects load distribution in the forearm. *J Hand Surg Am.* 1997;22(6):975-980.

8. Palmer AK, Werner FW. Biomechanics of the distal radioulnar joint. *Clin Orthop Relat Res.* 1984;(187):26-35.

9. Drobner WS, Hausman MR. The distal radioulnar joint. *Hand Clin.* 1992;8:631-644.

10. Hotchkiss RN. Fractures of the radial head and related instability and contracture of the forearm. *Instr Course Lect.* 1998;47:173-177.

11. Bong MR, Egol KA, Leibman M, Koval K. A comparison of immediate postreduction splinting constructs for controlling intial displacement of fractures of the distal radius: a prospective randomized study of long-arm versus short-arm splinting. *J Hand Surg.* 2006;31A:766-770.

12. Cai XZ, Yan SG, Giddins G. A systematic review of the nonoperative treatment of nightstick fractures of the ulna. *Bone Joint J.* 2013;95-B:952-959.

13. Moss JP, Bynum DK. Diaphyseal fractures of the radius and ulna in adults. *Hand Clin.* 2007;23:143-151.

14. Bado J. The Monteggia lesion. *Clin Orthop Relat Res.* 1967;50:71-86.

15. Calfee R, Wilson J, Wong A. Variations in the Anatomic Relations of the Posterior Interosseous Nerve Associated with Proximal Forearm Trauma. *J Bone Joint Surg Am.* 2011;93:81-90.

16. Eathiraju S, Dorth DN, Mudgal CS, Jupiter JB. Monteggia fracture-dislocations. *Hand Clin.* 2007;23:165-177.

17. Atesok K, Jupiter J, Weiss AP. Galezzi fractures. *J Am Acad Orthop Surg.* 2011;19:623-633.

18. Eberl R, Singer G, Schalamon J, Petnehazy T, Hoellwarth ME. Galeazzi lesions in children and adolescents: treatment and outcome. *Clin Orthop Relat Res.* 2008;466(7):1705-1709.

19. Mikic ZD. Galeazzi fracture dislocations. *J Bone Joint Surg Am.* 1975;57(8):1071-1080.

20. Jupiter JB, Kellam JF. Diaphyseal fractures of the forearm. In: Browner BD, Jupiter JB, Levine AM, Trafton PG, Krettek C, eds. *Skeletal Trauma.* Philadelphia, PA: Saunders Elsevier; 2009:1478-1481.

21. Komura S, Nonomura H, Satake T, Yokoi T. Bilateral Galeazzi fracture-dislocations: a case report of early rehabilitation. *Strateg Trauma Limb Reconstr.* 2012;7(2):99-104.

22. Gwinn DE, O'Toole RV, Eglseder WA. Early motion protocol for select Galeazzi fractures after radial shaft fixation. *J Surg Orthop Adv.* 2010;19:104-108.

23. Grassmann JP, Hakimi M, Gehrmann SV, et al. The treatment of the acute essex-lopresti injury. *Bone Joint J.* 2014;96-B:1385-1391.

24. Matson AP, Ruch DS. Management of the Essex-Lopresti injury. *J Wrist Surg.* 2016;5:172-178.

25. Adams JE, Osterman MN, Osterman AL. Interosseous membrane reconstruction for forearm longitudinal instability. *Tech Hand Up Extrem Surg.* 2010;14(4):222-225.

26. Morrey BF, Askew LJ, Chao EY. A biomechanical study of normal functional elbow motion. *J Bone Joint Surg Am.* 1981;63A:872-877.

SUGGESTED READINGS

Adams JE, Culp RW, Osterman AL. Interosseous membrane reconstruction for the Essex-Lopresti injury. *J Hand Surg Am.* 2010;35(1):129-136.

Adams JE, Steinmann SP, Osterman AL. Management of injuries to the interosseous membrane. *Hand Clin.* 2010;26(4):543-548.

Brin YS, Palmanovich E, Bivas A, et al. Treating acute Essex-Lopresti injury with the TightRope device: a case study. *Tech Hand Up Extrem Surg.* 2014;18(1):51-55.

Duckworth AD, Watson BS, Will EM, et al. Radial shortening following a fracture of the proximal radius. *Acta Orthop*. 2011;82:356-359.

Edwards GS Jr, Jupiter JB. Radial head fractures with acute distal radioulnar dislocation: Essex-Lopresti revisited. *Clin Orthop*. 1988;234:61-69.

Hausmann JT, Vekszler G, Breitenseher M, et al. Mason type-I radial head fractures and interosseous membrane lesions: a prospective study. *J Trauma*. 2009;66:457-461.

Jungbluth P, Frangen TM, Arens S, Muhr G, Kälicke T. The undiagnosed Essex-Lopresti injury. *J Bone Joint Surg Br*. 2006;88-B:1629-1633.

Marcotte AL, Osterman AL. Longitudinal radioulnar dissociation: identification and treatment of acute and chronic injuries. *Hand Clin*. 2007;23(2):195-208.

Matthias R, Wright TW. Interosseous membrane of the Forearm. *J Wrist Surg*. 2016;5:188-193.

Morrey BF, Chao EY, Hui FC. Biomechanical study of the elbow following excision of the radial head. *J Bone Joint Surg Am*. 1979;61-A: 63-68.

Neuber M, Joist A, Joosten U, Rieger H. Consequences and possible treatment of distal radio-ulnar dislocation after Essex-Lopresti lesion. *Unfallchirug*. 2000;103:1093-1096.

Rettig ME, Raskin KB. Galeazzi fracture-dislocation: a new treatment-oriented classification. *J Hand Surg Am*. 2001;26(2):228-235.

Ring D, Jupiter J, Waters P. Monteggia fractures in children and adults. *J Am Acad Orthop Surg*. 1998;6:215-224.

Ring D, Rhim R, Carpenter C, Jupiter JB. Isolated radial shaft fractures are more common than Galeazzi fractures. *J Hand Surg Am*. 2006;31(1):17-21.

Sabo MT, Watts AC. Reconstructing the interosseous membrane: a technique using synthetic graft and endobuttons. *Tech Hand Up Extrem Surg*. 2012;16(4):187-193.

Schneiderman G, Meldrum RD, Bloebaum RD, Tarr R, Sarmiento A. The interosseous membrane of the forearm: structure and its role in Galeazzi fractures. *J Trauma*. 1993;35(6):879-885.

Skahen JR III, Palmer AK, Werner FW, Fortino MD. Reconstruction of the interosseous membrane of the forearm in cadavers. *J Hand Surg Am*. 1997;22(6):986-994.

Soubeyrand M, Oberlin C, Dumontier C, Belkheyar Z, Lafont C, Degeorges R. Ligamentoplasty of the forearm interosseous membrane using the semitendinosus tendon: anatomical study and surgical procedure. *Surg Radiol Anat*. 2006;28(3):300-307.

Stabile KJ, Pfaeffle J, Saris I, Li ZM, Tomaino MM. Structural properties of reconstruction constructs for the interosseous ligament of the forearm. *J Hand Surg Am*. 2005;30(2):312-318.

Tomaino MM, Pfaeffle J, Stabile K, Li ZM. Reconstruction of the interosseous ligament of the forearm reduces load on the radial head in cadavers. *J Hand Surg Br*. 2003;28(3):267-270.

Trousdale RT, Amadio PC, Cooney WP, Morrey BF. Radio-ulnar dissociation. A review of twenty cases. *J Bone Joint Surg Am*. 1992;74(10):1486-1497.

16

Distal Radius Fractures: Postsurgical Care and Rehabilitation

Ryan Martyn
Matthew S. Hoehn

EPIDEMIOLOGY

Distal radius fractures (DRFs) are one of the most common fractures in adults. Fractures of the distal radius occur more often in older women as a result of low-energy trauma, such as falls from standing height.[1] Data from the National Hospital Ambulatory Care Survey showed an incidence on 643,097 DRFs in the United States, representing 44% of hand and forearm fractures.[2] In 2007, Medicare made $170 million in DRF attributable payments with a mean payment of $1983 per patient.[3] The incidence of DRFs has increased, affecting predominantly postmenopausal women.[4] The increased incidence of these fractures may be due to increased longevity, increased working ages, and better reporting. In Sweden, the incidence of distal forearm fractures was found to have increased 23% from 1999 to 2010[5] and has nearly doubled the incidence from 1953-1957 to 1980-1981.[6] A survey in Japan showed a statistically significant increase in the incidence of DRFs among women, but not men, from 164.9 per 100,000 person years in 1986 to 211.4 in 1995.[7] Postmenopausal women are particularly prone to sustaining these fractures. Thompson et al reported that the incidence of DRFs rose from 10 per 10,000 population per year among premenopausal women to 120 per 10,000 population per year.[4] DRFs can lead to increased morbidity, deformity, and pain.[8] Complications from DRFs include persistent neuropathies, finger stiffness, disuse atrophy, and complex regional pain syndrome. These complications are often difficult to treat but may be avoided by proper treatment principles. Understanding these fractures is crucial for healthcare providers as they are common and can have adverse outcomes if poorly managed.

FUNCTIONAL ANATOMY AND KINEMATICS

The wrist is a unique and highly complex joint. An understanding of its functional anatomy is crucial for the treatment of injuries involving the wrist. Although many individuals can maintain activities of daily living with altered wrist anatomy secondary to trauma or degeneration, outcomes related to function and pain depend largely on restoring native anatomy and maintaining normal movement of the wrist. A knowledgeable provider can help guide treatment during the rehabilitative stage of treatment by facilitating restoration of native anatomy. An anatomical understanding of the wrist is of little consequence to the practicing physician without the complimentary knowledge of functionality. The column and row theory of the wrist provide such functional knowledge of the wrist to guide the provider as to what position to immobilize the patient in. Similarly, knowledge of the column and row theory may alert the physician to pay attention to certain fracture characteristics that may predispose a patient to malunion or post-traumatic arthritis. Finally, an understanding of the functional movement of the wrist is imperative when transitioning patients from the immobilization phase to the mobilization phase of treatment.

The wrist is composed of the distal radius, distal ulna, eight carpal bones, and five metacarpals. The distal radius is triangularly shaped with the scaphoid facet separated from the lunate facet by a sagittal ridge. Although the wrist is generally considered to be one joint, it is composed of 20 small articulations. Movement between bones of the wrist is variable and complex. At the most basic level, the wrist bones form a series of arches, with two transverse arches formed by the carpal bones proximally and the metacarpal

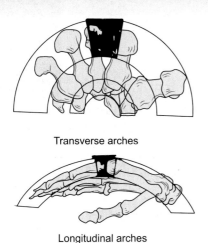

Transverse arches

Longitudinal arches

FIGURE 16.1 The wrist bones form a series of arches. (Modified from Tang JB. General concepts of wrist biomechanics and a view from other species. *J Hand Surg Eur Vol.* 2008;33(4):519-525.)

heads distally. Longitudinal arches are formed by the bones of the rays[9] (**Figure 16.1**). The structure and function of the wrist can be further conceptualized as being composed of columns, rows, or a combination of both.[10]

Originally proposed by Navarro in 1921, the column theory of the wrist divides the wrist into three columns[11,12] (**Figure 16.2**). Several modifications have been made to the column theory, largely to account for the motion of the proximal row during radial and ulnar deviation. Many classifications for DRFs have been created but are beyond the scope of this chapter. A fragment-specific classification has been elucidated by Medoff, which is based on a functional understanding of the column theory. The fragment-specific classification includes the radial column, dorsal ulnar column, volar ulnar corner, volar rim, and free intra-articular fragment (**Figure 16.3**).[13,14] The number of fragments correlates with outcomes, including grip strength, range of motion (ROM), pain, and patient-reported outcomes.[15]

The radial column consists of the radial styloid and scaphoid facet.[16] The radial column has many important functions. It serves as a buttress to prevent radial translation of the carpus, holds the carpus out to length radially, and functions as a platform when the wrist is load bearing in ulnar deviation, such as when using a walker.[14] Several important ligaments attach to the radial column. The brachioradialis inserts 17 mm from the tip of the styloid and can create a deforming force in distal radius by contributing to the loss of radial height.[17,18] The loss of radial height increases the load across the ulna and lunate facet and can lead to painful loss of motion at the distal radial-ulnar joint (DRUJ), impingement of the triangular fibrocartilage complex (TFCC), and subluxation of the ulnar head.[16,18] The long radiolunate ligament and the radioscaphocapitate ligament attach on the radial column. The long radiolunate ligament provides constraint against ulnar or distal translocation of the lunate.[19] The radioscaphocapitate supports the scaphoid waist and prevents the carpus from translating ulnarly.[14,20] Fractures through the radial column warrant special attention during the postoperative period, especially comminuted fractures treated nonoperatively, as these fractures are unstable. Radial column fractures with tenuous fixation or treated nonoperatively should be immobilized in slight ulnar deviation with a thumb spica.[14]

The central column contains the lunate facet and sigmoid notch of the distal radius.[13] The lunate facet projects volarly making it susceptible to shear fractures. The primary role of the central column is load transmission from the carpus to the forearm, with approximately 80% of load being transferred to radius with axial loading in an ulnar-neutral wrist.[14,20-22] The treating provider should be attentive to injury to the central column as it contains the volar rim and the dorsal ulnar corner of the distal radius. The volar rim is the attachment site of the short radiolunate ligament. When the volar rim is fractured, volar displacement of the carpus can occur. The dorsal ulnar corner is the attachment for the

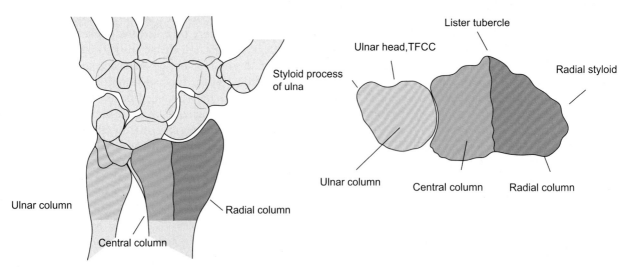

FIGURE 16.2 The wrist seen as three columns. (Modified from Rikli DA, Regazzoni P. Fractures of the distal end of the radius treated by internal fixation and early function. *J Bone Joint Surg Br.* 1996;78:588-592.)

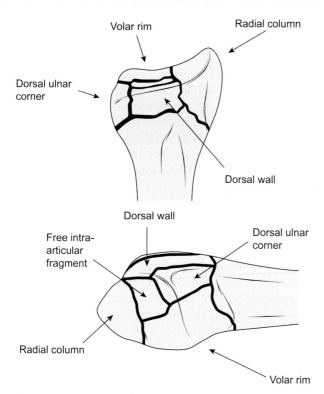

FIGURE 16.3 A fragment-specific classification that co-relates to outcomes. (Modified from Rhee PC, Medoff RJ, Shin AY. Complex distal radius fractures: an anatomic algorithm for surgical management. *J Am Acad Orthop Surg.* 2017;25(2):77-88.)

dorsal radioulnar ligament. When fractured, disruption of the DRUJ may occur, which can adversely affect normal wrist supination and pronation.[14] In DRFs involving the volar rim or the dorsal ulnar corner that are managed nonoperatively or have questionable fixation, the provider should splint the patient in neutral rotation.

The ulnar column consists of the distal ulna, TFCC, and the DRUJ.[16] The function of the ulnar column is to provide stability to the DRUJ and distal forearm motion. The DRUJ is the articulation between the ulnar head and the sigmoid notch of radius. This joint allows the radius to rotate around the ulna and creates stability between the ulna and radius. The TFCC, joint capsule, interosseous membrane, pronator quadratus, and ECU are important stabilizers of the DRUJ. Injuries to the ulnar column may lead to ulnar-sided pain, loss of supination and pronation, and instability of the DRUJ. Loss of radial height and dorsal tilt increase load across the ulna.[13,14,16] Fractures involving the ulnar head, dorsal ulnar corner of the radius, and injuries resulting in DRUJ instability should be immobilized in supination, particularly in fractures treated via closed means.

The row theory of the wrist was introduced in 1926 by Destot.[23,24] The row theory is important for providers to understand as it provides a functional framework for the anatomy and kinematics of the proximal row, which is frequently injured in DRFs. Injury to the ligaments of the proximal row may be overlooked acutely but may become more manifest during the postimmobilization period. The

proximal row consists of the scaphoid, lunate, and triquetrum. No tendon inserts on the bones of the proximal row. The scaphoid moves independent of the proximal row, serving as a link between the proximal row and distal row.[24,25] The proximal row moves relatively independently between the fixed articular surface of the radius and the distal row. Because no ligaments attach to the proximal row, the motion is dependent on the forces from surrounding articulations.[19] This motion was elucidated by Landsmeer in 1961 when he coined the term "intercalated segment."[24,26] Stability of the proximal row is dependent on the contour of the distal radius. The distal row consists of the trapezium, capitate, and hamate. There is little motion between bones of the distal row, while there is significant motion between bones of the proximal row. The pisiform is unique in that it is contained within the flexor carpi ulnaris tendon. The pisiform functions as a sesamoid similar to the patella by increasing the flexion force and stability.[27,28] However, in an evolutionary context, the pisiform bone is not a sesamoid, but more akin to a vestigial calcaneus as evidenced by its prominence among quadrupedal animals.[9,28]

Two important ligaments stabilize the proximal row and link the motion among the scaphoid, lunate, and triquetrum. The articulation between scaphoid and lunate is stabilized by the scapholunate (SL) ligament, while the articulation between the lunate and triquetrum is stabilized by the lunotriquetral (LT) ligament. The SL ligament has a volar part, dorsal part, and a proximal fibrocartilaginous membrane that unites the two.[19,29] The LT ligament also has three parts consisting of a volar ligament, dorsal ligament, and a connecting fibrocartilaginous membrane. The dorsal SL ligament is stronger than the volar SL ligament while the volar LT ligament is stronger than the dorsal LT ligament.[29] Injuries to the SL ligament are common after DRFs and may lead to SL dissociation, scaphoid-lunate advanced collapse. Gapping at the SL interval on a posteroanterior x-ray, an SL angle over 60° as viewed on a lateral x-ray, and continued pain or clunking sensation with hand use should alert the provider that there is likely an SL injury and further intervention may be necessary.[29]

The motion of the wrist is complex and the subject of much debate. Understanding the functional planes of motion of the wrist is important for management of wrist injuries acutely and during the rehabilitation period. Motion is usually described in terms of radial-ulnar inclination and flexion-extension. Radial-ulnar inclination is now the favored term as an alternative to radial-ulnar deviation according to the Nomenclature Committee of the International Federation of Societies for Surgery of the Hand.[30] The complexity of the human wrist anatomy and kinematics nearly precludes the usage of terminology that reduces its movement to orthogonal planes. Activities of daily living, especially activities requiring precision and power, do not occur in mere linear sagittal and coronal planes, but rather in an oblique manner from radial deviation-extension to ulnar deviation-flexion.

This motion, commonly called the dart thrower's motion, is a uniquely human trait not shared among other primates.[9,31] The dart thrower's plane of motion likely represents an adaptive trait that conferred an evolutionary advantage to early humans giving them an advantage in precisely throwing stones and using clubs as tools or weapons.[24,31] During the dart thrower's motion, the proximal row stays still while most of motion occurs through the midcarpal joint.[32-34] However, when there is disruption of the SL ligament, the dart thrower's motion can induce gapping between the scaphoid and lunate.[35] The most important tendons that facilitate the dart thrower's motion are the extensor radialis longus and the flexor carpi ulnaris.[36] Utilization of the dart thrower's motion during rehabilitation of DRFs has been advocated; however, caution should be maintained if there is an SL injury.

RADIOGRAPHIC PARAMETERS

The treating provider must obtain x-ray images during the initial stages of DRFs. Weekly x-rays should be obtained during the first 3 weeks for DRFs being treated nonoperatively.[13] A minimum of two of view are acceptable in the majority of cases in identifying and assessing DRFs. Elbow and forearm images are warranted in identifying more proximal injuries. Advanced imaging, such as computed tomography and magnetic resonance imaging, provide much greater detail and are useful adjuncts for surgical planning, but rarely necessary in the postoperative period. Two-view wrist x-rays are necessary for assessment of radial inclination (normal: 19°-29°), radial height (normal: 11-12 mm), and volar tilt (normal: 11°-14.5°).[37] In complex DRFs, other x-ray views can assist the provider in characterizing the fracture pattern.

ASSOCIATED INJURIES

Soft-tissue disruption and chondral injuries are common after injury to the distal radius. Damage to the surrounding soft tissues can contribute to pain, swelling, stiffness, and functional deficits. Lindau et al reported 82% of patients had traumatic TFCC injuries and 78% with tears. Ulnar styloid fractures increased the risk of TFCC injury.[38] Another study looked at 89 patients with DRFs who underwent arthroscopic treatment. TFCC injury was present in 59% of cases, scapholunate interosseous ligament (SLIL) injury was found in 54.5%, and lunotriquetral interosseous ligament (LTIL) injury was found in 34.5%. The authors found 81% of patients had some intracarpal soft-tissue injury.[39] Concomitant carpal fractures occur frequently with DRFs, with scaphoid fractures being the most common. Younger males involved in high-energy trauma should raise the suspicion of an associated carpal fracture and may warrant a CT.[40] During the postimmobilization period, disproportional pain should raise the suspicion of an associated injury.

TREATMENT

DRFs can be managed operatively or nonoperatively. There are various methods of operative fixation, including open reduction internal fixation, external fixation, closed reduction with pinning, or a combination of these methods. Open reduction internal fixation with volar locking plates has become increasingly popular. Nonoperative methods of DRF management often entail closed reduction with subsequent immobilization. The advantages and disadvantages of surgical versus nonsurgical treatment and the various forms of surgical management are areas of continued research and debate. Despite multiple studies, there is no consensus regarding how best to treat DRFs, especially in older adults. The decision to operate should be a shared decision with the patient and surgeon. There are numerus subjective and objective measurements to assess outcomes, with inherent discrepancies between outcome measures. Subjective and objective measures should be used in conjunction when assessing functional outcomes.[41]

The goals of surgery are to restore volar tilt, radial height, radial length, and articular surface. The benefits of internal fixation include earlier ROM and anatomic reduction. The surgeon should strive to achieve anatomical reduction at the time of surgery, as outcomes are positively associated with improvement of articular step-off, decreasing gap between fragments, and restoring radial height.[15,42] Volar locking plates allow better restoration of the articular surface and volar tilt. The American Academy of Orthopaedic Surgeons guidelines from 2010 recommend surgical fixation for fractures with postreduction radial shortening over 3 mm, intra-articular step off over 2 mm, and dorsal tilt over 10°. It is also recommended to use rigid immobilization instead of removable splints for fractures treated nonoperatively, beginning early wrist motion following fixation, and giving prophylactic vitamin C.[43]

Despite internal fixation techniques and technology, the majority of elderly patients with DRFs are treated nonoperatively with good results.[44] In 2007, 74% of the Medicare population that were treated for DRFs were treated nonoperatively.[45] Diaz-Garcia et al conducted a large, systematic review of outcomes and complications in treating DRFs in patients over 60 and found no difference in functional outcomes between those treated with surgery and those treated with cast immobilization, despite worse radiographic outcomes in those treated with cast immobilization.[46] Furthermore, more complications were found with those treated operatively.[46] A 2003 Cochrane review analyzed 48 randomized clinical trials involving DRFs in adults comparing different surgical interventions in the treatment of DRFs including external fixation, open reduction and internal fixation, and insertion of bone scaffolding materials. These interventions were compared to nonoperative management. The authors concluded that there is insufficient evidence to suggest that surgical intervention of most fractures will consistently offer better long-term results.[47]

Given that many fractures are treated nonoperatively, providers should be aware of fracture characteristics that may be unstable or displace after closed reduction. LaFontaine identified several factors that were associated with secondary displacement of DRFs treated nonoperatively: dorsal angulation over 20°, dorsal comminution, intra-articular fractures, associated ulna fractures, and age over 60. The more factors that are present, the more likely the risk of secondary displacement even if there is satisfactory reduction.[48] Mackenney analyzed approximately 4000 DRFs and found that patient age, metaphyseal comminution, and ulnar variance were consistent predictors of radiographic outcome.[49] Elderly patients are at particular risk for secondary displacement if they are reduced first.[50,51] Reduction is not always necessary. Neidenback et al examined 83 elderly patients with DRFs and found no difference between radiographic parameters and functional ROM between those that underwent closed reduction and those that did not. Patients without closed reduction had better patient-reported outcomes.[52] The treating physician should consider patient functional demands and pain level, even when radiographic parameters are not restored. In elderly patients, radiographic parameters at the time of union following closed treatment or operatively treated fractures do not always predict functional outcomes.[44,53,54]

COMPLICATIONS

Complications following DRFs are relatively common with a reported incidence of up to 80%.[55] Providers treating DRFs during the postoperative period should be aware of the potential complications associated with these injuries. The mechanism and severity of injury, number of manipulations, type of fixation, surgeon experience, pre-existing nerve dysfunction, and patient characteristics are factors that can contribute to adverse outcomes. Following operative fixation with volar locking plates, flexor and extensor tendon irritation is the most common complication[56,57] followed by flexor pollicis longus tendon rupture, extensor pollicis longus tendon rupture, carpal tunnel syndrome, complex regional pain syndrome (CRPS), and screw malposition.[56] Other common complications include loss of motion, reduced arc of wrist flexion and extension, and reduced forearm rotation.[46] Fall from a height and injury to the ipsilateral side are positive predictors of early complications such as screw misplacement or loss of fixation. High-volume surgeons and surgeons using unfamiliar plates predict late complications such as tendon irritation, malunion, or DRUJ complications.[57] CRPS is a contentious postoperative complication given its subjective nature and loose diagnostic criterion. CRPS is diagnosed exclusively based on clinical signs and symptoms of erythema, edema, pain, and sympathetic nerve dysfunction. The diagnosis of CRPS is contradictory in that the criterion for CRPS includes no other explanation for the symptoms. Bot and Ring proposed that CRPS should be referred to as

disproportionate pain and disability, which is best treated with the cognitive behavioral therapy.[58] Despite the lack of consensus as to what CRPS is or whether CRPS is an actual entity, several studies have shown that the use of vitamin C prophylactically is associated with a lower risk of developing CRPS.[59-61]

REHABILITATION

The orthopaedic literature is replete with discussion on the surgical management of DRFs but is relatively sparse in terms of rehabilitation. The rehabilitation of DRFs is of equal importance to the surgical management of these common injuries. The goals of rehabilitation should be discussed with the patient and realistic expectations should be discussed. The general goals of rehabilitation after DRFs include setting expectations for realistic outcomes and determining what type of interventions should be utilized, why they should be utilized, and for how long. Restoration of ROM, grip, weight bearing activities, and decreasing pain are the goals of the therapist in the postoperative or postimmobilization period. Many types of interventions are available during the postoperative period including supervised physical therapy, home therapy, strengthening exercise, ice pack, transcutaneous electrical nerve stimulation (TENS), heat application, and various splints.

The timing of when to start therapy has been debated. There is evidence to support that patients do not need to begin early motion after a wrist fracture has been fixed.[62-64] Lozano-Calderon examined 60 patients with DRFs that were fixed with volar locking plates. Half were randomized to early mobilization at 2 weeks, the other half were randomized to motion at 6 weeks. No differences in patient-reported outcomes or objective measures were found.[63] Accelerated rehabilitation programs that emphasize wrist and forearm passive ROM and strengthening at 2 weeks, versus the traditional 4 weeks, have been shown to have an earlier return to function for patients when compared to traditional programs.[65] The timing of when to start early motion should be determined by the patient, his or her activity level, and the amount of pain.

If early motion and strengthening are begun on a patient, knowledge of the forces that the implant can tolerate is essential. There is a linear relationship between the amount of grip force and the force experienced by the distal radius. Putnam et al reported that for each 10 N of grip force, 52 N go across the radius and ulna with 51% of the force, or 26 N, going through the distal radius. If, during power grip, all the force goes through the radius, 52 N go across the radius for each 10 N of grip force.[66] Depending on the position of the wrist, 2410 N can be transmitted through the distal radius with the male average grip strength of 463 N.[66,67] Other studies have shown that approximately 80% of the force with axial loading is transmitted through the radius, which would equate to 41.6 N for every 10 N of grip force. According to Putnam et al, grip force during rehabilitation should not exceed 159 N, depending on the type of fixation used.[66] Dahl et al evaluated eight volar locking plates in a biomechanical study that reproduced the forces seen in early fracture healing. They found that all plates tested had ultimate yield strengths of 1000 to 2000 N after cyclic loading at loads up to 300 N, suggesting that all plates tested can provide adequate strength for early postoperative rehabilitation.[68]

The decision to pursue formal therapy with a certified hand therapist or self-direct therapy should be based on patient characteristics and the ability to perform home therapy. After open reduction and internal fixation with a volar locking plate, formal occupational therapy is not necessary. Instructions for a home exercise program can be more effective than a formal therapy.[69,70] In a randomized control trial involving 94 patients with DRFs treated with volar locking plates, patients who received instructions for independent exercises did better than those who received formal physical therapy.[71]

EDEMA

Edema is the body's normal response to injury. Continued edema can have negative effects on the ROM and function.[72] Edema that is controlled early can minimize subsequent scar formation that can interfere with the normal gliding of tendons and nerves.[73] Initial therapy for edema should consist of elevation, ice pack, retrograde massage, compressive dressings and garments, and active motion, which can be started in the immobilization period.[74] Edema management may also include electrical stimulation and manual edema mobilization (MEM). Electrical stimulation has shown positive results in edema reduction after an acute injury.[75,76] Stralka et al conducted a study on the use of high-voltage pulsed direct current in reducing chronic hand edema in conjunction with a wrist orthosis that demonstrated significant decreases for hand edema and pain following treatment.[77] TENS, which is based on the modified gate control theory, can be used for treatment of pain.[76] TENS when used in conjunction with ice pack can have effects on both edema and pain management.[78] Patients who have edema beyond the normal acute phase that is not reducing with the usual acute-phase treatment methods may benefit from MEM, which includes the use of exercises, light skin-tractioning massage techniques following the lymphatic pathways, and the use of low-compression garments.[72,73] Patients that this may be appropriate for are those with a healthy lymphatic system that is temporarily overloaded.[73] Knygsand-Roenhoej and Maribo compared MEM and traditional techniques in edema management in patients with a fractured distal radius. They found that MEM resulted in fewer sessions to decrease subacute hand/arm edema compared with using traditional edema reduction techniques.[79] In addition to helping with edema, cyclic pneumatic soft-tissue compression during the immobilization period has been shown to lead to faster

improvement in muscle strength compared to patients not using compression devices.[80]

MOTION

It is important to begin motion exercises immediately in the postoperative period, including finger, elbow, and shoulder motion. Finger stiffness is a common complication following DRFs. This difficult problem can largely be avoided by beginning early ROM exercises. Regardless of the fixation method, finger motion should be started as soon as possible. Patients will often exhibit catastrophic thinking that may preclude them from moving their fingers. The provider should help patients overcome the inherent trepidation that moving their fingers will cause further damage to their DRF.[58]

STIFFNESS AFTER IMMOBILIZATION

Preventing stiffness should be a major part of the management of DRFs. A period of immobilization in a splint or cast will be required after DRFs. Immobilization in the context of tissue repair after trauma predisposes to contracture formation.[81-83] Collagen provides most of the tensile strength of tissue. Although these fibers are inelastic, movement between the collagen fibers imparts elasticity to the tissue.[81] Normal motion occurs when these strong, dense connective tissue structures glide relative to one another.[81,83] Stiffness is caused by the fixation of the tissue layers so that the usual elastic relational motion is restricted by crosslinks binding the collagen fibers together.[81] Collagen is being absorbed and laid down again constantly and new bonding patterns are created.[81] When tissue is injured, it creates a relatively extended period of heightened collagen synthesis, degradation, and deposition.[81,82] Tissue can adaptively shorten when immobilized, which can lead to stiffness.[83] Available knowledge of the phases of tissue repair and healing supports an early initiation of rehabilitation in patients.[82] The best method of preventing stiffness is early management of edema, immobilization only if needed, and early ROM as soon as possible.

Adhesions of tendons can frequently occur after trauma affecting the hand. Most of the literature on tendon gliding is from tendon repairs. The flexor digitorum profundus (FDP) and the flexor digitorum superficialis (FDS) enter the hand by passing through the carpal tunnel. They have a synovial sheath and utilize a pulley system. Good finger motion and hand function are dependent on gliding of these tendons as well as differential gliding of these tendons.[84] Damage to the gliding surfaces after fracture or surgical fixation can interfere with tendon excursion and lead to adhesions.[84,85] Wehbe and Hunter studied flexor tendon gliding of the hand in vivo from the results of their studies and they came up with three positions of the hand that provided maximum differential gliding. The three positions of the hand can be utilized for tendon gliding exercises to prevent adhesions and/or restore

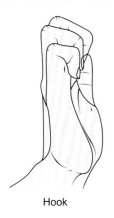 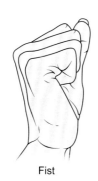 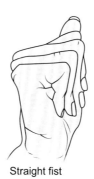

Hook   Fist   Straight fist

FIGURE 16.4 Three positions of the hand for tendon gliding exercises. (Modified from Wehbe MA. Tendon gliding exercises. *Am J Occup Ther.* 1987;41:164-167.)

motion.[84] The three positions of the hand in tendon gliding exercises include hook fist, full fist, and straight fist (**Figure 16.4**). The straight fist, with the MCP joints and PIP joints flexed but the DIP joints extended, elicits maximum FDS glide in relation to surrounding structures. The full fist, with the MCP, PIP, and DIP joints flexed, elicits maximum FDP glide in relation to surrounding structures.[86,87] In the hook fist, with the MCP joints extended while the IP joints flex, maximum differential gliding between the two tendons is achieved.[84,86,88]

STAGES OF THERAPY FOR DRF

The focus of DRF rehabilitation is to manage pain and allow the patient to regain motion, strength, and most importantly function.[74] Management of DRFs can be divided into three stages: protective, restoration of motion, and strengthening/return of function.

PROTECTIVE

The patient may see a therapist within 1 week and be provided with home instructions. Instructions should contain ROM, edema control, and pain management. ROM to be completed should include uninvolved joints including fingers, elbow, and shoulder. Finger ROM should include tendon gliding exercises.[86] Education on edema and pain management should include elevation above the heart and use of cold packs. Retrograde massage and compression wraps may also be used to control edema, as needed.[89]

RESTORATION OF MOTION AFTER THE IMMOBILIZATION PERIOD

This period begins when the immobilization period is over. Orthosis that allows full finger motion may be worn between exercises initially. Orthosis, whether custom or prefabricated, should be modified as needed for changes in edema. The provider should continue with ROM exercises from the protective stage and begin active motion of the wrist and forearm. ROM to include wrist flexion and extension, radial and ulnar deviation, and forearm supination

and pronation. Attention should be paid to wrist extension and supination and pronation motions that have been most difficult to restore after DRF.[86] Restoration of these motions has been correlated with higher function as measured by DASH scores.[90] Active wrist extension with finger flexion should be emphasized as wrist extension without the use of the finger extensors can be difficult to restore. Wrist extension without assistance from finger extensors is important for grip strength and overall hand function.[86] Exercises can be completed with ten repetitions, three to four times per day. Passive ROM of the wrist and forearm may be completed when fracture healing permits. Joint mobilizations may also be used for joint stiffness, but care should be taken with intra-articular fractures.[86] Application of heat can have beneficial results on pain and motion. Some modalities for heat include moist heat packs and paraffin. Heat can allow patients to participate in rehabilitation with more comfort and can also be easily utilized in the patient's home exercise program. Passive stretches can be performed when fracture healing is deemed appropriate. Stretches should be held for 30 seconds and completed several times a day but literature varies on what is the most appropriate dose.[91] The use of a dynamic or static progressive orthosis can be used for deficits in ROM of the fingers, wrist, and forearm when plateaus are reached before functional motion.[90] Sufficient fracture healing must be determined for use of orthosis.

STRENGTHENING/RETURN OF FUNCTION

Strengthening can start when fracture healing is determined appropriate. Strengthening typically begins around 8 weeks. Exercises should progress from light grip to wrist isometrics, to progressive resisted exercises and, finally, closed chain exercises including weight bearing.[74]

SPLINTING FOR ROM DEFICITS

Most patients after a DRF recover adequate ROM and function in a relatively brief period.[90] Patients whose ROM plateaus before reaching functional levels may benefit from either a dynamic or static progressive orthosis to help restore motion. Splinting is based on the concept that an adequate level of stress, applied over extended periods of time, will stimulate the connective tissue growth and reorganization needed to achieve permanent lengthening.[90,92] Dynamic splints are made of a stable static base and an elastic mobilizing component.[83,93] Static progressive orthosis is similar in design to a dynamic splint, but it utilizes nonelastic materials like straps and turnbuckles. Static progressive orthoses are typically better when there is a "hard-end feel" to ROM.[86] Static progressive orthoses use the principle of low-load prolonged stretch (LLPS). LLPS is more effective than high-load brief stress.[94] Dynamic or static progressive orthosis for wrist and forearm motion can be fabricated or commercially made ones are available. Wearing times of 30 to 60 minutes three times per day have shown good results for both wrist and forearm ROM.[90,92] Dynamic and static progressive splints also can be effective in treating a stiff hand that continues after a DRF.[93]

SPECIAL CONSIDERATIONS FOR FRACTURE FIXATION TYPE

EXTERNAL FIXATION

The complications most commonly seen are pin-site infection, edema, first web space tightness, and intrinsic tightness of the digits.[86] Patients should be educated on keeping the pin sites dry and clean because the pin is a conduit of infection.[95]

VOLAR PLATING

Earlier ROM may begin at the wrist if chosen by the surgeon. Some accelerated rehabilitation protocols have wrist ROM starting before 2 weeks.[63,65] If early motion is suggested by the surgeon, then a wrist orthosis should be worn between therapy sessions until 6 weeks.[86] Scar management may need to be addressed including desensitization, scar massage, and use of elastomer putty or gel sheets as needed.

DORSAL PLATING

ROM of the wrist after dorsal plating may be started earlier then nonoperative or with external fixation. Scar management, as with volar plating, may need to be addressed.[96]

PROTOCOLS

OPEN REDUCTION INTERNAL FIXATION

Immobilization

- 0 to 2 weeks immobilization with a splint or cast. Exception is extreme osteopenia, where prolonged casting of up to 6 weeks may be indicated.
- Patient educated on immediate finger ROM and elevation above heart and ice pack for edema control.
- Wound check at 2 weeks.

Patient to visit therapist at 2 weeks for further education on finger and wrist active range of motion (AROM) and passive range of motion (PROM) of digits including tendon gliding exercises. ROM education also to include elbow and shoulder motion for prevention of stiffness.

Restoration of Motion

- Cast removal and therapy visit at 2 weeks.
- Therapy visit to include thorough education on hep, which includes continuing of finger ROM and starting AROM of wrist and forearm. ROM education also to include elbow and shoulder motion for prevention of stiffness.
- Wrist cock-up prefabricated or custom to be worn between exercises for two -four additional weeks then weaned.
- Compression glove issued for assistance with edema control.
- Education on scar massage and use of heat prior to exercises.
- Active assisted range of motion (AAROM) for wrist and forearm at 6 weeks.
- Light grip strengthening with putty to start at 4-6 weeks.
- PROM for wrist and forearm started at 7-8 weeks.

Strengthening/Return TO Function (8-12 weeks)

- Wrist and forearm strengthening started.
- Progress weight bearing as tolerated.
  Static progressive orthosis if ROM plateaus.

NONOPERATIVE

Immobilization

- Immobilization for 4 to 6 weeks (long arm cast initially if forearm rotation needs to be immobilized).
- Immediate education on finger A/PROM including tendon gliding exercises. Elbow and shoulder ROM for prevention of stiffness. Edema control including elevation above heart and fisting.

Restoration of Motion

- Therapy visit day of cast removal. Therapy to include thorough education on hep, which includes continuing of finger ROM and starting A/AAROM of wrist and forearm.
- Wrist cock-up prefabricated or custom may be worn for additional 1 to 2 weeks with activity if needed.
- Compression glove issued for assistance with edema control.
- PROM of wrist and forearm initiated at 8 to 10 weeks.

Strengthening/Return to Function

- Light grip strengthening initiated at 6 to 8 weeks.
- Initiation of progressive resistive exercises at 8 to 10 weeks.
- Progress weight bearing as tolerated at 8 to 10 weeks.
- Static progressive orthosis prn if motion plateaus.

REFERENCES

1. Alffram PA, Bauer GC. Epidemiology of fractures of the forearm. A biomechanical investigation of bone strength. *J Bone Joint Surg Am.* 1962;44-A:105-114.
2. Chung KC, Spilson SV. The frequency and epidemiology of hand and forearm fractues in the United States. *J Hand Surg.* 2001;26(5):908-915.
3. Shauver MJ, Yin H. Current and future national costs to medicare for the treatment of distal radius fracture in the elderly. *J Hand Surg.* 2011;36(8):1282-1287.
4. Thompson PW, Taylor J, Dawson A. The annual incidence and seasonal variation of fractures of the distal radius in men and women over 25 years in Dorset, UK. *Injury.* 2004;35(5):462-466.
5. Jerrhaq D, Englund M, Karlsson MK, Rosengren BE. Epidemiology and time trends of distal forearm fractures in adults – a study of 11.2 million person-years in Sweden. *BMC Musculoskelet Disord.* 2017;18(1):240.
6. Bengner U, Johnell O. Increasing incidence of forearm fractures. A comparison of epidemiologic patterns 25 years apart. *Acta Orthop Scand.* 1985;56(2):158.
7. Hagino H, Yamamoto K, Ohshiro H, Nakamura T, Kishimoto H, Nose T. Changing incidence of hip, distal radius, and proximal humerus fractures in Tottori Prefecture, Japan. *Bone.* 1999;24(3):265-270.
8. Edwards BJ, Song J, Dunlop DD, Fink HA, Cauley JA. Functional decline after incident wrist fractures - study of osteoporotic fractures: prospective cohort study. *BMJ.* 2010;341:c3324.
9. Tang JB. General concepts of wrist biomechanics and a view from other species. *J Hand Surg Eur Vol.* 2008;33(4):519-525.
10. Craigen MA, Stanley JK. Wrist kinematics row, column or both? *J Hand Surg Eur Vol.* 1995;20(2):165-170. https://sciencedirect.com/science/article/pii/s0266768105800440. Accessed April 3, 2018.
11. Taleisnik J. The ligaments of the wrist. *The J Hand Surg Am.* 1976;1:110-118.
12. Navarro A. *Luxaciones del carpo.* Lima, Peru: An Fac Med; 1921:113-141.
13. Medoff RJ. Distal radius fractures: Classification and management. In: Skirven TM, ed. *Rehabilitation of the hand and upper extremity.* 6th ed. Philidelphia: Mosby Inc; 2011:941-948.
14. Rhee PC, Medoff RJ, Shin AY. Complex distal radius fractures: an anatomic algorithm for surgical management. *J Am Acad Orthop Surg.* 2017;25(2):77-88.
15. Trumble TE, Schmitt SR, Vedder NB. Factors affecting functional outcome of displaced intra-articular distal radius fractures. *J Hand Surg Eur Vol.* 1994;19(2):325-340. https://ncbi.nlm.nih.gov/pubmed/8201203. Accessed February 13, 2018.
16. Rikli DA, Regazzoni P. Fractures of the distal end of the radius treated by internal fixation and early function. *J Bone Joint Surg Br.* 1996;78:588-592.
17. Koh S, Andersen CR. Anatomy of the distal brachioradialis and its potential relationship to distal radius fracture. *The J Hand Surg Am.* 2006;31(1):2-8.
18. Fernandez DL. Radial osteotomy and Bowers arthroplasty for malunited fractures of the distal end of the radius. *J Bone Joint Surg Am.* 1988;70:1538-1551.
19. Kijima Y, Viegas SF. Wrist anatomy and biomechanics. *J Hand Surg Am.* 2009;34(8):1555-1563.
20. Rikli DA, Honigmann P, Babst R, Cristalli A, Morlock M, Mittlmeier T. Intraarticular pressure measurement in the radioulnocarpal joint using a novel senosor: In vitro and in vivo results. *J Hand Surg Am.* 2007;32(1):67-75.
21. Palmer AK, Werner F. Biomechanics of the distal radioulnar joint. *Clin Orhop Relat Res.* 1984;187:26-35.
22. Trumble T, Glisson RR, Seaber AV, Urbaniak JR. Forearm force transmission after surgical treatment of distal radioulnar joint disorders. *J Hand Surg.* 1987;12(2):196-202.
23. Destot E. Injuries of the Wrist: A Radiological Study. *Clin Orthop Relat Res.* 2006;445:8-14.
24. Rohde RS, Crisco JJ, Wolfe SW. The advantage of thowing the first stone: how understanding the evolutionary demands of Homo sapiens is helping us understand carpal motion. *J Am Acad Orthop Surg.* 2010;18(1):51-58.
25. Moojen TM, Snel JG, Ritt MJPF, Kauer JMG, Venema HW, Bos KE. Three-dimensional carpal kinematics in vivo. *Clin Biomech.* 2002;17:506-514.
26. Landsmeer JM. Studies in the anatomy of articulation: I. The equilibrium of the "intercalated" bone. *Acta Morphol Neerl Scand.* 1961(3):287-303.
27. Moojen TH, Snel JG, Ritt MJ, Venema HW, den Heeten GJ, Bos KE. Pisiform kinmatics in vivo. *J Hand Surg.* 2001;26(5):901-907.
28. Shulman BS, Rettig M, Sapienza A. Management of Pisotriquetral Instability. *J Hand Surg (American ed).* 2018;43(1):54-60.
29. Garcia-Elias M, Lluch AL. Wrist instabilities, misalignments, and dislocations. In: Wolfe SW, Pederson WC, Kozin SH, Cohen MS. *Green's Operative Hand Surgery.* 7th ed. Philadelphia, PA: Elsevier; 2017:418-478.
30. Lluch AH. *Terminology for hand surgery.* In: *Nomenclature Committee of the International Federation of Societies for Surgery of the Hand.* London: Harcourt Health Sciences; 2011.
31. Wolfe SW, Crisco JJ, Orr CM, Marzke MW. The dart-throwing motion of the wrist: is it unique to humans? *J Hand Surg.* 2006;31:1429-1437.
32. Crisco JJ, Coburn JC, Moore DC, Akelman E, Weiss AP, Wolfe SW. In vivo radiocarpal kinematics and the dart thrower's motion. *J Bone Joint Surg.* 2005;87(12):2729-2740.
33. Ishikawa J, Cooney WP, Niebur G, An K-N, Minami A, Kaneda K. The effects of wrist distraction on carpal kinematics. *J Hand Surg.* 1999;24A:113-120.
34. Moritomo H, Apergis EP, Garcia-Elias M, Werner FW, Wolfe SW. International federation of societies for surgery of the hand 2013 committee's report on wrist dart-throwing motion. *J Hand Surg Am.* 2014;39(7):1433-1439.
35. Garcia-Elias M, Serrallach XA, Serra JM. Darth-throwing motion in patients with scapholunate instability: a dynamic four-dimensional computed tomography study. *J Hand Surg Eur Vol.* 2013;39(7):1433-1439.
36. Werner FW, Short WH, Palmer AK, Sutton LG. Wrist tendon forces during various dynamic wrist motions. *J Hand Surg Eur Vol.* 2010;35(4):628-632.
37. Levin LS, Rozell JC, Pulos N. Distal radius fractures in the elderly. *J Am Acad Orthop Surg.* 2017;25(3):179-187.
38. Lindau T, Arner M, Hagberg L. Intraarticular lesion in distal fractures of the radius in young adults. A descripitve arthroscopic study in 50 patients. *J Hand Surg.* 1997:638-643.
39. Ogawa T, Tanaka T, Yanai T, Kumagai H, Ochiai N. Analysis of soft tissue injuries associated with distal radius fractures. *Sports Med Arthrosc Rehabil Ther Technol.* 2013;5(1):19. https://link.springer.com/content/pdf/10.1186/2052-1847-5-19.pdf. Accessed February 14, 2018.
40. Komura S, Yokoi T. Incidence and characteristics of carpal fractures occurring concurrently with distal radius fractures. *J Hand Surg.* 2012;37(3):469-476.
41. Goldhahn J, Angst F, Simmen BR. What counts: outcome assessment after distal radius fractures in aged patients. *J Orthop Trauma.* 2008;22(8):S126-S130. https://ncbi.nlm.nih.gov/pubmed/18753889. Accessed April 14, 2018.
42. Altisimi M, Antenucci R, Fiacca C, Mancini GB. Long-term results of conservative treatment of fractues of the distal radius. *Clin Orthop.* 1986;206:202-210.
43. Lichtman DM, Bindra RR, Boyer MI, et al. Treatment of distal radius fractures. *J Am Acad Orthopaedic Surgeons,* 2010;18(3):180-189. https://ncbi.nlm.nih.gov/pubmed/20190108. Accessed February 18, 2018.
44. Burt T, Young GM. Outcome following nonoperative treatment of displaced distal radius fractures in low-demand patients older than 60 years. *J Hand Surg.* 2000;25:19-28.
45. Chung KC, Shauver MJ, Yin H, Birkmeyer JD. The epidemiology of distal radius fracture in the united states medicare population: level 2 evidence. *J Hand Surg.* 2010;35(10):24-25.
46. Diaz-Garcia RO. A systematic review of outcomes and complications of treating unstable distal radius fractures in the elderly. *J Hand Surg Am.* 2011;36(5):824-835.e2.
47. Handoll HHG, Madhok R. Surgical interventions for treating distal radius fractures in adults. *Cochrane Database Syst Rev.* 2003;3:CD003209.
48. LaFontaine M, Delince P, Hardy D, Simons M. Instability of fractures of the lower end of the radius: apropos of a series of 167 cases. *Acta Orthop Bel.* 1989;55(2):203-216.
49. Mackenney PJ, McQueen MM, Elton R. Prediction of instability in distal radial fractures. *J Bone Joint Surg.* 2006;88(9):1944-1951.
50. Makhni EC, Ewald TJ, Kelly S, Day CS. Effect of patient age on the radiographic outcomes of distal radius fractures subject to nonoperative treatment. *J Hand Surg.* 2008;33:1301-1308.
51. Nesbitt KS, Failla JM, Les CM. Assessment of instability factors in adult distal radius fractures. *J Hand Surg Eur Vol,* 2010;29(6):1128-1138. http://jhandsurg.org/article/s0363-5023(04)00531-3/fulltext. Accessed February 20, 2018.

52. Neidenbach P, Audige L, Wilhelmi-Mock M, Hanson B, De Boer P. The efficacy of closed reduction in displaced distal radius fractures. *Injury.* 2010;41(6):592-598. https://ncbi.nlm.nih.gov/pubmed/19959165. Accessed February 11, 2018.

53. Jaremko JL, Lambert RG, Rowe BH, Johnson JA, Majumdar SR. Do radiographic indicies of distal radius fracture reduction predict outcomes in older adults receiving conservative treatment? *Clin Radiol.* 2007;62:65-72.

54. Synn AJ, Makhni EC, Makhni MC, Rozental TD, Day CS. Distal radius fractures in older patients: is anatomic reduction necessary? *Clin Orthop Relat Res.* 2009;467(6):1612-1620. https://link.springer.com/article/10.1007/s11999-008-0660-2. Accessed February 14, 2018.

55. Chapman DR, Bennette JB, Bryan WJ, Tullos HS. Complications of distal radius fractures: pins and plaster treatment. *J Hand Surg.* 1982;7:509-512.

56. Arora R, Lutz M, Hennerbichler A, Krappinger D, Espen D, Gabl M. Complications following internal fixation of unstable distal radius fracture with a palmar locking-plate. *J Orthop Trauma.* 2007;21(5):316-322. https://ncbi.nlm.nih.gov/pubmed/17485996. Accessed February 14, 2018.

57. Soong M, van Leerdam R, Guitton TG, Got C, Katarincic J, Ring D. Fracture of the distal radius: risk factors for complications after locked volar plate fixation. *J Hand Surg.* 2011;36(1):3-9.

58. Bot AG. Recovery after fracture of the distal radius. *Hand Clinics.* 2012;28(2):235-243.

59. Aim F, Klouche S, Frison A, Bauer T, Hardy P. Efficacy of vitamin C in preventing complex regional pain syndrome after wrist fracture: A systematic review and meta-analysis. *Orthop Traumatol Surg Res.* 2017;103(3):465-470. https://sciencedirect.com/science/article/pii/s1877056817300555. Accessed May 8, 2018.

60. Zollinger PE, Tuinebreijer WE, Breederveld RS, Kreis R. Can vitamin C prevent complex regional pain syndrome in patients with wrist fractures? A randomized, controlled, multicenter dose-response study. *J Bone Joint Surg Am.* 2007;89(7):1424-1431. http://tdh.org.nz/assets/ed/misc/guidelines--protocols/canvitamincpreventcrps-zollingeretal8971424-jbjs.pdf. Accessed March 8, 2018.

61. Zollinger PE, Tuinebreijer WE, Kreis R, Breederveld RS. Effect of vitamin C on frequency of reflex sympathetic dystrophy in wrist fractures: a randomised trial. *Lancet.* 1999;354(9195):2025-2028. https://sciencedirect.com/science/article/pii/s0140673699030597. Accessed March 8, 2018.

62. Allain JL. Trans-styloid fixation of fractues of the distal radius: A prospective randomized comparison between 6- and 1-week postoperative immobilization in 60 fractures. *Acta Orthop Scand.* 1999;70(2):119-123.

63. Lozano-Calderon SS. Wrist mobilization following volar plate fixation of fractures of the distal part of the radius. *J Bone Joint Surg.* 2008;90(6):1297-1304.

64. McQueen MM, Hajducka C, Court-Brown CM. Redisplaced unstable fractures of the distal radius: a prospective randomised comparison of four methods of treatment. *J Bone Joint Surg Br Vol.* 1996;78:404-409.

65. Brehmer JL, Husband J. Accelerated rehabilitation compared with a standard protocol after distal radial fractures treated with volar open reduction and internal fixation: A prospective, randomized, controlled study. *J Bone Joint Surg Am.* 2014;96(19):1621-1630.

66. Putnam MD, Meyer NJ, Nelson EW, Gesensway D, Lewis JL. Distal radial metaphyseal forces in an extrinsic grip model: Implications for postfracture rehabilitation. *J Hand Surg.* 2000;25(3):469-475.

67. Mathiowetz V, Kashman N, Volland G, Weber K, Dowe M, Rogers S. Grip and pinch strength: normative data for adults. *Arch Phys Med Rehabil.* 1985;66(2):69-74.

68. Dahl WJ, Nassab PF, Burgess KM, et al. Biomechanical properties of fixed-angle volar distal radius plates under dynamic loading. *J Hand Surg.* 2012;37(7):1381-1387.

69. Krischak GD, Krasteva A, Schneider F, Gulkin D, Gebhard F, Kramer M. Physiotherapy after volar plating of wrist fractures is effective using a home exercise program. *Arch Phys Med Rehabil.* 2009;90(4):537-544.

70. Maciel JS, Taylor NF, McIlveen C. A randomised clinical trial of activity-focussed physiotherapy on patients with distal radius fractures. *Arch Orthop Trauma Surg.* 2005;125(8):515-520.

71. Souer JS, Buijze G, Ring D. A prospective randomized controlled trial comparing occupational therapy with independent exercises after volar plate fixation of a fracture of the distal part of the radius. *J Bone Joint Surg Am.* 2011;93(19):1761-1766.

72. Miller LK, Jerosch-Herold C, Shepstone L. Effectiveness of edema managment techniques for subacute hand edema: a systematic review. *J Hand Ther.* 2017;30(4):432-446.

73. Artzberger SM. Manual edema mobilization: An edema reduction technique for the orthopedic patient. In: Skirven TM, ed. *Rehabilitation of the hand and upper extremity.* 6th ed. Philadelphia, PA: Mosby Inc; 2011:868-881.

74. Michlovitz SL, LaStayo PC, Alzner S, Watson E. Distal radius fractures: therapy practice patterns. *J Hand Ther.* 2001;14(4):249-257. Retrieved 2 11, 2018, from http://sciencedirect.com/science/article/pii/s0894113001800028.

75. Bleakley C, McDonough S, MacAuley D. The use of ice in the treatment of acute soft-tissue injury: A systematic review of randomized controlled trials. *Am J Sports Med.* 2004;32(1):251-261.

76. Reed B. Effect of high voltage pulsed electrical stiumlation on microvascular permeability to plasma proteins: a possible mechanism in minimizing edema. *Phys Ther.* 1988;68:491-495.

77. Stralka SW, Jackson JA, Lewis AR. A randomized clinical trial of high voltage pulsed, direct current built into a wrist splint. *AAOHN J.* 1998;46:233-236.

78. Cheing GL, Wan JWH, Lo SK. Ice and pulsed electromagnetic field to reduce pain and swelling after distal radius fractures. *J Rehabil Med.* 2005;37(6):372-377.

79. Knygsand-Roenhoej K, Maribo T. A randomized clinical controlled study comparing the effect of modified manual edema mobilization treatment with traditional edema technique in patients with a fracture of the distal radius. *J Hand Ther.* 2011;24:184-194.

80. Challis MJ, Jull GJ, Stanton WR, Welsh MK. Cyclic pneumatic soft-tissue compression enhances recovery following fracture of the distal radius: a radomised controlled trial. *Aust J Physiother.* 2007;53(4):247-252.

81. Colditz J. Therapist's management of the stiff hand. In: Skirven TM, ed. *Rehabilitation of the hand and upper extremity.* 6th ed. Philadelphia, PA: Mosby Inc; 2011:868-881.

82. Glasgow C, Tooth LR, Fleming J. Mobilizing the stiff hand: Combining theory and evidence to improve clinical outcomes. *J Hand Ther.* 2010;23(4):392-401.

83. Yang G, McGlinn EP, Chung KC. Management of the stiff finger: evidence and outcomes. *Clin Plast Surg.* 2014;41(3):501-512.

84. Wehbe MA, Hunter JM. Flexor tendon gliding in the hand. Part I. In vivo excursions. *J Hand Surg.* 1985a;10(A):570-578.

85. Neal P. Anatomy and Kinesiology. In: Skirven TM, ed. *Rehabilitation of the Hand and Upper Extremity.* 6th ed. Philadelphia, PA: Mosby Inc; 2011:3-17.

86. Micholovitz SL, Festa L. Therapist's management of distal radius fractures. In: Skirven TM, ed. *Rehabilitation of the Hand and Upper Extremity.* 6th ed. Philadelphia, PA: Mosby Inc; 2011:949-962.

87. Wehbe MA, Hunter JM. Flexor tendon gliding in the hand. Part II. Diferential gliding. *J Hand Surg.* 1985b;10(A):575-578.

88. Wehbe MA. Tendon gliding exercises. *Am J Occup Ther.* 1987;41:164-167.

89. Sorensen MK. The edematous hand. *Phys Ther.* 1989;69:1059-1064.

90. Lucado AM, Li Z, Russell GB, Papadonikolakis A, Ruch DS. Changes in impairment and function after static progressive splinting for stiffness after distal radius fracture. *J Hand Ther.* 2008;21:319-325.

91. Youdas JW, Krause DA, Egan KS, Therneau TM, Laskowski ER. The effect of static stretching on the calf muscle-tendon unit on active ankle dorsiflexion range of motion. *J Orthop Sports Phys Ther.* 2003;33:408-417.

92. McGrath MS, Ulrich SD, Bonutti PM, Marker DR, Johanssen HR, Mont MA. Static progressive splinting for restoration of rotational motion of the forearm. *J Hand Ther.* 2009;22:3-8.

93. Glasgow C, Tooth LR, Fleming J, Peters S. Dynamic splinting for the stiff hand after trauma: predictors of contracture resolution. *J Hand Ther.* 2011;24:195-205.

94. Cyr LM, Ross RG. How controlled stress affects healing tissues. *J Hand Ther.* 1998;11(2):125-130.

95. Egol KA, Paksima N, Puopolo S, Klugman J, Hiebert R, Koval KJ. Treatment of external fixation pins about the wrist: a prospective, randomized trial. *J Bone Joint Surg.* 2006;88A:349-354.

96. Kamath AF, Zurakowski D. Low-profile dorsal plating for dorsally angulated distal radius fractures: an outcomes study. *J Hand Surg.* 2016;31A(7):1061-1067.

17

Hand Fractures

Michael Suk
Daniel S. Horwitz
Daniela Furtado Barreto Rocha
Mark S. Rekant

INTRODUCTION

Hand fractures include the metacarpals (long bones of the palm) and the phalanges (small bones of the fingers) (**Figure 17.1**). They are classified as intra-articular or extraarticular and as stable or unstable. Hand fractures are the most common fracture of the upper extremity. The most common hand fracture is a fracture at the neck of the fifth metacarpal also known as a "boxer's fracture," which results most often by punching a hard object with a closed fist.

The majority of hand fractures will heal well without surgical intervention. Nonoperative treatment may include therapeutic modalities (eg, heat, ice or ultrasound) and orthotics or devices that provide a range of controlled immobilization. The decision around the ideal course of action depends on the type and location of the fracture.

GENERAL PRINCIPLES

Following hand fractures, four phases of therapy have been described: protective, restorative, strengthening, and functional (**Table 17.1**).

Whether treated with or without surgical intervention, the general progression of most hand fractures follows a similar pattern. Early controlled mobilization of tissues surrounding a healing fracture has been shown to enhance fracture healing and improve both range of motion and function of the hand.[1]

Paralleling the astonishing and complex interactions governed by the hand, an extraordinary broad range of therapeutic strategies exists in its rehabilitation—ranging from heat and range-of-motion exercises to more complex splinting and tendon gliding modalities (**Figures 17.2-17.6**).[2]

Tables 17.2-17.6 provide algorithms for some of the most common fractures of the hand.

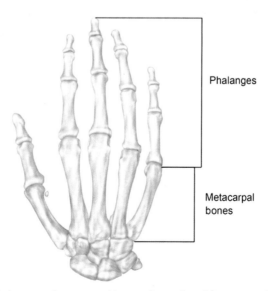

Phalanges

Metacarpal bones

FIGURE 17.1 Illustration showing the phalanges and metacarpal bones. (Reproduced from Sarwark JF, ed. *Essentials of Musculoskeletal Care.* 4th ed. Rosemont, IL: American Academy of Orthopaedic Surgeons; 2010.)

TABLE 17.1 Phases of Hand Fracture Therapy

Phases of Hand Fracture Therapy	Characteristics	Goal	Time Frame
Protective	Limited motion; immobilization	Control swelling and inflammation	0-2 wk Initial fracture to early signs of radiographic healing; or after early operative fixation
Restorative	Gentle active and passive range of motion	Gradual restoration of ROM	2-6 wk Look for clinical pain tolerance or progressive radiographic healing and stability
Strengthening	Exercise repetition, resistance, and duration	Focus on improving strength and endurance	Initiate between 8 and 12 wk
Functional	Exercise aimed at life, employment, or leisure skills	Return to activities of daily living, work, or leisure	Ongoing

ROM, range of motion.
Reproduced with permission from Michlovitz SL. Principles of hand therapy. In: Berger RA, Weiss AC, eds. Hand Surgery. *1st ed. Philadelphia, PA: Lippincott Williams and Wilkins; 2003:105-122.*

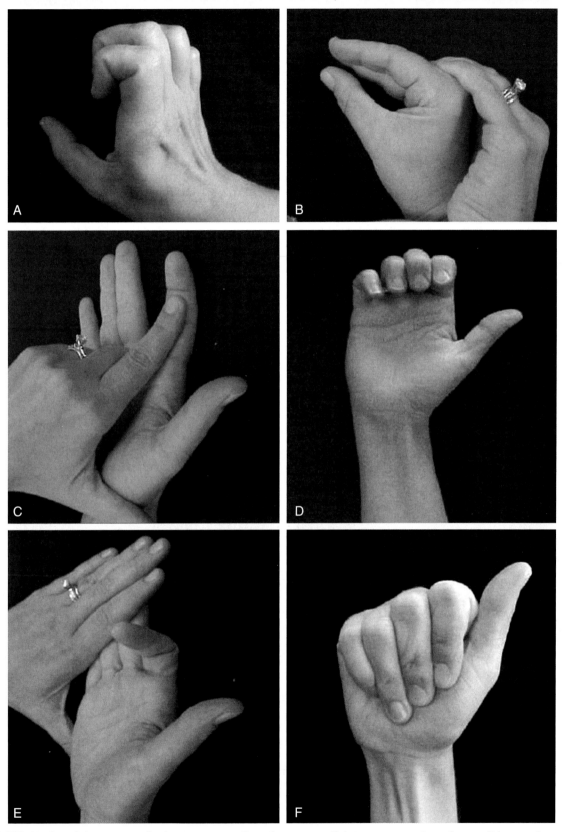

FIGURE 17.2 Tendon glide exercises: **A**, claw posture to allow the extensor digitorum communis tendon to glide over the metacarpal bone; **B**, intrinsic plus posture to achieve central slip/lateral bands to glide over the proximal phalanx; **C**, flexor digitorum profundus (FDP) blocking exercises to glide over the proximal phalanx; **D**, hook fist posture to promote selective FDP tendon glide; **E**, flexor digitorum sublimis (FDS) blocking exercise to glide FDS over the middle phalanx; **F**, sublimis fist posture to promote selective FDS tendon gliding. (Reproduced with permission from Hardy MA. Principles of metacarpal and phalangeal fracture management: a review of rehabilitation concepts. *J Orthop Sports Phys Ther.* 2004;34:781-799. doi:10.2519/jospt.2004.34.12.781. ©JOSPT®, Inc.)

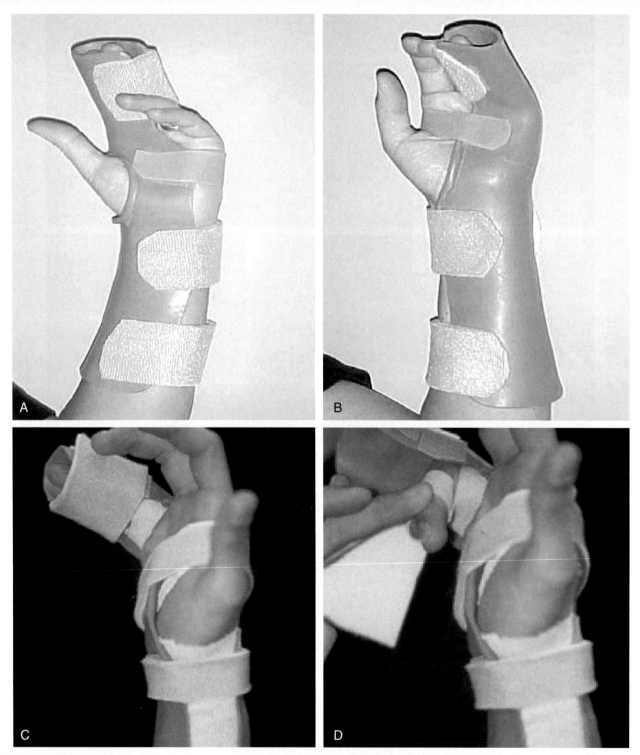

FIGURE 17.3 **A**, Radial gutter splint for fractures of the index or middle metacarpals; **B**, ulnar gutter splint for fractures of the ring or small metacarpals; **C**, serial reduction of splint to permit motion as fracture healing occurs; **D**, passive range of motion in splint. (Reproduced with permission from Hardy MA. Principles of metacarpal and phalangeal fracture management: a review of rehabilitation concepts. *J Orthop Sports Phys Ther.* 2004;34:781-799. doi:10.2519/jospt.2004.34.12.781. ©JOSPT®, Inc.)

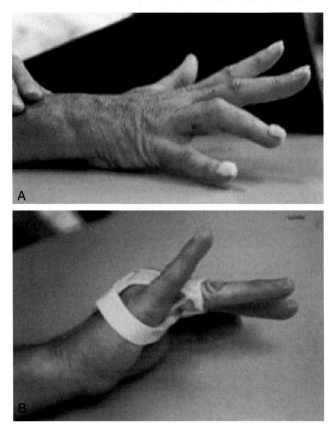

FIGURE 17.4 **A**, Pseudo-Boutonniere deformity of ring digit following proximal phalanx fracture; **B**, the blocking splint facilitates flexor and extensor tendon gliding at the proximal interphalangeal joint. (Reproduced with permission from Hardy MA. Principles of metacarpal and phalangeal fracture management: a review of rehabilitation concepts. *J Orthop Sports Phys Ther.* 2004;34:781-799. doi:10.2519/jospt.2004.34.12.781. ©JOSPT®, Inc.)

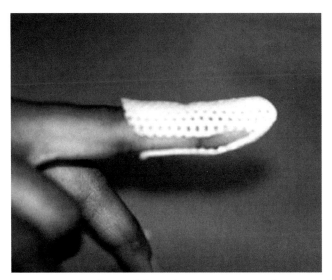

FIGURE 17.5 Tip protector splint to maintain distal interphalangeal joint extension and accommodate swelling for mallet fractures. (Reproduced with permission from Hardy MA. Principles of metacarpal and phalangeal fracture management: a review of rehabilitation concepts. *J Orthop Sports Phys Ther.* 2004;34:781-799. doi:10.2519/jospt.2004.34.12.781. ©JOSPT®, Inc.)

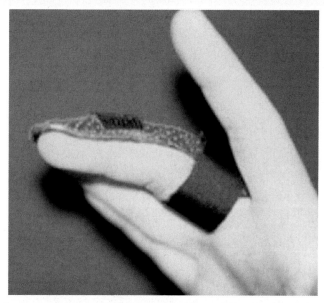

FIGURE 17.6 Volar plate avulsion fracture with extension block splint that limits full extension at the proximal interphalangeal joint (PIP); the degree of blocking is determined by fracture displacement with extension. The distal strap (not shown) is removed to allow PIP and distal interphalangeal joint flexion and extension. (Reproduced with permission from Hardy MA. Principles of metacarpal and phalangeal fracture management: a review of rehabilitation concepts. *J Orthop Sports Phys Ther.* 2004;34:781-799. doi:10.2519/jospt.2004.34.12.781. ©JOSPT®, Inc.)

TABLE 17.2

Metacarpal Shaft	Immobilization/Orthosis	AROM	PROM	Strengthening	Considerations
Nondisplaced/ stable	Removable, static radial/ ulnar gutter splint including MCP joint in 50°-70° of flexion for injured and adjacent joint	Immediate as tolerated Active flexion/ extension of MCP, avoid lateral stress	~4-6 wk with evidence of radiographic healing	~6-8 wk with evidence of radiographic healing	
Closed reduced/ stable	Removable, static radial/ ulnar gutter splint including MCP joint in 50°-70° of flexion for injured and adjacent joint	~2-3 wk Active flexion/ extension of MCP, avoid lateral stress	~5-6 wk with evidence of radiographic healing	~6-8 wk with evidence of radiographic healing	
CRPP	Removable, static radial/ ulnar gutter splint including MCP joint in 50°-70° of flexion for injured and adjacent joint	~2-3 wk Active flexion/ extension of MCP, avoid lateral stress	~5-6 wk with evidence of radiographic healing	~6-8 wk with evidence of radiographic healing	Initial splint may be bulky volar resting splint Removal of hardware ~ 4-6 wk
ORIF	Removable, static radial/ ulnar gutter splint including MCP joint in 50°-70° of flexion for injured and adjacent joint	~2-3 wk (begin at first follow-up visit) Active flexion/ extension of MCP, avoid lateral stress	~3-4 wk with evidence of radiographic healing	~6-8 wk with evidence of radiographic healing	Scar massage Tissue gliding

AROM, active range of motion; CRPP, closed reduction percutaneous pinning; MCP, metacarpophalangeal joint; ORIF, open reduction internal fixation; PROM, passive range of motion.
Data from Hays PL, Rozental TD. Rehabilitative strategies following hand fractures. Hand Clin. 2013;29(4):585-600. doi:10.1016/j.hcl.2013.08.011. PMID: 24209956.

TABLE 17.3

Proximal Phalanx Shaft	Immobilization/Orthosis	AROM	PROM	Strengthening	Considerations
Nondisplaced/ stable	Hand-based radial/ulnar gutter splint in PIP 20°-40° flexion and MCP 50°-70° flexion	Immediate as tolerated Buddy tape to adjacent digit	~4-6 wk with evidence of radiographic healing	~6-8 wk with evidence of radiographic healing	Edema control Joint blocking Tissue gliding
Closed reduced/ stable	Hand-based radial/ulnar gutter splint in PIP 20°-40° flexion and MCP 50°-70° flexion	Immediate as tolerated Buddy tape to adjacent digit	~4-6 wk with evidence of radiographic healing	~6-8 wk with evidence of radiographic healing	Edema control Joint blocking Tissue gliding
CRPP	Hand-based radial/ulnar gutter splint in PIP 20°-40° flexion and MCP 50°-70° flexion	~3-4 wk	~5-6 wk with evidence of radiographic healing	~6-8 wk with evidence of radiographic healing	Initial splint may be bulky volar resting splint Removal of hardware ~ 4-6 wk
ORIF	Hand-based radial/ulnar gutter splint in PIP 20°-40° flexion and MCP 50°-70° flexion	~2-3 wk (begin at first follow-up visit) Active flexion/ extension of MCP, avoid lateral stress	~3-4 wk with evidence of radiographic healing	~6-8 wk with evidence of radiographic healing	Scar massage Tissue gliding

AROM, active range of motion; CRPP, closed reduction percutaneous pinning; MCP, metacarpophalangeal joint; ORIF, open reduction internal fixation; PIP, proximal interphalangeal joint; PROM, passive range of motion.
Reproduced with permission from Gallagher KG, Blackmore SM. Intra-articular hand fractures and joint injuries: part II – therapist's management. In: Skirven TM, Osterman AL, Fedorczyk J, et al, eds. Rehabilitation of the Hand and Upper Extremity. *7th ed. Philadelphia, PA: Elsevier Mosby; 2021:322-344.*

TABLE 17.4

Middle Phalanx Shaft	Immobilization/ Orthosis	AROM	PROM	Strengthening	Considerations
Nondisplaced/ stable	Hand-based radial/ulnar gutter splint in PIP 20°-40° flexion and MCP 50°-70° flexion	Immediate as tolerated Buddy tape to adjacent digit	~4-6 wk with evidence of radiographic healing	~6-8 wk with evidence of radiographic healing	Edema control Joint blocking Tissue gliding
Closed reduced/ stable	Hand-based radial/ulnar gutter splint in PIP 20°-40° flexion and MCP 50°-70° flexion	Immediate as tolerated Buddy tape to adjacent digit	~4-6 wk with evidence of radiographic healing	~6-8 wk with evidence of radiographic healing	Edema control Joint blocking Tissue gliding
CRPP	Hand-based radial/ulnar gutter splint in PIP 20°-40° flexion and MCP 50°-70° flexion	~3-4 wk	~5-6 wk with evidence of radiographic healing	~6-8 wk with evidence of radiographic healing	Initial splint may be bulky volar resting splint Removal of hardware ~ 4-6 wk
ORIF	Hand-based radial/ulnar gutter splint in PIP 20°-40° flexion and MCP 50°-70° flexion	~2-3 wk (begin at first follow-up visit) Active flexion/extension of MCP, avoid lateral stress	~3-4 wk with evidence of radiographic healing	~6-8 wk with evidence of radiographic healing	Scar massage Tendon gliding

AROM, active range of motion; CRPP, closed reduction percutaneous pinning; MCP, metacarpophalangeal joint; ORIF, open reduction internal fixation; PIP, proximal interphalangeal joint; PROM, passive range of motion.

TABLE 17.5

Distal Phalanx Tuft	Immobilization/Orthosis	AROM	PROM	Strengthening	Considerations
Nondisplaced/stable	Static digital splint with DIP in full extension	Immediate as tolerated	~3-4 wk with evidence of radiographic healing	~4-6 wk with evidence of radiographic healing	Edema control Joint blocking
Closed reduced/stable	Static digital splint with DIP in full extension	Immediate as tolerated	~3-4 wk with evidence of radiographic healing	~4-6 wk with evidence of radiographic healing	Edema control Joint blocking
CRPP	Static digital splint with DIP in full extension	After removal of pins	After removal of pins with improving AROM	After removal of pins with restoration of AROM	

AROM, active range of motion; CRPP, closed reduction percutaneous pinning; DIP, distal interphalangeal joint; PROM, passive range of motion.

TABLE 17.6

PIP Joint Avulsion	Immobilization/Orthosis	AROM	PROM	Strengthening	Considerations
Volar plate Nondisplaced/stable	Buddy tape to adjacent digit	Immediate as tolerated	Advance as tolerated	~4-6 wk with improved motion	
Middle phalanx dorsal avulsion Nondisplaced/stable	Hand-based volar splint with PIP in extension	~3-4 wk with evidence of radiographic healing	~5-6 wk with improving AROM	~6-12 wk with restoration of AROM	Avoid development of late Boutonniere deformity
CRPP Middle phalanx dorsal avulsion Displaced/unstable	Hand-based volar splint with PIP in extension	After removal of pins	~4-6 wk with evidence of radiographic healing	After removal ~ 6-12 wk with restoration of AROM	
ORIF Middle phalanx dorsal avulsion Displaced/unstable	Hand-based volar splint with PIP in extension	~2-3 wk (begin at first follow-up visit)	~4-6 wk with evidence of radiographic healing	After removal ~ 6-12 wk with restoration of AROM	

AROM, active range of motion; CRPP, closed reduction percutaneous pinning; ORIF, open reduction internal fixation; PIP, proximal interphalangeal joint; PROM, passive range of motion.

POTENTIAL PROBLEMS WITH METACARPAL FRACTURES AND STRATEGIES FOR THERAPEUTIC INTERVENTION

Potential Problems	Prevention and Treatment
Dorsal hand edema	Coban wrap compression, ice, elevation, high-voltage stimulation
Dorsal skin scar contracture that prevents full fist	Silicone TopiGel, simultaneous heat and stretch with hand wrapped in a fisted position; friction massage
MP joint contracted in extension	Initially: position MP joint at 70° flexion in protective splint Late: dynamic or static progressive MP joint flexion splint
Adherence of EDC tendon to fracture with limited MP joint flexion	Initially: teach EDC glide exercises to prevent adherence; splint IP joint in extension during exercise to concentrate flexion power at MP joint Late: dynamic MP flexion splint; NMES of EDC with on > off cycle
Intrinsic muscle contracture secondary to swelling and immobilization	Initially: teach intrinsic stretch (intrinsic minus position) Late: static progressive splint in intrinsic minus position
Dorsal sensory radial/ulnar nerve irritation	Desensitization program; iontophoresis with lidocaine
Attrition and potential rupture of extensor tendon over prominent dorsal boss or large plate	Rest involved tendon; contact physician if painful symptoms with AROM persist
Scissoring/overlapping of digits with flexion	Slight: buddy tape to adjacent digit Severe: malrotation deformity requiring ORIF
Absence of MP head	Shortening of metacarpal; may not be functional problem
Absence of MP head and MP joint extension lag	Shortening of metacarpal with redundancy in extensor length; splint in extension at night; strengthen intrinsics abduction/adduction; NMES of intrinsics with off > on cycle
Absence of MP head with volar prominence and pain with grip	Neck fracture angulated volarly; minor: padded work glove; major: reduction of angulation required

AROM, active range of motion; EDC, extensor digitorum communis; IP, interphalangeal; MP, metacarpophalangeal; NMES, neuromuscular electrical stimulation; ORIF, open reduction internal fixation.

Reproduced with permission from Hardy MA. Principles of metacarpal and phalangeal fracture management: a review of rehabilitation concepts. *J Orthop Sports Phys Ther.* 2004;34:781-799. doi:10.2519/jospt.2004.34.12.781. ©JOSPT®, Inc.

POTENTIAL PROBLEMS WITH PHALANGEAL FRACTURES AND STRATEGIES FOR THERAPEUTIC INTERVENTION

Potential Problems	Prevention and Treatment
Loss of MP flexion	Circumferential PIP and DIP extension splint to concentrate flexor power at MP joint; NMES to interossei
Loss of PIP extension	Central slip blocking exercises; during the day MP extension block splint to concentrate extensor power at PIP joint; at night PIP extension gutter splint; NMES to EDC and interossei with dual channel setup
Loss of PIP flexion	Isolated FDP tendon glide exercises; during the day MP flexion blocking splint to concentrate flexor power at PIP joint; at night flexion glove; NMES to FDS
Loss of DIP extension	Resume night extension splinting; NMES to interossei
Loss of DIP flexion	Isolated FDP tendon glide exercises; PIP flexion blocking splint to concentrate flexor power at DIP joint; stretch ORL tightness; NMES to FDP
Lateral instability any joint	Buddy strap or finger hinged splint that prevents lateral stress
Impending Boutonniere deformity	Early DIP active flexion to maintain length of lateral bands
Impending swan neck deformity	FDS tendon glide at PIP joint and terminal extensor tendon glide at the DIP joint
Pseudoclaw deformity	Splint to hold MP joint in flexion with PIP joint full extensor glide
Pain	Resume protective splinting until healing is ascertained; address edema, desensitization program

DIP, distal interphalangeal; EDC, extensor digitorum communis; FDP, flexor digitorum profundus; FDS, flexor digitorum superficialis; MP, metacarpophalangeal; NMES, neuromuscular electrical stimulation; ORL, oblique retinacular ligament; PIP proximal interphalangeal.

Reproduced with permission from Hardy MA. Principles of metacarpal and phalangeal fracture management: a review of rehabilitation concepts. *J Orthop Sports Phys Ther.* 2004;34:781-799. doi:10.2519/jospt.2004.34.12.781. ©JOSPT®, Inc.

SUMMARY

The goal of rehabilitation of hand fractures is the establishment of stability allowing early range of motion. The joints of the hand are prone to stiffness and disability following injury. A wide variety of strategies are available to the surgeons and therapists that can achieve enhanced patient outcomes. A team approach that emphasizes frequent communication and consistent messaging is critical.[2] Managing patient expectations, whether tempering unrealistic goals or motivating progress, is another key factor to success.[3] Developing home programs using digital tools accompanied with explicit visual instructions can enhance patient compliance.[4]

REFERENCES

1. Feehan L. Early controlled mobilization of potentially unstable extra-articular hand fracture. *J Hand Ther.* 2003;16(2):161-170.
2. Gallagher KG, Blackmore SM. Intra-articular hand fractures and joint injuries: part II – therapist's management. In: Skirven TM, Osterman AL, Fedorczyk J, et al, eds. *Rehabilitation of the hand and upper extremity.* 7th ed. Philadelphia, PA: Elsevier Mosby; 2021:322-344.
3. Marks M, Herren DB, Vlieland TP, et al. Determinants of patient satisfaction after orthopedic interventions to the hand: a review of the literature. *J Hand Ther.* 2011;24:303-312.
4. Wakefield A, McQueen M. The role of physiotherapy and clinical predictors of outcome after fracture of the distal radius. *J Bone Joint Surg Br.* 2000;82B:972-976.

18

Injuries of the Pelvis

Mirza Shahid Baig
Daniela Furtado Barreto Rocha
Daniel S. Horwitz

INTRODUCTION

Pelvic injuries are a heterogeneous group of injuries that affect the bony pelvic ring (sacrum and innominate bones) and ligaments that hold it together. The incidence of these injuries is 0.82 per 100,000 and affect patients of all ages. The predominant age group affected is 18- to 44-year-olds.[1] Males are affected more often than females.

The pelvis contains the pelvic viscera and acts as a conduit to major vessels and nerves entering from the abdomen to the lower limbs. Injury to major vessels can result in life-threatening bleeding, and injuries to the nerves and viscera can result in lifelong morbidity.

MECHANISM OF INJURY

In the younger age group, most of these injuries occur due to high-energy trauma, whereas in the geriatric population, they occur as a result of low-energy trauma as the bone is weakened due to osteoporosis. Low-energy injuries often result in stable fractures, whereas high-energy injuries often disrupt the pelvic ring, resulting in unstable injuries. The most common mechanisms are motor vehicle-pedestrian accidents and motorcycle accidents.

It is essential to note the injury mechanism as the fracture patterns are determined by the magnitude and direction of forces acting on the pelvis at the time of injury. These forces are

1. Anteroposterior compression: This force causes the pelvis to open like a book, hinged at posterior sacroiliac ligaments (**Figure 18.1A**)
2. Lateral compression: This force results in pelvis collapse toward midline (**Figure 18.1B**)
3. Vertical shear: This force causes the displacement in the plane of sacroiliac joints (**Figure 18.1C**)

ANATOMY

The pelvis is a ring structure formed by one sacrum and two innominate bones, connected anteriorly at symphysis pubis and posteriorly at sacroiliac joints by ligaments. The bony components provide structure while the stability is mainly provided by the ligaments connecting them (**Figure 18.2**). These ligaments can be divided into two groups.

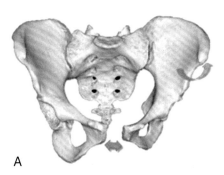
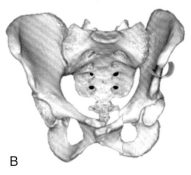
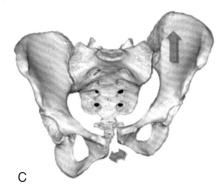

A   B   C

FIGURE 18.1 Trauma mechanisms of pelvic ring injuries. **A**, Anteroposterior compression causing symphysis diastasis and widening of the anterior part of the sacroiliac. **B**, Lateral compression causing fractures of the ilio- and ischiopubic rami, overlapping dislocation of the symphysis and anterior sacral fracture-impaction. **C**, Vertical shear causing symphysis and sacroiliac diastasis. (Reprinted with permission from Moliere S, Dosch JC, Bierry G. Pelvic, acetabular and hip fractures: What the surgeon should expect from the radiologist. *Diagn Interv Imaging*. 2016;97:711, with permission from Elsevier.)

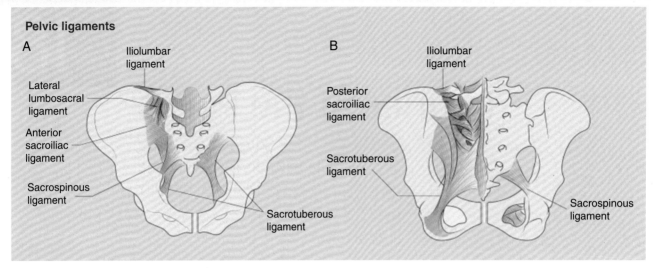

FIGURE 18.2 Pelvic ligaments. Anterior (**A**) and posterior (**B**) view of the pelvis with attached ligaments. (Reprinted with permission from Popescu M, Kassam A-AM. Pelvic injuries. *Surgery (Oxford)*. 2018;36:348, with permission from Elsevier.)

ANTERIOR GROUP

1. Symphyseal ligaments

POSTERIOR GROUP

1. *Sacroiliac ligaments*: These ligaments stabilize the sacroiliac joint and consist of anterior sacroiliac ligament, interosseous sacroiliac ligament, and posterior sacroiliac ligament (short and long).
2. *Sacrotuberous ligament*: It goes from the posterior iliac spine and posterolateral aspect of sacrum to the ischial tuberosity. In association with interosseous ligament and posterior sacroiliac ligament, this ligament is vital in maintaining the vertical stability of the pelvis.
3. *Sacrospinous ligament*: It goes from lateral margin of sacrum and coccyx to the ischial spine.
4. *Iliolumbar ligaments*: These are bilateral and run from tip of the fifth lumbar transverse process to iliac crest.
5. *Lateral lumbosacral ligament*: It goes from transverse process of the fifth lumbar vertebra to the ala of sacrum.

The posterior ligaments play a vital role in imparting stability to the pelvic ring. They collectively form the posterior tension band of the pelvis and resist the deforming forces. The transversely placed ligaments, short posterior sacroiliac, anterior sacroiliac, iliolumbar, and sacrospinous, withstand rotational forces, whereas the vertically placed ligaments, long posterior sacroiliac, sacrotuberous, and lateral lumbosacral ligaments, resist vertical shear forces. These ligaments acting together assure a stable posterior pelvis.[2]

The pelvic cavity is divided into false (upper) and true (lower) pelvis by the pelvic brim. The pelvic brim consists of sacral promontory, iliopectineal line, pubic crest, and upper portion of the pubic symphysis. The pelvic cavity contains and supports the bladder, rectum, anal canal, reproductive tracts, numerous blood vessels, and nerves. Due to proximity of these structures to the pelvic ring, visceral injuries must be considered and ruled out in all pelvic injuries.

CLASSIFICATION OF PELVIC FRACTURES

Numerous attempts have been made for classifying these injuries. There are two significant pelvic fracture classification system that we would like to discuss briefly here:

1. Tile classification
2. Young and Burgess classification

TILE CLASSIFICATION (FIGURE 18.3)[3]

Type A: Stable pelvic ring
  A1: Pelvic ring is not involved (avulsions, iliac wing or crest fractures).
  A2: Minimally displaced fractures
Type B: Rotationally unstable but vertically stable pelvic ring
  B1: Open book
  B2: Lateral compression, ipsilateral
  B3: Lateral compression, contralateral, or bucket handle-type injury
Type C: Rotationally and vertically unstable pelvic ring
  C1: Unilateral
  C2: Bilateral
  C3: Associated with an acetabular fracture

YOUNG AND BURGESS CLASSIFICATION (FIGURE 18.4)[4]

This is the most widely used classification system of pelvic fracture. It is based on the mechanism of injury. Four major types have been described:

1. Lateral compression (LC I-III)
2. Anteroposterior compression (APC I-III)
3. Vertical shear
4. Combined mechanism

Lateral compression is the most common pattern observed. It results from internal rotation force on the hemipelvis, which

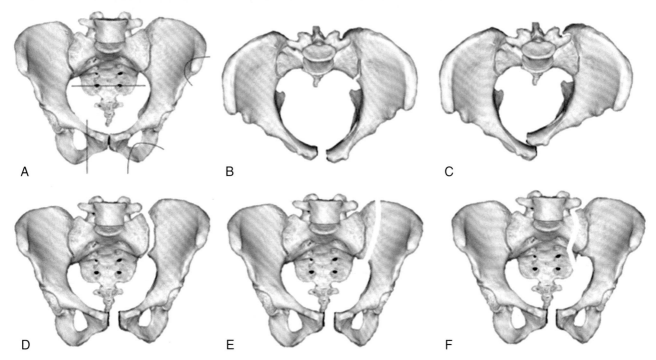

FIGURE 18.3 Main types of pelvic ring fractures based on the Tile/AO classification. **A**, Stable fracture (type A); (**B**) unstable fracture in rotation with unilateral open book fracture (type B1); (**C**) unstable type B fracture in rotation with unilateral compression (type B2); (**D**) completely unstable fracture (type C) with posterior ligament injury; (**E**) type C with transiliac fracture; and (**F**) type C with transsacral fracture. (Reprinted with permission from Moliere S, Dosch JC, Bierry G. Pelvic, acetabular and hip fractures: What the surgeon should expect from the radiologist. *Diagn Interv Imaging.* 2016;97:712, with permission from Elsevier.)

sustains the force of impact. As a result of this force, anteriorly, rami fracture and, posteriorly, sacral impaction and iliac wing fractures can occur. Depending on the posterior lesion, these injuries are further subclassified into three groups:

a. LC I: Sacral fracture on side of the impact
b. LC II: Crescent fracture on side of the impact (fracture-dislocation of the iliac wing through the sacroiliac joint)
c. LC III: LC I or LC II on the side of impact with contralateral open book injury.

Anteroposterior compression (APC) injury is caused by severe external rotation force acting on the pelvis. Symphysis pubis fails first (APC I), and sequentially, sacrotuberous and sacrospinous and anterior sacroiliac ligaments fail (APC II). With continuing external rotational force, failure of intra-articular and posterior sacroiliac ligaments result in APC III pattern.

Vertical shear injuries occur due to cephalad force and are most commonly seen in falls from height. Combined mechanism fractures show features of two or more patterns mentioned above.

TREATMENT

NONOPERATIVE

Historically pelvic injuries have been treated nonoperatively in traction and immobilization. In recent times, with an increase in knowledge of pelvic biomechanics, availability of quality implants, and improved surgical techniques, many surgeons are attempting operative treatment. However, there is still a role for nonoperative management in many pelvic injuries. The indications are as follows:

1. Stable pelvic ring injuries (most LC I and APC I)
2. Comorbidities that preclude surgical treatment
3. Inadequate bone stock which compromises screw purchase

OPERATIVE

Indications for anterior ring stabilization[5]:

1. Symphyseal dislocations showing greater than 2.5 cm diastasis
2. Augmentation of posterior fixation in vertically displaced pelvic injuries
3. Locked symphysis
4. Bilateral superior and inferior rami fractures

Indications for posterior ring stabilization:

1. Disruption of the sacroiliac joint and anterior and posterior ligaments
2. Any posterior ring injury with vertical displacement
3. Complete sacral fractures
4. Lumbopelvic disassociation
5. Open fractures with visceral injury (absolute indication)

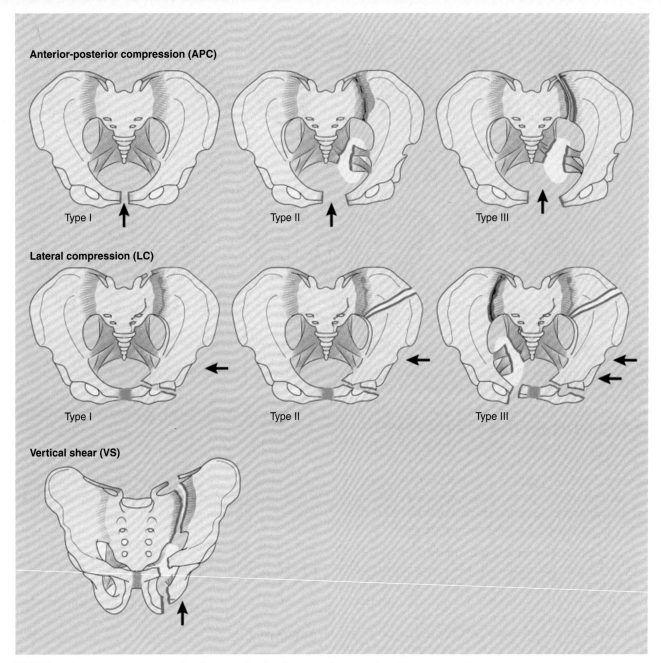

FIGURE 18.4 Young and Burgess classification of pelvic fractures. (Reprinted with permission from Popescu M, Kassam A-AM. Pelvic injuries. *Surgery (Oxford)*. 2018;36:349, with permission from Elsevier.)

OPERATIVE TECHNIQUES

External Fixation

This is mostly used as a resuscitative fixation to control pelvic bleeding, and sometimes it can be used for definitive fixation of anterior pelvic injuries, especially in those with bladder rupture.

The frame is constructed with the help of two to three 5-mm threaded Schanz pins placed 1 cm apart along the iliac crest directed toward the supra-acetabular region (**Figure 18.5**).

Hanover frame: In this construct, single Schanz pins are inserted in the supra-acetabular area in AP direction,[6]and these pins are biomechanically superior.[7]

Internal Fixation

Internal fixation is superior to external fixation in resisting vertical displacement of the hemipelvis. The selection of surgical approach and technique is based on factors like patient condition, of soft tissues, associated injuries, availability of implants, and surgeon's skill.

Methods of internal fixation of anterior ring:

1. Symphysis diastasis: Open reduction and internal fixation (ORIF) with plate fixation (**Figure 18.6C**).
2. Rami fractures: ORIF with pelvic reconstruction plates or percutaneous stabilization with screw fixation using either antegrade or retrograde technique.

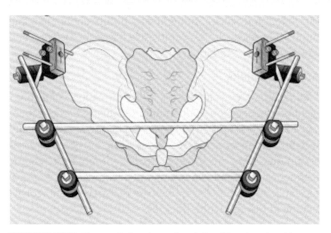

FIGURE 18.5 External fixation of pelvis. (Reprinted with permission from Popescu M, Kassam A-AM. Pelvic injuries. *Surgery (Oxford)*. 2018;36:351, with permission from Elsevier.)

Methods of internal fixation of posterior ring:

1. Sacroiliac joint dislocation: ORIF with iliosacral screw placement is usually done (**Figure 18.6C**). Other options include plating.[8]
2. Sacral fractures: These fractures are approached via posterior approach. The fixation depends on the unilateral or bilateral nature of the injury and is carried out with iliosacral screw fixation, plating, and sacral bars.
3. Iliac wing fractures: These fractures can be approached using either anterior or posterior approaches. The fixation is achieved using lag screws and neutralization plates.

REHABILITATION PROTOCOL

The main goal of rehabilitation is to facilitate an optimal return of function by improving pain, strength, flexibility,

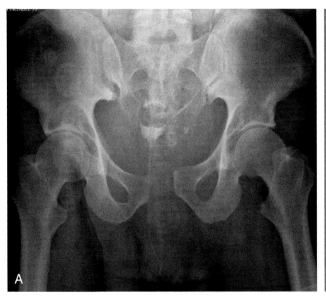

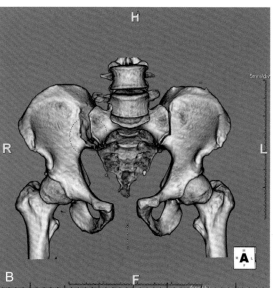

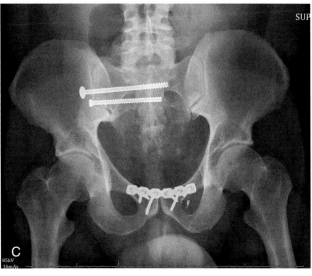

FIGURE 18.6 A, Anteroposterior (AP) radiograph showing symphyseal widening (anterior injury) and right sacroiliac joint disruption (posterior injury to the pelvic ring). **B**, Three-dimensional (3D) computed tomographic (CT) image showing symphyseal widening and right sacroiliac joint disruption as depicted by dotted arrow and circle, respectively. **C**, Postoperative AP radiograph of the same patient with internal fixation-symphyseal plate anteriorly and iliosacral screw posteriorly.

and hip and leg motion. It also aims at shortening the time needed for recovery. The main factor driving the rehabilitation protocol is the stability of the pelvis.

Patients with pelvic fractures are usually victims of polytrauma, and associated nonorthopaedic injuries like head, thoracic, and abdominal trauma dictate mobilization whereas the associated lower limb trauma dictates weight-bearing. Assuming that there are no factors mentioned above inhibiting mobility and weight-bearing, the following is a guideline to rehabilitation.

STABLE INJURIES

0 to 8 Weeks

An ice pack is used for controlling edema. Weight-bearing as tolerated can be started in stable pelvic ring injuries with assisted devices. Radiographic evaluation of the fracture must be performed for the first few weeks after the patient has been immobilized to ensure no displacement of fracture fragments. Active, assisted, and gentle passive range of motion exercises at hip, knee, and ankle.

8 to 12 Weeks

Weight-bearing is progressively increased to achieve full weight-bearing at 12 weeks. Continuation of range of motion at ankle, knee, and hip—gentle passive, assisted, and active. As part of gait training, the patient is initially made to walk between parallel bars and later progressed to walk with a walker or cane.

Above 12 Weeks

Full weight-bearing. Progressive resisted strengthening of muscles of the hip and knee. Cycling and swimming are encouraged to improve hip range of motion and increase the strength and conditioning of hip and trunk muscles.

UNSTABLE INJURIES

0 to 2 Weeks

An ice pack is used for controlling edema. The patient should be mobilized from bed to chair on the next day of surgery, assuming there are no injuries that would prevent it. Toe-touch weight-bearing on the side of injury with the help of ambulatory devices. Radiographic evaluation should be carried out to check for the displacement of fracture fragments post mobilization. Active range of motion at the knee (flexion and extension) and ankle (dorsiflexion and plantarflexion) are encouraged.

2 to 8 Weeks

The patient is evaluated after two weeks for wound status and suture removal. Toe-touch weight-bearing and ambulation with assistive devices. Isometric exercises of the gluteal, lumbar, abdominal, and lower extremity muscles.

8 to 12 Weeks

X-rays are performed and evaluated for healing. Toe-touch weight-bearing with assistive devices. Range of motion at

hip, knee, and ankle. Strengthening of hip, abdominal, and lumbar muscles. Proprioceptive exercises for balance and gait training are started.

Above 12 Weeks

Radiographs are evaluated for callus formation. With bone healing evidence on radiographic evaluation, the patient can be progressed to weight-bearing as tolerated until full weight-bearing is achieved. Progressive resistive exercises at hip and knee are incorporated in the physical therapy regime. Cycling and swimming are encouraged to improve hip range of motion and to increase the strength and conditioning of hip and trunk muscles.

SPECIAL CONSIDERATIONS

GENITOURINARY DYSFUNCTION

Urogenital injuries can occur due to direct damage to urogenital structures from an associated pelvic fracture or indirectly from damage to their neurovascular supply.

Sexual dysfunction presents as retrograde ejaculation and impotence in men, while in women, dyspareunia (painful intercourse) is expected due to vaginal dryness. In men, medical treatment with phosphodiesterase 5 inhibitors like sildenafil is tried initially, and if that fails, a penile implant can be offered.

Urethral injury is more common in males and can result in stricture formation. Urethral strictures are treated with repeat dilations.

NERVE INJURIES

The presence of nerve injuries can profoundly affect rehabilitation in pelvic fractures. Unstable pelvic fractures and medial sacral fractures are associated with a high incidence of neurological injuries. Less commonly, nerve injury may also result from iatrogenic damage during iliosacral screw placement, reduction maneuvers, and implant placement. Lumbosacral plexus and nerve roots (especially L5 and S1) are affected more commonly.

POLYTRAUMA

High-energy pelvic fractures are associated with polytrauma, which can have a profound effect on rehabilitation. Injuries of the brain, spinal cord, and associated fractures of lower limbs significantly impede the rehabilitation process by affecting the patient's ability to mobilize and bear weight.

REFERENCES

1. Yoshihara H, Yoneoka D. Demographic epidemiology of unstable pelvic fracture. 2014;76(2):8-13.
2. Vukicevic S, Marusic A, Stavljenic A, Vujicic G, Skavic J, Vukicevic D. Holographic analysis of the human pelvis. *Spine (Phila Pa 1976)*. 1991;16(2):209-214.

3. Tile M. Pelvic ring fractures: Should they be fixed? *J Bone Joint Surg Br.* 1988;70(1):1-12.

4. Young JW. Pelvic fractures: Value of plain radiography in early assessment and management. *Radiology.* 1986;160(2):445-451.

5. Matta JM. Indications for anterior fixation of pelvic fractures. *Clin Orthop Relat Res.* 1996;(329):88-96.

6. Gänsslen A, Pohlemann T, Krettek C. A simple supraacetabular external fixation for pelvic ring fractures. *Oper Orthop Traumatol.* 2005;17:296-312.

7. Fangio P, Asehnoune K, Edouard A, Smail N, Benhamou D. Early embolization and vasopressor administration for management of life-threatening hemorrhage from pelvic. 2005;58:978-984.

8. Krappinger D, Larndorfer R, Struve P, et al. Minimally invasive transiliac plate osteosynthesis for type C injuries of the pelvic ring : A clinical and radiological follow-up. *J Orthop Trauma.* 2007;21(9):595-602.

19

Acetabular Fractures

Geoffrey P. Wilkin
Lindsay E. Hickerson
Diederik O. Verbeek
David L. Helfet

ANATOMY

The acetabulum is a concave surface on the hemipelvis that is formed at the confluence of the ilium, ischium, and pubis. Prior to skeletal maturity, the triradiate cartilage connects these three bones in a "T"-shaped configuration. During embryonic and childhood development, the acetabulum deepens and grows from the triradiate cartilage in response to a well-centered femoral head.[1] At 14 to 16 years of age, the triradiate cartilage closes and the three bones of the hemipelvis fuse to give the acetabulum its final adult shape.

Articular cartilage covers the majority of the acetabular surface in a horseshoe configuration. The most medial/inferior portion of the acetabulum (the cotyloid fossa) is devoid of articular cartilage and is the site of attachment for the ligamentum teres. The cartilage-covered areas of the acetabulum articulate with the femoral head to form the hip joint.

The ball and socket configuration of the hip joint allows for a mobile, yet very stable joint. The bony anatomy provides a highly congruent fit for the femoral head in the acetabulum and provides much of the hip's inherent stability. This bony stability is enhanced by the acetabular labrum that attaches peripherally on the acetabular rim. The labrum deepens the acetabulum[2] and forms a suction seal that contains the synovial fluid and generates negative intra-articular pressure to resist joint distraction.[3] The highly congruent and stable nature of the acetabular-labral complex allows uniform force distribution across the articular cartilage. The near-perfect sphericity of the articular surface permits the hip to rotate around a single center of rotation throughout much of its range of motion (ROM) so that the cartilage is subjected to minimal shear stresses.

After a fracture of the acetabulum, restoration of a smooth joint surface is critical. If residual irregularities in the articular surface remain, these areas are subject to increased stress with weight bearing and will lead to cartilage degeneration. Similarly, if the congruency of the acetabulum is not recreated, the femoral head may translate within the acetabulum rather than rotating around a single center of rotation. This translation leads to elevated shear stresses on the cartilage that can cause premature cartilage degeneration.

BIOMECHANICS

Two thick corridors of bone, termed the anterior and posterior columns, support the acetabulum in an inverted "Y" configuration. A third corridor of bone, the sciatic buttress, extends from the supra-acetabular region to the sacroiliac joint (**Figure 19.1**). The sciatic buttress transmits force from the acetabulum to the axial skeleton with weight bearing.

Two liplike projections of the acetabular rim extend anteriorly and posteriorly and form the anterior and posterior walls, respectively. The posterior wall is larger than the anterior wall and plays a much greater role in hip stability, particularly when the hip is in a flexed position.

Acetabular fractures occur when the femoral head is forcefully driven into the acetabulum. The position of the hip and the angle of force application will determine the ultimate fracture pattern. For example, a force applied along the axis of the femoral shaft to a flexed hip, as when a car passenger's knee impacts a dashboard, will result in a posteriorly directed force that typically results in a posterior wall fracture (or another "posterior" pattern). Conversely, a fall backward onto the greater trochanter, with the hip extended and externally rotated, results in an anteriorly directed force and typically results in an anterior column fracture (or another "anterior" pattern). There are an infinite number of potential hip positions and force vectors that can occur at the time of injury, so each fracture pattern will be slightly different, though surgeons tend to classify fracture patterns into defined groups based on locations of the major fracture lines.

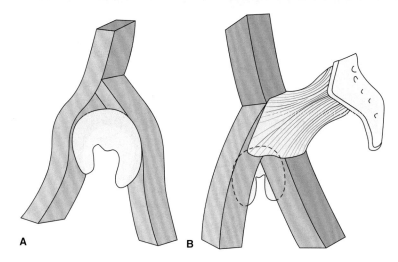

FIGURE 19.1 A, Diagram of the two columns supporting the two columns of the inverted Y. **B,** The two columns are linked to the sacral bone by the sciatic buttress. The two thick corridors of bone, termed the anterior and posterior columns, support the acetabulum in an inverted "Y" configuration. A third corridor of bone, the sciatic buttress, extends from the supra-acetabular region to the sacroiliac joint. (From Tile M, et al. *Fractures of the Pelvis and Acetabulum—Principles and Methods of Management-Acetabulum.* New York: Thieme; 2015.)

FRACTURE CLASSIFICATION

The Letournel-Judet classification is the most widely used classification system for describing acetabular fractures. This system first broadly divides the fracture patterns into five "elementary" or simple patterns and five "associated" or complex patterns. All the "simple" patterns are defined by a single primary fracture line, whereas the "associated" patterns all have two or more primary fracture lines. The complete classification system is shown in **Table 19.1** and **Figure 19.2**.

An alternative way to group fracture patterns is by the direction of greatest displacement. This grouping can help the surgeon decide on the optimal surgical approach (posterior, anterior, or combined), and the choice of surgical approach will often dictate a certain postoperative rehabilitation protocol.

EPIDEMIOLOGY

Acetabular fractures are usually the result of higher energy injuries in younger patients, with motor vehicle collisions being the most common mechanism of injury. However, in keeping with the change in general population demographics, the average age of patients sustaining acetabular fracture has been steadily increasing. Patients over age 60 are making up a larger proportion of the patients sustaining these injuries.

Ferguson et al[4] reviewed a large single-surgeon database of patients treated for displaced acetabular fractures covering the years 1980 to 2007. During the first half of the review period (1980-1994), the average patient age was 38 years and 10% of the patients were over 60 years old. In the second half of the study period (1994-2007), the mean age had increased to 45 years and 24% of patients were over age 60. In patients under 60 years, motor vehicle collisions accounted for 66% of all injury mechanisms, whereas in patients over age 60, falls were the most frequent mechanism of injury (50%). Due to the higher energy mechanisms of injury in younger patients, the rate of associated injuries was also higher (20% vs 10%) when compared to older patients.

NONOPERATIVE TREATMENT

Before modern surgical techniques were commonplace, most acetabular fractures were treated nonoperatively. Methods ranged from simple bed rest, to various methods of traction and bracing. However, due to the limited ability to restore congruence of the hip joint with closed means, functional outcomes were poor in the majority of patients.

As surgical techniques for open reduction of acetabular fractures improved, it became clear that patients who had their joint congruity sufficiently restored had improved long-term functional outcomes compared to nonoperative treatment. As a result, most displaced acetabular fractures are now managed operatively. However, there are still certain circumstances when nonoperative treatment may be chosen.

The main fracture patterns suitable for nonoperative treatment are:

• Fractures with minimal displacement of the weight-bearing articular surface (<2 mm).

TABLE 19.1 The Letournel-Judet Classification of Acetabular Fractures

Elementary (Simple) Fracture Patterns	Associated (Complex) Fracture Pattern
Posterior wall	Posterior column/posterior wall
Posterior column	Transverse/posterior wall
Anterior wall	T-type
Anterior column	Anterior column or wall/posterior hemitransverse
Transverse	Both columns

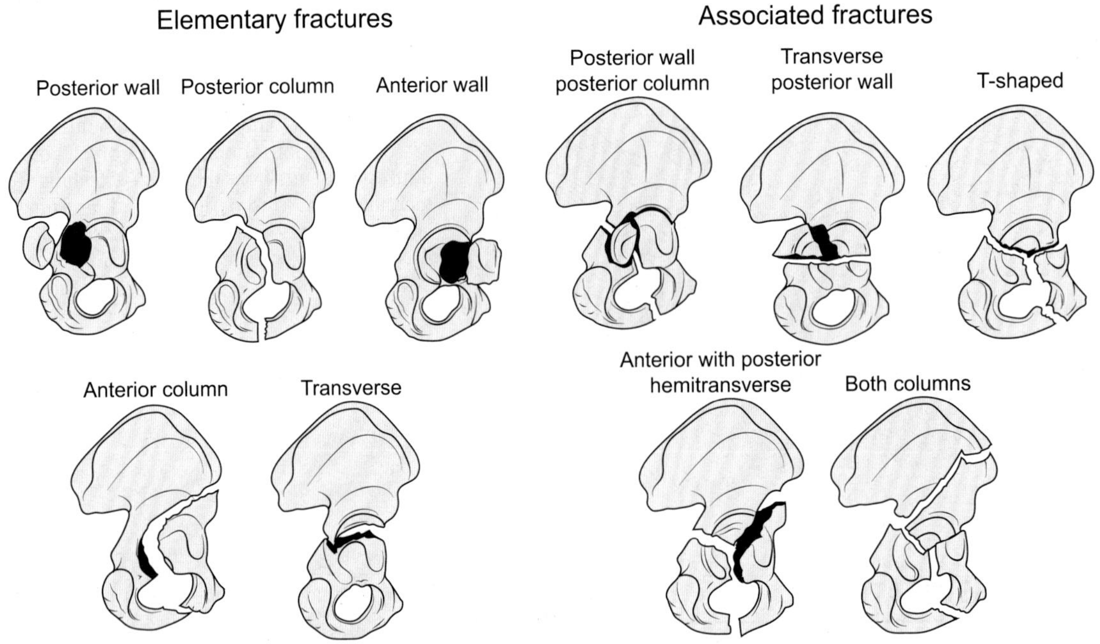

Elementary fractures

Posterior wall   Posterior column   Anterior wall

Anterior column   Transverse

Associated fractures

Posterior wall
posterior column   Transverse
posterior wall   T-shaped

Anterior with posterior
hemitransverse   Both columns

FIGURE 19.2 The Letournel-Judet classification of acetabular fractures. (Redrawn with permission from Pagenkopf E, Grose A, Partal G, Helfet DL. Acetabular fractures in the elderly: treatment recommendations. *HSS J.* 2006;2(2):161-171. doi:10.1007/s11420-006-9010-7.)

- Fracture patterns that do not involve the main superior weight-bearing dome such that a sufficiently large intact superior weight-bearing region remains with the femoral head congruent under this fragment.[5]
- Small posterior wall fractures with no evidence of hip instability on static or dynamic stress x-rays.[6]
- Both column fracture pattern with secondary congruence in a low-demand patient.[7]
  - In this pattern, since no articular fragments remain attached to the intact pelvis, the fragments may remain congruent with the femoral head, but with the entire joint in a nonanatomic position. Though congruency of the joint is maintained, the alteration in hip center may lead to abductor dysfunction and/or leg length discrepancy.

Furthermore, certain patient-related factors may cause the surgeon to elect for nonoperative treatment with or without a planned delayed hip arthroplasty procedure. Some of these conditions include:

- patients with severe medical comorbidities that preclude a major pelvic surgery,
- patients with very low preoperative functional demands (ie, wheelchair ambulators), and
- patients with cognitive impairment, psychiatric illness, or substance dependence conditions that will significantly interfere with compliance with postoperative precautions.

OPERATIVE TREATMENT

Most displaced acetabular fractures will require operative intervention. In the majority, that will mandate an open reduction and internal fixation (**Figures 19.3** and **19.4**). As

previously mentioned, the goals of surgery are to anatomically restore the articular surface and to restore stability to the hip joint. However, in certain situations, acute total hip arthroplasty may be selected as an alternative.[8] Regardless of the treatment method selected, the following are generally accepted indications for surgical treatment[9]:

- >2 mm displacement in the weight-bearing region of the acetabulum,
- evidence of hip instability/subluxation on static or dynamic stress x-rays,
- large posterior wall fractures, and
- incarcerated intra-articular fragments.

Different surgical approaches can be used to access and reduce the main fracture fragments, and the choice of approach will depend on the fracture pattern and direction of displacement.

For patterns with primarily posterior displacement, a posterior (Kocher-Langenbeck) approach is required. This approach divides the gluteus maximus muscle and allows direct access to the posterior column and posterior wall by dividing and reflecting the piriformis, obturator internus, and gemelli muscles off the proximal femur. A trochanteric osteotomy may also be combined with this approach to aid with exposure in certain fracture patterns. The Kocher-Langenbeck approach allows direct visualization of the sciatic nerve, though it puts the nerve at risk for injury. The superior gluteal neurovascular bundle is also at risk. The proximity of the femoral head blood supply during this approach also increases the risk of femoral head avascular necrosis.

For anterior fracture patterns, the two approaches used most commonly are the ilioinguinal approach and the anterior intrapelvic (modified Stoppa) approach. The ilioinguinal

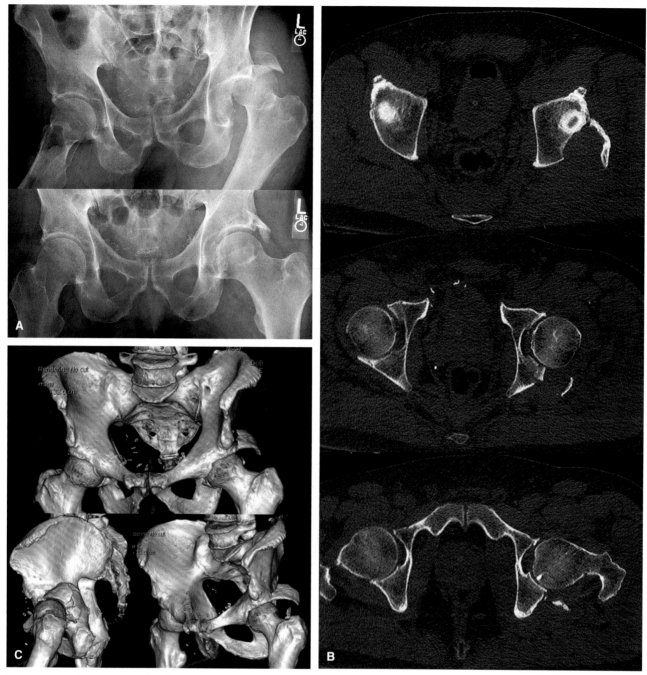

FIGURE 19.3 A, Case example of a posterior wall type acetabular fracture; top image illustrates the fracture and dislocated hip in the prereduction anteroposterior (AP) radiograph and the bottom image demonstrates the post–hip reduction AP radiograph. **B**, Axial-plane CT imaging further delineates the posterior wall fracture pattern and displacement. **C**, 3D CT reformats further illustrate the fracture pattern.

approach gains access to the pelvis by elevating the abdominal wall musculature off the iliac crest and dividing the abdominal muscles just proximal to the inguinal ligament. The bony pelvis is then accessed through three "windows": (1) lateral to the iliopsoas muscle/femoral nerve, (2) medial to the iliopsoas muscle/femoral nerve and lateral to the femoral artery, vein, and genitofemoral nerve, and (3) medial to the femoral artery, vein, genitofemoral nerve, and lateral to the inguinal canal contents (spermatic cord in males, round ligament in females). The femoral, lateral femoral cutaneous,

and obturator and genitofemoral nerves are all encountered during this approach and thus are at risk for injury. The femoral vessels are also at risk for injury or thrombosis.

The anterior intrapelvic (modified Stoppa) approach gains access to the pelvis via a midline approach.[10] Typically, a horizontal skin incision is made over the pubic symphysis and the rectus abdominis is split vertically along the linea alba. This gives access to the retroperitoneal space and the bladder is retracted posteriorly. Dissection can then be carried laterally along the pelvic brim and down the inner surface of

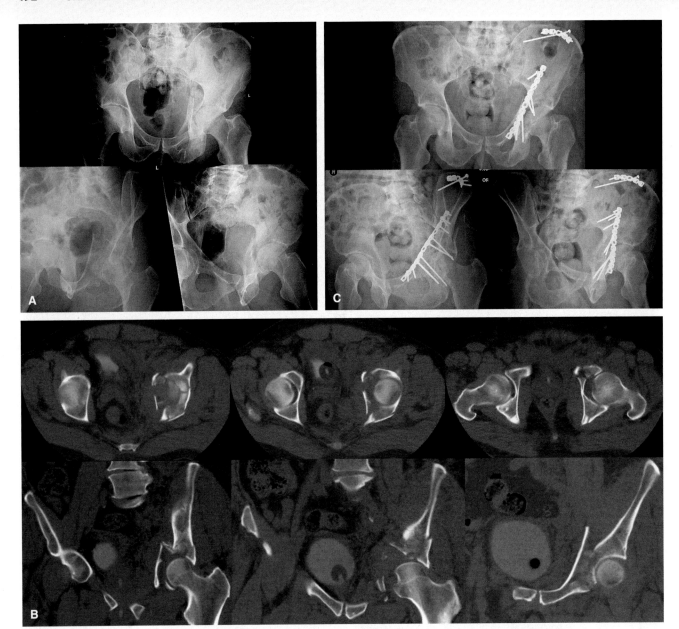

FIGURE 19.4 A, Case example of an associated both column type acetabular fracture; images from counterclockwise from top show the AP, obturator oblique, and iliac oblique radiographic views. **B**, CT scan imaging further delineates the associated both column fracture margins, displacement, and comminution of the dome of the acetabulum. **C**, Radiographic images from counterclockwise from top show the AP, obturator oblique, and iliac oblique radiographic views following open reduction and internal fixation performed through the lateral two windows of the ilioinguinal surgical approach. Radiographs demonstrate an acceptable reduction and placement of hardware.

the pelvis to expose the fracture fragments. An advantage of this approach is that it does not require direct visualization and dissection of the femoral neurovascular structures. This approach also allows more direct access to the medial aspect of the acetabulum. However, access to the iliac wing is limited and this approach must frequently be combined with the lateral window of an ilioinguinal approach to access all the fracture lines.

Alternative approaches such as the extended iliofemoral or the triradiate approach may be used for select cases. In addition, a fracture pattern may necessitate two separate approaches, performed either concurrently during the same surgery, sequentially on the same operative day, or in a staged fashion under separate anesthetics.

COMMON REHABILITATION PROTOCOLS

THERAPEUTIC INTERVENTIONS: POSTOPERATIVE ACETABULUM FRACTURE

These are general guidelines. Consult with surgeon regarding specifics of the rehabilitation expectations.

0 to 8 Weeks

Toe touch weight bearing (TTWB) (TT/20 lbs)*, ice pack for edema. Return to clinic at 2 weeks for wound check and suture removal after which scar massage can start. Use assisted device (walker or crutches) 100% of the time. Train for safe sleep habits and toileting.

SPECIAL CONSIDERATIONS

For acetabular fractures with a posterior wall component, emphasize posterior hip precautions for 6 weeks, which are typically no flexion of hip beyond 90°, no internal rotation of hip/leg beyond neutral, and no cross body adduction of leg unless further specified by physician. Patients may be prescribed a knee immobilizer or abduction hip wedge for added protection if patient and fracture characteristics warrant. Anterior wall fractures (**Figure 19.5A-C**) are uncommon and often more unstable, secondary to comminution. For anterior wall fractures, essentially the opposite precautions are in place (no hip extension, no external rotation beyond neutral, and no adduction beyond neutral). A hip flexion orthosis may help.

A trochanteric slide (**Figure 19.6**) may be necessary to access the superior aspect of acetabulum from a Kocher-Langenbeck approach (posterior approach). If this is performed, the osteotomy of the greater trochanter needs to heal and active abduction restrictions may be in place for 6 weeks by the surgeon (**Figure 19.7**).

8 to 12 Weeks

At 8 weeks, patients can usually begin progressive weight bearing through the operative leg until full weight bearing at 12 weeks. Train with foot on a scale for biofeedback to "feel" what 20 to 40 pounds is like. Patients usually tolerate gentle ROM (abduction, adduction, flexion, extension, internal rotation, and external rotation) of the hip, active, active assisted, and gentle passive. Pool gait training with the height of water at or above the nipple line may be of great benefit.

At full weight bearing, patients may transition to a cane in the opposite hand, assuming they are able to maintain a minimally antalgic gait pattern.

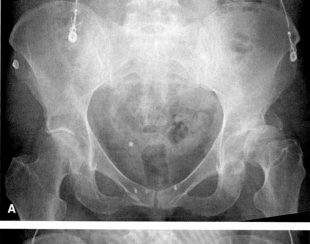
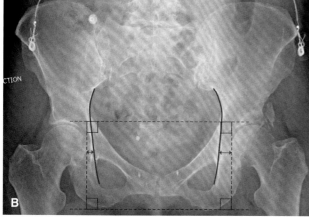
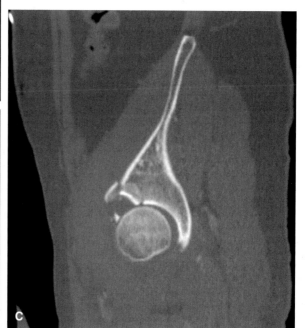

FIGURE 19.5 A, Anteroposterior (AP) radiograph of a pelvis with a left-sided anterior wall fracture and anterior hip dislocation. Anterior dislocations are rare and present with external rotation of the femur (note lesser trochanter larger thus externally rotated) and hip extension. **B**, Postreduction AP radiograph of left anterior hip dislocation. Ongoing external rotation of the femur and increased distance of the femoral head to the ilioischial line suggest subluxation. **C**, Sagittal view of CT scan after closed reduction of anterior wall acetabular fracture demonstrating impaction of the acetabulum and ongoing subluxation of the hip joint as the prior radiograph suggested.

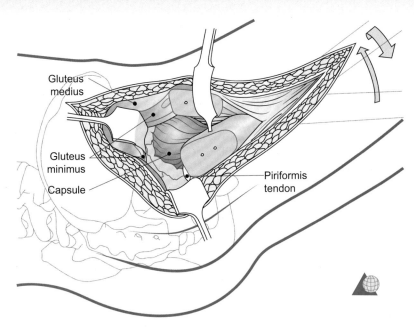

FIGURE 19.6 Illustration of a trochanteric slide. Here the patient is positioned lateral and the greater trochanter is osteotomized and slid anterior via a posterior approach. This osteotomy increases visibility to the superior and anterior acetabulum. It is a digastric osteotomy with gluteus medius muscle attached proximally and the vastus lateralis attached distally and these opposing muscle forces aid it its stability. The osteotomy is repaired with various means (screws/wires) at the end of the case; however, most surgeons will protect the osteotomy until healed with restriction of active hip abduction. (Reprinted with permission Mayo K, Oransky M, Rommens P, Sancineto C, *AO Surgery Reference: Acetabulum – Trochanter Flip Extension*, edited by Trafton P. Copyright by AO Foundation, Switzerland, AO Surgery Reference, Available at www.aosurgery.org.)

12 Weeks +

After full weight bearing has begun, progressive resisted activities focusing on abductor strength are added. Avoid impact activities until advised by the surgeon. Encourage low impact activities that improve hip ROM and strength such as stationary cycling, elliptical, and swimming.

OBSTACLES TO REHABILITATION

HETEROTOPIC OSSIFICATION

The more contused the muscle from injury and surgical intervention, especially the Kocher-Langenbeck and extensile approaches, the more likely the development of

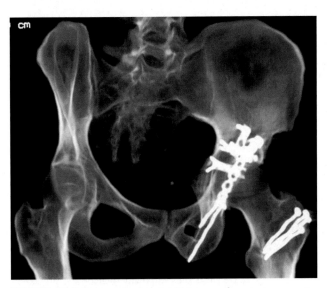

FIGURE 19.7 Volume-rendered CT image of posterior-superior wall acetabular fracture status postfixation demonstrating trochanteric osteotomy fixation and hardware superior to joint.

excess bone formation within the muscles within the zone of injury. Heterotopic ossification (HO) more frequently occurs in polytraumatized patients with a head injury. HO typically is a late presentation (2-6 months) and takes months to mature on radiographs. That is too long to wait if excision is mandated, that is, if there is a functional loss of ROM. The HO can safely be removed sooner using bone alkaline phosphatase and erythrocyte sedimentation rate as markers of bone activity. Upon HO excision, exquisite care should be made to the surrounding neurovascular structures as they can become incarcerated in bone.

AVASCULAR NECROSIS

Death of the femoral head from lack of blood supply can be caused by the injury, a dislocation, the surgical approach, and the host. This can lead to increasing pain during rehabilitation and loss of ROM. There is a two-year window for this to potentially develop after an injury.

INFECTION

Infection is characterized by a wound that has erythema, drainage, and heat. Patient's postinjury and postsurgical pain levels typically do not improve or get worse. The organism needs to be aggressively identified and in most cases, this includes surgical debridement.

SUBLUXATION/DISLOCATION

The goal of acetabular surgery is to restore a concentric hip joint in comparison to the contralateral hip if healthy. The Judet radiograph views of the *pelvis* will demonstrate side-by-side 45° oblique views for comparison. Should the joint not be concentrically reduced, the patient can feel the hip "give way" or in more severe cases dislocate. This typically will progress to posttraumatic arthritis.

IMPACTION FRACTURES

Visible on a preoperative computed tomography (CT) scan, an impaction fracture of the femoral head (**Figure 19.8**) or the acetabulum (**Figure 19.5C**) is often secondary to dislocation of the hip at the time of injury. This is common with posterior wall fractures that present dislocated and "anterior" column fractures in the elderly. The most common acetabular fracture is a posterior wall fracture in the young and in the elderly and for this reason among others (osteonecrosis, comminution), the posterior wall fractures do not do as well long term as other types of acetabular fractures despite anatomic to good intraoperative fracture reductions.

POSTTRAUMATIC CHONDROLYSIS (EARLY)/ ARTHRITIS (LATE)

Characterized by pain and stiffness. Chondrolysis is diagnosed on radiographs with joint space narrowing and often progresses to arthritis in the posttraumatic setting.

LOOSE BODIES/LABRAL TEAR

This typically presents with mechanical symptoms such as grinding, locking, and catching. Often times, the injury will cause intra-articular loose bodies which are visible on a CT scan (**Figure 19.9**). Should these loose bodies not be removed during surgery, the patient could have postoperative pain related to free fragments in the weight bearing zone of the acetabulum. Labral tears may have been visualized and fixated during operative fixation or visualized and deemed not fixable and excised. This soft-tissue fixation

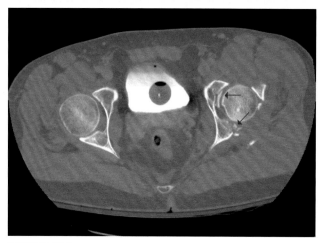

FIGURE 19.9 Axial CT of comminuted posterior wall acetabular fracture with several intra-articular fragments.

takes as long as the bone to heal often and is protected by avoiding extreme ROMs.

*TTWB: Place foot on ground but not transfer weight to the leg. This does not imply placing "toes" on the ground, which increases risk of equinus contracture at the ankle and hip flexion contracture. This is also known as TDWB or touch down weight bearing.

**No flexion of hip beyond 90°, internal rotation of leg, and cross body adduction of leg.

SPECIAL CONSIDERATIONS

NERVE INJURIES

Nerve injuries can significantly complicate the rehabilitation of acetabular fracture patients. The severity of injury can vary greatly and patients may exhibit signs of a pure sensory, motor, or combined neurologic deficit[11] Approximately 7% of (nonoperatively or operatively treated) patients with an acetabular fracture have a nerve injury on hospital discharge.[12] The majority of injuries (57%) occur as a result of the initial trauma owing to displacement of the acetabular fracture fragments or femoral head.[11] Less commonly (19%), the nerve injury presents as a complication from operative treatment of acetabular fractures (iatrogenic injury). Depending on the acetabular fracture type and the surgical approach, a variety of nerves are at risk.

The most common nerve injury associated with acetabular fractures is an injury to the sciatic nerve.[11] This large nerve exits the pelvis through the sciatic foramen and travels down the back of the leg. The sciatic nerve consists of the tibial and the common fibular (peroneal) nerve divisions. It is particularly at risk in patients with an acetabular fracture type that involves the posterior column and in patients with posterior hip dislocations. The most common fracture types associated with sciatic nerve injury are posterior wall (with or without a transverse component) and associated both column fractures.

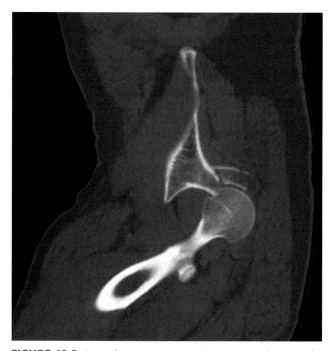

FIGURE 19.8 Sagittal reconstruction CT prior to reduction of a large posterior wall acetabular fracture demonstrating dislocation and femoral head impaction onto the acetabulum.

The surgical approach that puts the sciatic nerve at particular risk for iatrogenic injury is that of Kocher-Langenbeck. Most commonly, this injury results from excessive retraction or compression on the nerve in an attempt to obtain a reduction or adequate exposure. Iatrogenic injury to the sciatic nerve is rarely a result of a direct surgical injury or transection.

Patients with sciatic nerve injuries typically present with symptoms of an L5 nerve root deficit. This includes complaints of a foot drop with an inability to dorsiflex the foot and great toe. Management involves splinting and use of a brace to maintain a neutral position of the ankle along with ROM exercises.

The extent of initial sciatic nerve palsy, ranging from limited weakness to complete paralysis, is an important determinant for the chances of recovery. The majority (up to 71%) of sciatic nerve injuries with L5 nerve root palsies will have significant or complete recovery of foot dorsiflexion.[11] It is important to note that recovery from sciatic nerve injuries can take a prolonged period of time and improvement has been described up to 3 years from injury.[13]

A much less common nerve injury is injury to the femoral nerve. Injury to this nerve is typically associated with the ilioinguinal approach. The femoral nerve lies on the psoas muscle and can get injured when the nerve is retracted along with the psoas muscle. Symptoms include muscle weakness or paralysis of the quadriceps muscle resulting in an inability to extend the knee.

Other nerves that can potentially get injured in acetabular fracture patients include the obturator nerve, which is particularly at risk with the modified Stoppa and ilioinguinal approach. Injury to this nerve may result in weakness of the hip adductor muscles. In addition, the superior gluteal nerve can get injured, typically with the Kocher-Langenbeck approach, resulting in gluteal weakness. An important sensory nerve that is injured relatively frequently with the ilioinguinal approach is the lateral femoral cutaneous nerve. This nerve provides sensation to the lateral aspect of the proximal thigh. Injury generally results in hyposensitivity in this area, but some patients complain of painful hypersensitivity, a condition known as meralgia paresthetica.

MULTITRAUMA

Acetabular fractures may be associated with other traumatic injuries that can have a significant impact on recovery. It is important to recognize that acetabular fractures in the elderly tend to be a distinctly different entity from those occurring in the younger population. Elderly patients generally sustain isolated acetabular fractures resulting from low-impact falls. However, younger patients are more likely to have high-energy acetabular fractures with multiple associated injuries.

Of particular importance in that regard are traumatic brain and spinal cord injuries, both of which can have a profound and long-term effect on rehabilitation in acetabular fracture patients. In terms of associated musculoskeletal injuries, it is critical to consider injuries to the lower as well as the upper extremities. In determining the weight-bearing status of acetabular fracture patients, the presence of injuries to the lower extremities is of obvious importance. However, injuries to the upper extremities can also have a considerable impact on the patient's ability to mobilize. In some patients with upper extremity injuries, walking aids like platform walkers can be used to help off-load the lower extremities and facilitate early mobilization.

REFERENCES

1. Ponseti IV. Growth and development of the acetabulum in the normal child. Anatomical, histological, and roentgenographic studies. *J Bone Joint Surg.* 1978;60:575-585.
2. Tan V, Seldes RM, Katz MA, Freedhand AM, Klimkiewicz JJ, Fitzgerald RHJ. Contribution of acetabular labrum to articulating surface area and femoral head coverage in adult hip joints: an anatomic study in cadavera. *Am J Orthop.* 2001;30(11):809-812.
3. Crawford MJ, Dy CJ, Alexander JW, et al. The 2007 Frank Stinchfield Award. The biomechanics of the hip labrum and the stability of the hip. *Clin Orthop Relat Res.* 2007;465:16-22.
4. Ferguson TA, Patel R, Bhandari M, Matta JM. Fractures of the acetabulum in patients aged 60 years and older: an epidemiological and radiological study. *J Bone Joint Surg Br.* 2010;92(2):250-257.
5. Olson SA, Matta JM. The computerized tomography subchondral arc: a new method of assessing acetabular articular continuity after fracture (a preliminary report). *J Orthop Trauma.* 1993;7(5):402-413.
6. Grimshaw CS, Moed BR. Outcomes of posterior wall fractures of the acetabulum treated nonoperatively after diagnostic screening with dynamic stress examination under anesthesia. *J Bone Joint Surg Am.* 2010;92(17):2792-2800.
7. Gänsslen A, Hildebrand F, Krettek C. Conservative treatment of acetabular both column fractures: does the concept of secondary congruence work? *Acta Chir Orthop Traumatol Cech.* 2012;79(5):411-415.
8. Mears DC, Velyvis JH. Acute total hip arthroplasty for selected displaced acetabular fractures: two to twelve-year results. *J Bone Joint Surg Am.* 2002;84-A(1):1-9.
9. Tornetta P. Displaced acetabular fractures: indications for operative and nonoperative management. *J Am Acad Orthop Surg.* 2001;9(1):18-28.
10. Archdeacon MT, Kazemi N, Guy P, Sagi HC. The modified Stoppa approach for acetabular fracture. *J Am Acad Orthop Surg.* 2011;19(3):170-175.
11. Bogdan Y, Tornetta P III, Jones C, et al. Neurologic injury in operatively treated acetabular fractures. *J Orthop Trauma.* 2015;29(10):475-478.
12. Lehmann W, Hoffmann M, Fensky F, et al. What is the frequency of nerve injuries associated with acetabular fractures? *Clin Orthop Relat Res.* 2014;472(11):3395-3403.
13. Letournel E, Judet R. *Fractures of the Acetabulum.* 2nd ed. New York, NY: Springer; 1993.

20

Rehabilitation After Geriatric Hip Fracture

Michael P. Campbell
Stephen L. Kates

INTRODUCTION

Data show that fragility fractures, and specifically hip fractures, are a growing problem facing our society today. We need to continue to focus on improving our quality of care for patients with these fractures and refining our rehabilitation methods in order to maximize recovery. The goal of rehabilitation is to help patients reach their preinjury level of function and to mitigate the circumstances that led to the injury. This includes osteoporosis treatment, adequate nutrition, and instituting an exercise program to maximize mobility.

PREOPERATIVE ASSESSMENT OF FUNCTION

Geriatric hip fractures are treated surgically in a large majority of cases, unless there are underlying comorbidities that prevent operative intervention. The most common treatment methods are intramedullary nails and lateral screw and side plates (**Figure 20.1**). Restoration of height, alignment, acceptable and reduction is crucial to rapid and successful healing. A detailed history must be taken to identify the mechanism by which the injury occurred, past medical history to identify illnesses that may affect treatment or determine need for preoperative optimization, and a detailed social history. Preoperative function will determine the ultimate outcome. This includes the place of residence, ability to ambulate, cognitive status, and frailty.

With a detailed social history, one can determine the patient's preinjury level of activity and independence. Obtaining this information can be difficult if the patient has memory loss, delirium, or pain from narcotic medications administered in the Emergency Department. Important information concerning function is use of any assistive devices prior to injury, the preinjury ambulatory status (community ambulator vs household ambulator vs bedbound), and whether the patient lived independently or required significant assistance with activities of daily living and instrumental activities of daily living.

A detailed social history can be difficult to obtain if the patient has underlying memory loss or has acute delirium associated with hip fracture and pain medication. It is important to locate the family of the patient if not present, in order to corroborate the information obtained from the patient. If the patient is unable to provide information about the event, it is vital to obtain information from family members. Additionally, it must be determined if there are advance directives in place. These should be recorded in the medical record.[1]

Frailty is a patient's vulnerability to adverse outcomes. It can be measured by the Fried Frailty Index, which has been shown to predict hospitalization, disability, and death.[2] This has been modified to allow for limitations in patients' status postfracture fixation. The index evaluates shrinking, exhaustion, slowness, weakness, and physical activity. For each criterion, a patient is rated 0 if it is not present and 1 if present indicating that a person is frail for that criterion. A total score of 3 or more determines that a person is frail. Also, there is consideration that cognitive impairment contributes to frailty. It has been found that patients with frailty have an increased complication rate and length of stay. Cognitive frailty contributes to an increased complication rate.[3]

With a detailed social history, a preinjury level of function can be determined as well as frailty scoring. This may affect surgical treatment.[4] With this information, a goal can be set with rehabilitation to restore the patients to their preinjury level of functioning and independence.

EARLY POSTOPERATIVE REHABILITATION

After surgical fixation of a hip fracture, rehabilitation begins. The goal of surgery is to allow the patient to bear weight immediately. Older adults, in most cases, cannot limit weight bearing nor follow restrictions. Thus, it is necessary to choose a surgical construct that will allow the patient to be full weight bearing immediately postoperatively.[4]

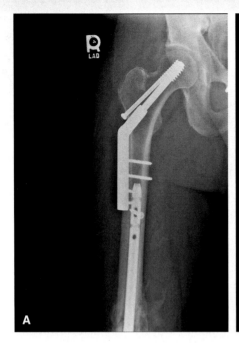

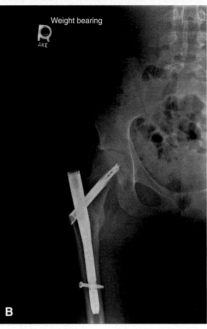

FIGURE 20.1 The image on the left shows a dynamic hip screw construct. The radiograph on the right demonstrates a short intramedullary nail.

Part of early rehabilitation includes adequate pain control and delirium prevention. With increased preoperative and postoperative pain, there is increased risk for development of delirium.[5] The presence of delirium may prevent a patient from working with physical therapy. With delays in physical therapy, a patient can quickly become deconditioned. Deconditioning makes it more difficult for patients to reach a preinjury level of function. Every day that a patient remains in bed takes at least a week to recover.[6]

Enhanced recovery pathways can improve patient outcomes. These have been shown to reduce complications, shorten length of stays, improve patient satisfaction, and reduce costs in elective total joint replacement.[7,8] These include surgical site infection prevention, venous thromboembolism reduction, and enhancing mobility. These pathways can be translated to the geriatric hip fracture population to improve recovery.[10,11]

The patient should be mobilized to stand and walk with a walker as soon as possible after surgery. Ideally, this will be achieved within 24 hours, with the goal of having the patient ambulate on the day of surgery.[4] There are many assistive devices that can be utilized to help with ambulation. These include standard walker, front-wheeled walker, rollator, axillary crutches, Lofstrand crutches, platform crutches, high roller, and canes.

As mentioned earlier, the patient's preinjury level of function is the rehabilitation goal. From the Cochrane database review of 19 trials in 2011, there was insufficient evidence to determine the best strategies for mobilizing patients after hip fracture surgery.[9]

Following the acute postoperative period, when the patient is medically stable, treatment includes a focus on discharge planning. Will the patient require further rehabilitation in the inpatient setting? Can the patient return to his or her prior living situation with a focused outpatient physical therapy regimen?[13]

A Cochrane review from 2009 looked at 13 trials involving 2498 patients who underwent hip fracture surgery. The intervention that was reviewed was multidisciplinary rehabilitation compared to usual care in an inpatient rehabilitation setting or an ambulatory setting or both. No statistically significant difference was found between intervention and controls for poor outcome (defined as outcomes of death or deterioration in residential status, generally the requirement for institutional care), mortality, or hospital readmission. There was a tendency for a better overall result in patients receiving multidisciplinary inpatient rehabilitation. These results were not statistically significant though.[14]

Home-based exercise programs have been shown to improve rehabilitation after formal hip fracture rehabilitation has ended. In a study, 232 patients were randomized to receive functionally oriented exercises taught by a physical therapist in their home for 6 months versus a control group who did not. The intervention group showed improved physical function in both patient-reported and physical performance measures.[15]

Posthospitalization rehabilitation thus needs to be planned using an individualized approach based upon the patient's preinjury level of function, progression with acute postoperative rehabilitation, and the patient's available social supports.

RESTORATIVE REHABILITATION

Rehabilitation focuses on muscle strength, balance, and fall prevention. These can all be improved by a well-designed exercise and physical training interventions.[10-12]

MAXIMIZING RECOVERY

It has been reported that recovery after hip fracture varies by functional domain. Depression, cognitive function, and upper extremity activities of daily living reach maximum recovery within 4 months of fracture. After a hip fracture, balance and gait can take up to 9 months to recover.[16]

Many elderly patients that sustain hip fractures have underlying osteoporosis. Treatment options include vitamin D and calcium supplementation, weight-bearing exercise, smoking cessation, and reduction in alcohol intake. Additionally, there is pharmacologic treatment. If a patient is currently being treated for osteoporosis, the treatment regimen needs to be reassessed. If a patient is not receiving treatment, a treatment regimen should be instituted.[17]

Proper nutrition is vital to maximizing recovery. It allows for better wound healing and a better recovery. Malnutrition contributes to frailty.[18] A diet should consist of small portions with high caloric content. Patients should be fed orally and may require assistance with feeding. Foods must be easily chewable because of poor dentition that is often found in the geriatric population. Nutritional supplementation can be utilized. Assistance from a dietician can be helpful.[4]

In order to improve a patient's prognosis, it is important to identify additional interventions that may contribute to recovery. Identifying and fixing cataracts can improve an elderly patient's visual acuity and help to prevent falls that may lead to geriatric hip fractures.[19] Identifying and treating painful knees and feet can improve a patient's ability to ambulate and also prevent future falls. It is important to recognize and treat cognitive dysfunction that may come from prolonged delirium or depression. Depression can augment symptoms of cognitive impairment and reduce a patient's capacity to participate in rehabilitation.[20] Finally, maximizing a patient's medication regimens can avoid other potential problematic detractors from rehabilitation, including orthostatic hypotension, arrhythmias, Parkinson disease, etc. A comprehensive geriatric assessment reduces the incidence of delirium after hip fracture, which has been shown to improve outcomes.[20]

Finally, continued exercise to improve strength, balance, and fall prevention is key to maximizing rehabilitation and preventing future falls that could result in fragility fractures.

OUTCOMES

Geriatric hip fracture represents a serious public health issue, and the prevalence continues to grow as our population ages. Despite adequate surgical treatment of these fractures, many patients are unable to return to their preinjury level of function, often resulting in a loss of independence, as well as an economic impact on the patient and his or her family due to the need for increased assistance.[21]

The in-hospital mortality of a hip fracture ranges from 2.3% to 13.9%, and 6-month mortality rates range from 12% to 23%.[22] When compared to patients receiving elective total hip arthroplasty, there is a 6- to 15-fold increased mortality risk.[23] Patients with hip fracture have significantly increased risk of mortality that persists for several years following the index fracture. The greatest risk of death is within the first 6 months following the index fracture. This mortality increases with increasing age. It is unclear the extent that underlying comorbidities contribute to mortality associated with hip fractures.[24] It has been shown that comanagement of hip fracture patients with a dedicated geriatrics team reduces overall mortality and decreases length of stay at acute care facilities.

Following hip fracture, elderly patients often experience loss of independence and function. One study showed that the proportion of patients living in nursing homes increased from 15% to 30% after sustaining a hip fracture. Of those patients living at home prior to the index fracture, 6% of those <75 years compared with 33% >85 years resided in a nursing home after the index fracture. Of the patients, 28% lost their ability to cook their own dinner.[3] This can have significant implications for the patients and their family.

SUMMARY

Patients that have experienced a hip fracture require appropriate postsurgical rehabilitation. This may be done in a facility or at home effectively. It is vital that patients be allowed to perform weight bearing as tolerated during the course of the rehabilitation with appropriate devices. Appropriate attention should be given to addressing cognitive issues such as delirium and medication side effects that may impair rehabilitation. During the rehabilitation phase, both osteoporosis prevention and fall prevention should be addressed to lessen the likelihood of additional factures. Despite appropriate rehabilitation, many patients are not restored to their preinjury level of function.

REFERENCES

1. Mears S, Kates S, Ahmed O, Bass J, Tyler W. A guide to improving the care of patients with fragility fractures, edition 2. *Geriatr Orthop Surg Rehabil.* 2015;6(2):58-120.
2. Fried LP, Tangen CM, Walston J, et al. Frailty in older adults: evidence for a phenotype. *J Gerontol A Biol Sci Med Sci.* 2001;56(3):M146-M156.
3. Kistler EA, Nicholas JA, Kates SL, Friedman SM. Frailty and short-term outcomes in patients with hip fracture. *Geriatr Orthop Surg Rehabil.* 2015;6(3):209-214.
4. Koval KJ, Sala DA, Kummer FJ, Zuckerman JD. Postoperative weight-bearing after a fracture of the femoral neck or an intertrochanteric fracture. *J Bone Joint Surg Am.* 1998;80(3):352-356.
5. Juliebo V, Bjoro K, Krogseth M, et al. Risk factors for preoperative and postoperative delirium in elderly patients with hip fracture. *J Am Geriatr Soc.* 2009;57(8):1354-1361.
6. Kortebein P, Symons TB, Ferrando A, et al. Functional impact of 10 days of bed rest in healthy older adults. *J Gerontol A Biol Sci Med Sci.* 2008;63:1076-1081.
7. Liu VX, Rosas E, Hwang J, et al. Enhanced recovery after surgery program implementation in 2 surgical populations in an integrated health care delivery system. *JAMA Surg.* 2017;152(7):e171032.
8. Childers CP, Siletz AE, Singer ES, et al. Surgical technical evidence review for elective total joint replacement conducted for the AHRQ safety program for improving surgical care and recovery. *Geriatr Orthop Surg Rehabil.* 2018;9:2151458518754451.
9. Handoll HHG, Sherrington C, Mak JCS. Interventions for improving mobility after hip fracture surgery in adults. *Cochrane Database Syst Rev.* 2011;3:CD001704. doi:10.1002/14651858.CD001704.pub4.

10. Liu CJ, Latham NK. Progressive resistance strength training for improving physical function in older adults. *Cochrane Database Syst Rev.* 2009;3:002759.

11. Howe TE, Rochester L, Jackson A, Banks PM, Blair VA. Exercise for improving balance in older people. *Cochrane Database Syst Rev.* 2007;4:004963.

12. Cameron ID, Murray GR, Gillespie LD, et al. Interventions for preventing falls in older people in nursing care facilities and hospitals. *Cochrane Database Syst Rev.* 2010;1:CD005465.

13. Beaupre LA, Jones CA, Saunders LD, Johnston DW, Buckingham J, Majumdar SR. Best practices for elderly hip fracture patients. *J Gen Intern Med.* 2005;20:1019-1025.

14. Handoll HHG, Cameron ID, Mak JCS, Finnegan TP. Multidisciplinary rehabilitation for older people with hip fractures. *Cochrane Database Syst Rev.* 2009;4:CD007125.

15. Latham NK, Harris BA, Bean JF, et al. Effect of a home-based exercise program on functional recovery following rehabilitation after hip fracture: A randomized clinical trial. *J Am Med Assoc.* 2014;311:700-708.

16. Magaziner J, Hawkes W, Hebel R, et al. Recovery from hip fracture in eight areas of function. *J Gerontol A Biol Sci Med Sci.* 2000;55A(9):498-507.

17. Beaupre LA, Binder EF, Cameron ID, et al. Maximizing functional recovery following hip fracture in frail seniors. *Best Pract Res Clin Rheumatol.* 2013;27:771-788.

18. Kaiser MJ, Bandinelli S, Lunenfeld B. Frailty and the role of nutrition in older people: a review of the current literature. *Acta Biomed.* 2010;81(suppl 1):37-45.

19. Clemson L, Mackenzie L, Roberts C, et al. Integrated solutions for sustainable fall prevention in primary care, the iSOLVE project: a type 2 hybrid effectiveness-implementation design. *Implement Sci.* 2017;12:12.

20. Shields L, Henderson V, Caslake R. Comprehensive geriatric assessment for prevention of delirium after hip fracture: a systematic review of randomized controlled trials. *J Am Geriatr Soc.* 2017;65:1559.

21. Hektoen LF, Saltvetd I, Sletvold O, et al. One-year health and care costs after hip fracture for home-dwelling elderly patients in Norway: results from the trondheim hip fracture trial. *Scand J Public Health.* 2016;44(8):791-798.

22. Boddaert J, Cohen-Bittan J, Khiami F, et al. Postoperative admission to a dedicated geriatric unit decreases mortality in elderly patients with hip fracture. *PLoS One.* 2014;9(1):e83795.

23. Cram P, Lu X, Kaboli PJ, et al. Clinical characteristics and outcomes of medicare patients undergoing total hip arthroplasty, 1991-2008. *J Am Med Assoc.* 2011;305(15):1560-1567.

24. Abrahamsen B, van Staa T, Ariely R, et al. Excess mortality following hip fracture: a systematic epidemiological review. *Osteoporos Int.* 2009;20:1633.

21

Femoral Shaft Fractures

Adam P. Schumaier
Michael T. Archdeacon

INTRODUCTION

The femoral shaft is the region between the lesser trochanter and the metaphyses. The incidence of femoral shaft fractures in Western countries ranges from 10 to 19 per 100,000 person years.[1-5] They frequently occur in young men following high-energy trauma or older women following a fall.[3,4] Surgical fixation with intramedullary nails (IMNs) has become the standard of care. Modern nails and soft-tissue friendly approaches allow early weight bearing and recovery with few major complications.[6] Union can be achieved in greater than 97% of cases.[7-10]

Despite the high union rate, a significant number of patients will have some residual disability.[11,12] Pain and functional deficits are attributed to soft-tissue injury from both the initial trauma and the surgery.[13] The common sequela of femoral IMN fixation includes hip abductor weakness, knee extensor weakness, and gait abnormalities.[14] Weakness of the hip abductors (10%-20%) can lead to a Trendelenburg gait (14%), while knee extensor weakness can lead to a quadriceps avoidance gait.[15-18] Hip pain (4%-40%), thigh pain (8%-10%), and knee pain (10%-55%)[17-19] are relatively common following intramedullary stabilization of femur fractures. Formalized rehabilitation protocols have been demonstrated to improve outcomes for many orthopaedic procedures including total joint replacement,[20,21] spine surgery,[22,23] and sports medicine procedures.[24,25] In regard to femur fractures, there is sparse literature regarding the impact of formal rehabilitation[26,27]; however, the authors have more than 15 years of experience with the described protocol and are advocates of formal rehabilitation after femur fractures.

GENERAL PRINCIPLES

The goals of rehabilitation are to facilitate fracture consolidation and return the patients to their preinjury functional status. Return to work and driving are debated topics; however, in the experience of the authors, driving should not be resumed until the patient can ambulate without assistive aids. Each clinic visit should include assessments of pain and swelling, which may be present for up to a year. Additionally, a distal neurosensory exam should be performed (**Table 21.1**). As pain subsides, active and passive range of motion (ROM) at the knee and hip should be assessed (**Table 21.2**). Throughout follow-up, full-length anteroposterior and lateral femur x-rays should be assessed for angulation, shortening, rotation, and callus formation/healing at the fracture site (**Figure 21.1**).[28,29]

Fractures are expected to show early stability by 4 weeks with union by 16 weeks, but the duration varies.[28] The duration of therapy can extend to 18 weeks but varies substantially as patients progress at different rates and require different levels of supervision and instruction. The rehabilitation protocol should focus on recognized deficits. The described protocol consists of three phases focusing on (1) early weight bearing, (2) strengthening, and (3) return to preinjury function. Each phase has specific goals, and the program consists of both inpatient and outpatient services. Every patient will have different needs, so that the program will be modified based on communication between the surgeon and the therapist. Some patients may require additional, activity-specific therapy following conclusion of the three phases.

TABLE 21.1 Distal Neurosensory Exam

Nerve	Motor	Sensation
Deep peroneal	Dorsiflexion, EHL	First/second web space
Superficial peroneal	Eversion	Dorsum of foot
Tibial	Plantar flexion, inversion	Medial/plantar foot
Sural		Lateral foot

EHL, extensor hallucis longus.

TABLE 21.2 Hip and Knee Range of Motion (in Degrees)

	Normal	Functional
Knee		
Flexion	135	110
Extension	0 to 5	0
Hip		
Flexion	130	90-110
Hyperextension	20	0-5
Abduction	40	0-20
Adduction	30	0-20
Internal rotation	30	0-20
External rotation	50	0-15

PHASE I (0-4 WEEKS)

Phase I generally lasts for 4 weeks and begins immediately postoperative. Twice daily inpatient physical therapy is ideal in order to facilitate discharge. Outpatient therapy is performed 2 to 3 d/wk depending on patient needs and resources. Some patients will master the exercises very quickly and transition to independent therapy at home until they progress to the next phase. The major targets of Phase I are knee extensor strength, hip abductor strength, and early gait training. These goals are accomplished primarily with light ROM, isometrics, and weight bearing-as-tolerated (WBAT) gait with walker or crutches as needed. Immediate WBAT gait is encouraged but may be limited by pain. Multiple studies have found that early weight bearing is safe and facilitates fracture healing.[30,31] Patients can be taught a three-point gait, where the crutches go first and are then followed by the affected extremity (second) and the unaffected extremity (third).

In addition to encouraging weight bearing, the primary focus should be knee extension and hip abduction. Knee extension should be pursued aggressively following surgery to prevent flexion contractures; the goal should be full, active extension prior to discharge. This can be accomplished with a combination of stretching, elevation, passive/active ROM exercises, and strengthening. Stretching of the posterior muscles consists of seated hamstring and gastrocnemius towel stretches. Edema may limit knee extension, so the lower extremity should be elevated by heel propping for 10 minutes three to four times per day. Heel propping also provides a long-duration stretch with a low load on the posterior knee. ROM exercises can begin with active knee extension in a seated position without added weight. Quadriceps strengthening can occur simultaneously with hip exercises, which are described below.

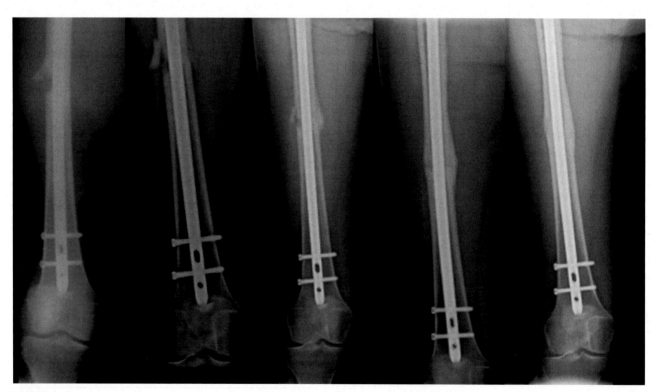

FIGURE 21.1 Anteroposterior x-rays demonstrating the progressive healing of a femoral shaft fracture treated with an intramedullary nail (from left to right: postoperative, 5 weeks, 15 weeks, 32 weeks, and 52 weeks). Callus is visible at 5 weeks, and the fracture line is resolving by 15 weeks. An external callus is all that remains visible by 52 weeks.

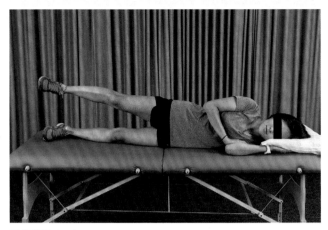

FIGURE 21.2 Hip abduction in the lateral decubitus position while simultaneously performing a full, isometric quadriceps contraction. Patients should be able to perform this exercise prior to initiating Phase II. (From Brody L, Hall C. *Therapeutic Exercise*. 4th ed. Philadelphia, PA: Wolters Kluwer; 2017.)

In early Phase I, hip exercises are done in a non–weight bearing position and consist of simple flexion, extension, and abduction exercises. Throughout these hip exercises, the patient should maintain a strong quadriceps contraction with the knee fully extended (**Figure 21.2**). In addition to proximal hip and knee strength, gastrocnemius and soleus strength should be addressed with resistive band exercises at the ankle. Contracting these muscles can help prevent venous stasis and phlebitis. Ankle ROM exercises should be done in sagittal, coronal, and transverse planes.

Weight bearing and gait training should progress throughout Phase I. Patient comfort with weight bearing can be facilitated with standing exercises, weight-shifting practice, and resistive band ankle training. At the first outpatient visit, standing hip flexion, hip abduction, and knee flexion can be initiated while using an assistive device such as a cane. Toe raises and mini-squats can begin with handheld assist at a table (**Figure 21.3**). Weight shifting can progress to gait training with assistive devices. For example, patients can walk over cones with the purpose of normalizing the gait pattern and encouraging knee flexion during the swing phase. Attention should be paid to normalizing the temporal and spatial parameters of gait, such as stride length, which has been linked to long-term outcomes.[32]

For progression from Phase I to Phase II, the patient should demonstrate 50% weight bearing and fair strength of the quadriceps and hip abductors. Weight bearing can be measured with a bathroom scale. Fair quadriceps strength consists of demonstrating a superior patellar glide, and fair hip abductor strength is being able to abduct the lower extremity while lying in a lateral decubitus position.

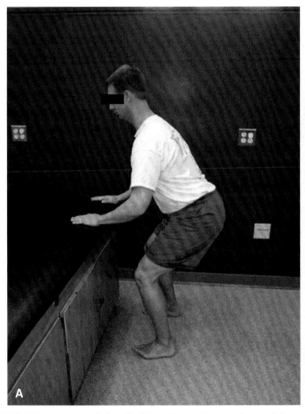
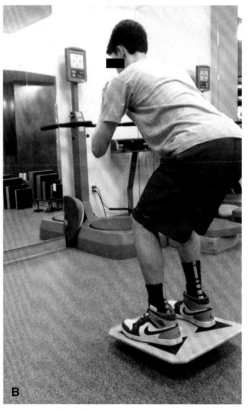

FIGURE 21.3 Mini-squat with handheld assist to allow early quadriceps activation (**A**). This activity can progress by increasing depth, removing the handheld assist, and eventually adding an unstable platform (**B**). (Left image from Lotke P, Abboud J, Ende J, *Lippincott's Primary Care Orthopaedics*. 1st ed. Philadelphia, PA: Wolters Kluwer; 2008; right image from Cordasco F, Green D, *Pediatric and Adolescent Knee Surgery*. 1st ed. Philadelphia, PA: Wolters Kluwer; 2015.)

Throughout Phase I, neuromuscular reeducation with electrical stimulation (NMES) and cryotherapy may be useful supplements. NMES can help regain volitional control of the quadriceps muscles, and cryotherapy can help manage effusion and edema. These therapies can continue into Phase II if necessary.

PHASE II

Phase II progresses to a more aggressive focus on strengthening with outpatient physical therapy two or three times per week as needed. Phase I exercises are increased in intensity with an additional attention to fitness and balance. Strength training of the knee and hip should be done with increased ROM and resistance. At this phase, knee extensions should be performed from 90° to 30° and include ankle weights (**Figure 21.4**). Added weight can begin with 2 pounds.

Once the patient can perform three sets of 10 repetitions, weight should be added in 1 pound increments. Similarly, ankle weights can be added to knee flexion exercises, which should be performed from 0° to 90° (**Figure 21.4**). Hip strengthening should consist of standing hip flexion and abduction with a resistive band (**Figure 21.5**).

Weight bearing is continued as tolerated and may progress to a single crutch if needed. Toe raises, mini-squats, and wall slides can be done without assistive devices. If there is suspicion for injury at the patellofemoral joint, full extension and deep flexion should be avoided during these exercises. In the absence of crepitation and anterior knee pain, progression should continue. Once adequate knee flexion is achieved, fitness conditioning with a stationary bicycle can begin. A self-selected intensity is acceptable, but the duration of bicycling should progressively increase.

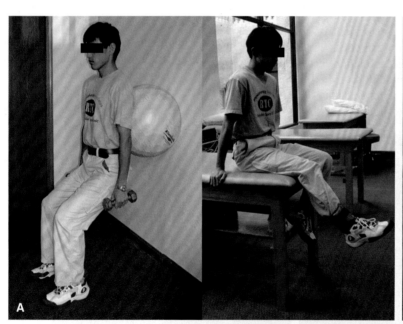
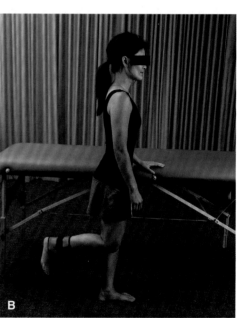
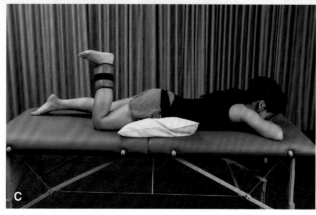

FIGURE 21.4 Ankle weights can be used to increase intensity of knee extension exercises (**A**). Similarly, knee flexion exercises can be performed while standing (**B**) or lying prone (**C**). (Top left image from Copyright © 2018 from *Conditioning for Strength and Human Performance*, 3rd edition by Chandler TJ, Brown LE. Reproduced by permission of Taylor and Francis Group, LLC, a division of Informa plc; top right and bottom images from Brody L, Hall C. *Therapeutic Exercise*. 4th ed. Philadelphia, PA: Wolters Kluwer; 2017.)

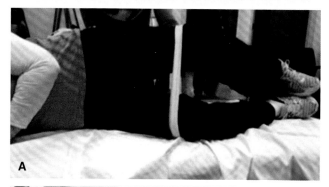

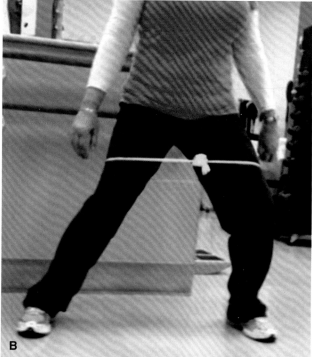

FIGURE 21.5 Resistance band sidestepping provides a functional hip abductor exercise. This can be performed while squatting at variable depth to recruit the quadriceps. (From Callaghan J. Rosenburg AG, Rubash HE, et al. *The Adult Hip (Two Volume Set).* 3rd ed. Philadelphia, PA: Wolters Kluwer; 2015.)

Toward the end of Phase II, proprioceptive and gait training activities can be advanced. Proprioceptive activities include balance boarding, marching on a mini trampoline, and weight bearing progressive resistance exercises on an unstable surface. Sustained-hold activities on the balance board can last for 10 to 30 seconds. Toe raises and mini-squats can also be performed on the unstable platform in three sets of 10 repetitions (**Figure 21.3**). Gait training should include sidestepping and assisted backward walking. A ROM that allows performance of all activities of daily living should be attained. Progression to Phase III requires full weight bearing, good quadriceps strength (4+/5), fair to good hip abductor strength (4/5), and minimal effusion.

PHASE III

Phase III typically focuses on advancing strength, balance, and conditioning with a goal of return to preinjury activities. Strengthening exercises from Phase II should be done at full weight bearing and continue to increase in resistance. The patient should begin single leg exercises, including step-ups, half-lunges, and mini-squats. These can start with three sets of 10 repetitions, and the intensity can be increased with hand weights and added repetitions. Balance activities should also progress to single-leg in this phase, beginning on a stable platform and progressing to an unstable platform. These can begin with 10 repetitions of 10-20 seconds and then advance to 30 seconds. Conditioning should include a treadmill with progressively increasing speed and duration. A typical progression on the treadmill starts at a normal walking pace, about three miles per hour, and advances in 1/3 to 1/2 mph increments every 3 to 5 days depending on the ability, stamina, and tolerance of the patient. When the desired pace of gait is achieved, incline grade can then be incrementally increased in order to increase stamina and endurance during gait. Similarly, the speed and duration of bicycling can be increased.

Phase III typically concludes when the patient returns to the preinjury activity level; however, this becomes fairly patient-specific and may ultimately be determined by insurance restrictions on therapy visits. This should be targeted to the patient's goals and may require an integrated work or return to sport program. After formal therapy, patients should be able to demonstrate the following: (1) normal gait pattern without signs of Trendelenburg gait and (2) quadriceps, knee flexor, and hip abductor strength of 5/5 or 85% to 90% of the contralateral side. Following discharge, patients should focus on global lower extremity strength and continue home exercise therapy using the same exercises performed in clinic. Self-selected gait speed should continue increasing and should approach a normal speed.[33] Most patients can be expected to return to work around 6 months and continue gaining function up to 2 years postoperatively.[14,34]

OTHER CONSIDERATIONS

Some additional circumstances deserve special attention. Patients with significant soft-tissue damage or bilateral injuries may require adaptation of the protocol; however, a goals-based progression focused on advancing weight bearing status should always be pursued. With modern IMN techniques, morbidly obese patients and those with segmental bone loss should still be allowed full weight bearing. Patients treated with plates or external fixation should be toe-touch weight bearing until fracture callus is visible. Multiple injured patients may be functionally limited, but parts of the protocol may remain useful; stretching, ROM, and reeducation can be performed by most patients (**Table 21.3**).

TABLE 21.3 Rehabilitation Protocol

	Phase I	Phase II	Phase III
Criteria	Immediately postoperative	50% weight bearing, minimal effusion, fair hip abductor strength, fair quadriceps strength	100% weight bearing, minimal effusion, fair to good hip abductor strength, good quadriceps strength
Weight bearing	WBAT (walker or crutches if needed)	WBAT (single crutch if needed, progress to no assistive devices)	WBAT, no assistive device
ROM	Hip, knee, ankle passive ROM/ active ROM in all planes	Continue as indicated	Continue as indicated
Stretching	Hamstrings, gastrocnemius, soleus (seated)	Continue as indicated	Continue as indicated
Strengthening			
• Hip	NWB (non–weight bearing) flexion, extension, abduction	Standing abduction and flexion, progress to ankle weights or tension band	Continue Phase II at full weight bearing with increased intensity
• Knee	NWB isometric quadriceps contractions during hip exercises	Extension from 90° to 30°, progress to ankle weights or tension band, flexion with ankle weights or tension band	Continue Phase II at full weight bearing with increased intensity
• Ankle	NWB plantar flexion, dorsiflexion, eversion, inversion with resistive band	Continue as indicated	Continue as indicated
• Multijoint	None	Toe raises, heel raises, mini-squats, wall sits	Single leg step-ups (forward and lateral), mini-squats, lunges
Balance and gait	Cup walking, weight shifting, gait retraining with focus on normalizing temporal and spatial parameters	Sidestepping, backward walking	Single leg stable platform, progress to an unstable platform
Conditioning	None	Stationary bicycling, pool therapy	Treadmill walking, jogging, stationary bicycling, activity-specific conditioning
Modalities	Elevation, cryotherapy, NMES	Continue as indicated	Continue as indicated

Adapted with permission from Paterno MV, Archdeacon MT. Is there a standard rehabilitation protocol after femoral intramedullary nailing? J Orthop Trauma. 2009;23(5):S39-S46.

REFERENCES

1. Fakhry SM, Rutledge R, Dahners LE & Kessler D Incidence, management, and outcome of femoral shaft fracture: a statewide population-based analysis of 2805 adult patients in a rural state. *J Trauma*. 1994;37:255-260.
2. Salminen ST, Pihlajamäki HK, Avikainen VJ, Böstman OM. Population based epidemiologic and morphologic study of femoral shaft fractures. *Clin Orthop*. 2000:241-249.
3. Court-Brown CM, Caesar B. Epidemiology of adult fractures: a review. *Injury*. 2006;37:691-697.
4. Weiss RJ, Montgomery SM, Al Dabbagh Z, Jansson K-A. National data of 6409 Swedish inpatients with femoral shaft fractures: stable incidence between 1998 and 2004. *Injury*. 2009;40:304-308.
5. Arneson TJ, Melton LJ, Lewallen DG, O'Fallon WM. Epidemiology of diaphyseal and distal femoral fractures in Rochester, Minnesota, 1965-1984. *Clin Orthop*. 1988:188-194.
6. Rockwood CA, Bucholz RW, Court-Brown CM, Heckman JD, Tornetta P. *Rockwood and Green's fractures in adults*. Wolters Kluwer Health/ Lippincott Williams & Wilkins; 2010.

7. Canadian Orthopaedic Trauma Society. Nonunion following intramedullary nailing of the femur with and without reaming. Results of a multicenter randomized clinical trial. *J Bone Joint Surg. Am.* 2003;85-A:2093-2096.
8. Winquist RA, Hansen ST. Comminuted fractures of the femoral shaft treated by intramedullary nailing. *Orthop Clin North Am.* 1980;11:633-648.
9. Wiss DA, Brien WW, Stetson WB. Interlocked nailing for treatment of segmental fractures of the femur. *J Bone Joint Surg Am.* 1990;72:724-728.
10. Wolinsky PR, McCarty E, Shyr Y, Johnson K. Reamed intramedullary nailing of the femur: 551 cases. *J Trauma*. 1999;46:392-399.
11. Bednar DA, Ali P. Intramedullary nailing of femoral shaft fractures: reoperation and return to work. *Can J Surg*. 1993;36:464-466.
12. Jurkovich G, Mock C, MacKenzie E, et al. The Sickness impact profile as a tool to evaluate functional outcome in trauma patients. *J Trauma*. 1995;39:625-631.
13. Hennrikus WL, Kasser JR, Rand F, Millis MB, Richards KM. The function of the quadriceps muscle after a fracture of the femur in patients who are less than seventeen years old. *J Bone Joint Surg Am.* 1993;75:508-513.

14. Paterno MV, Archdeacon MT, Ford KR, Galvin D, Hewett TE. Early rehabilitation following surgical fixation of a femoral shaft fracture. *Phys Ther.* 2006;86:558-572.

15. Kapp W, Lindsey RW, Noble PC, Rudersdorf T, Henry P. Long-term residual musculoskeletal deficits after femoral shaft fractures treated with intramedullary nailing. *J Trauma.* 2000;49:446-449.

16. Karumo I. Intensive physical therapy after fractures of the femoral shaft. *Ann Chir Gynaecol.* 1977;66:278-283.

17. Bain GI, Zacest AC, Paterson DC, Middleton J, Pohl AP. Abduction strength following intramedullary nailing of the femur. *J Orthop Trauma.* 1997;11:93-97.

18. Ostrum RF, Agarwal A, Lakatos R, Poka A. Prospective comparison of retrograde and antegrade femoral intramedullary nailing. *J Orthop Trauma.* 2000;14:496-501.

19. Leggon RE, Feldmann DD. Retrograde femoral nailing: a focus on the knee. *Am J Knee Surg.* 2001;14:109-118.

20. Quack V. Ippendorf AV, Betsch M, et al. Multidisciplinary rehabilitation and fast-track rehabilitation after knee replacement: faster, better, cheaper? A survey and systematic review of literature. *Rehabil.* 2015;54:245-251.

21. Labraca NS, Castro-Sánchez AM, Matarán-Peñarrocha GA, et al. Benefits of starting rehabilitation within 24 hours of primary total knee arthroplasty: randomized clinical trial. *Clin Rehabil.* 2011;25:557-566.

22. Oosterhuis T, Costa LO, Maher CG, et al. Rehabilitation after lumbar disc surgery. *Cochrane Database Syst Rev.* 2014;2014:CD003007. doi:10.1002/14651858.CD003007.pub3.

23. Ozkara GO, Ozgen M, Ozkara E, Armagan O, Arslantas A, Atasoy MA. Effectiveness of physical therapy and rehabilitation programs starting immediately after lumbar disc surgery. *Turk Neurosurg.* 2015;25:372-379.

24. Kruse LM, Gray B, Wright RW. Rehabilitation after anterior cruciate ligament reconstruction: a systematic review. *J Bone Joint Surg Am.* 2012;94:1737-1748.

25. Malempati C, Jurjans J, Noehren B, Ireland ML, Johnson DL. Current rehabilitation concepts for anterior cruciate ligament surgery in athletes. *Orthopedics.* 2015;38:689-696.

26. Edgren J. Salpakoski A, Sihvonen SE, et al. Effects of a home-based physical rehabilitation program on physical disability after hip fracture: a randomized controlled trial. *J Am Med Dir Assoc.* 2015;16:350. e1-357.e1.

27. Zhang B, Dai M, Tang Y, Zou F, Liu H, Nie T. Influence of integration of fracture treatment and exercise rehabilitation on effectiveness in patients with intertrochanteric fracture of femur. *Zhongguo Xiu Fu Chong Jian Wai Ke Za Zhi.* 2012;26:1453-1456.

28. Hoppenfeld S, Murthy VL. *Treatment and Rehabilitation of Fractures.* Philadelphia, PA: Lippincott Williams & Wilkins; 2000.

29. Child Z. *Basic Orthopedic Exams.* Philadelphia, PA: Wolters Kluwer/Lippincott Williams & Wilkins; 2007.

30. Arazi M, Oğün TC, Oktar MN, Memik R, Kutlu A. Early weight-bearing after statically locked reamed intramedullary nailing of comminuted femoral fractures: is it a safe procedure? *J Trauma.* 2001;50:711-716.

31. Brumback RJ, Toal TR, Murphy-Zane MS, Novak VP, Belkoff SM. Immediate weight-bearing after treatment of a comminuted fracture of the femoral shaft with a statically locked intramedullary nail. *J Bone Joint Surg Am.* 1999;81:1538-1544.

32. Archdeacon M, Ford KR, Wyrick J, et al. A prospective functional outcome and motion analysis evaluation of the hip abductors after femur fracture and antegrade nailing. *J Orthop Trauma.* 2008;22:3-9.

33. Perry J, Burnfield JM. *Gait Analysis: Normal and Pathological Function.* Thorofare, NJ: SLACK; 2010.

34. Kempf I, Grosse A, Beck G. Closed locked intramedullary nailing. Its application to comminuted fractures of the femur. *J Bone Joint Surg. Am.* 1985;67:709-720.

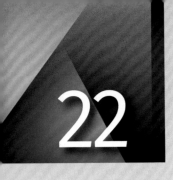

22

The Knee

Paul Henkel
James P. Stannard
Brett D. Crist

ANATOMY OF THE KNEE (FIGURE 22.1)

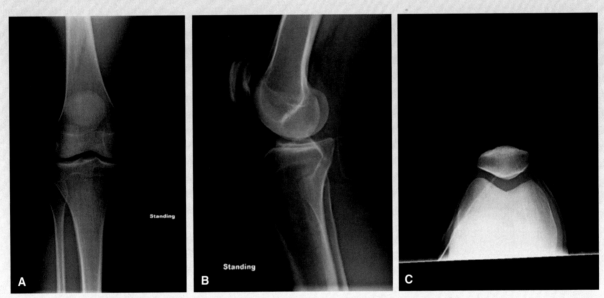

FIGURE 22.1 AP (**A**), Lateral (**B**), and Patellofemoral View (**C**) radiographs of a right knee.

DISTAL FEMUR (SEE FIGURE 22.1A–C)

Distally, the femur transitions from a cylindrical diaphysis to a trapezoid containing the trochlea and two condyles. The posterior aspect of the condyles is wider than the anterior distal femur, creating a slope of approximately a 25° medially and 15° laterally.[1]

The anterior compartment of the thigh includes the quadriceps femoris muscle, which is composed of four heads: the rectus femoris superficially, vastus lateralis, vastus intermedius, and vastus medialis deeper. The articularis genu is a separate muscle group that works in concert with the quadriceps extensor apparatus. The lateral and medial intermuscular septa separate the anterior and posterior compartments. The posterior compartment consists of the biceps femoris, semimembranosus, and semitendinosus. The biceps femoris

inserts on the head of the fibula and lateral condyle of the tibia. The semimembranosus inserts on to the medial condyle of the tibia. The semitendinosus inserts onto the medial surface of the tibia via the pes anserinus.

Fractures of the supracondylar area of the femur involve the length superior to the joint line that is equal to the width of the condyles. Muscular attachments cause femoral shortening and extension with displacement of the distal fragment (**Figure 22.2**). If there is intercondylar fracture involvement, the individual condyles will malrotate in the sagittal plane due to the attachment of the collateral ligaments.[1]

PATELLA

The patella is the largest sesamoid bone in the body and is divided into the superior and inferior poles. The quadriceps tendon inserts superiorly and the patella tendon inserts inferiorly. The articular surface consists of a larger lateral facet and a smaller medial facet that are separated by a vertical ridge (**Figure 22.3**).

The medial and lateral retinacula are formed by the aponeurotic fibers of the quadriceps muscles and stabilize the patella in the femoral trochlear groove. In the setting of a patella fracture, the retinaculum may still allow active knee extension.[2] Patella

fractures displace due to the quadriceps tendon pulling the superior fragments cephalad, while the patella tendon remains static maintaining the position of the inferior pole fragments.

During skeletal development, ossification centers may fail to fuse and lead to a bi- or tripartite patella that can often be mistaken for a fracture. This is usually bilateral, with the most common finding as a bipartite patella with segmentation in

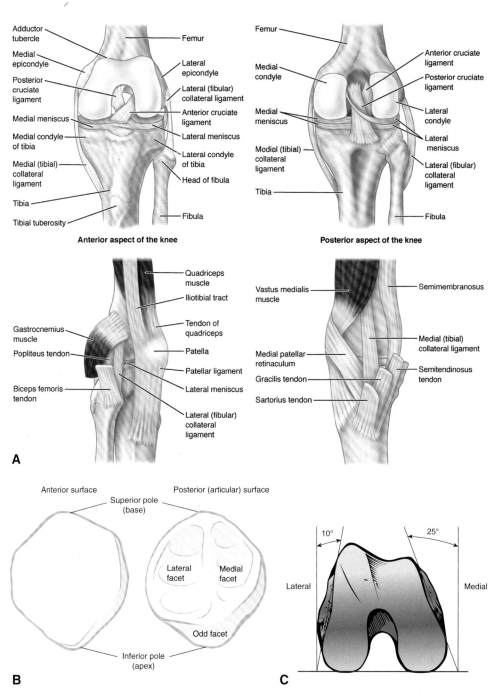

FIGURE 22.2 A, Knee soft-tissue structures. **B**, Patellar anatomy. **C**, Distal femur anatomy. (A, Reproduced with permission from Anderson MK. *Foundations of Athletic Training: Prevention, Assessment and Management.* 6th ed. Wolters Kluwer Health; 2016. B, Redrawn with permission from Wiesel SW. *Operative Techniques in Orthopaedic Surgery.* 2nd ed. Philadelphia: Wolters Kluwer; 2016. C, Redrawn with permission from Collinge CA, Wiss DA. Distal femur fractures. In: Tornetta P III, Ricci WM, Ostrum RF, et al, eds. *Rockwood and Green's Fractures in Adults.* Vol 2. 9th ed. Philadelphia: Wolters Kluwer; 2020:2430-2471.)

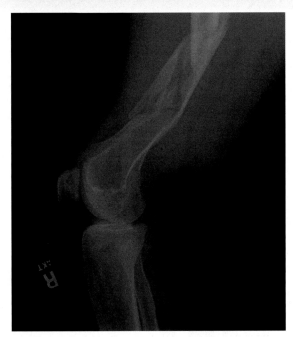

FIGURE 22.3 Distal femur fracture. Deforming forces include Hamstring and quadriceps musculature that shorten the fracture, while gastrocnemius muscles extend the distal femur.

the superolateral quadrant. These are generally asymptomatic and found incidentally on knee radiographic evaluation. However, with trauma, these may become symptomatic and should be considered as a source of pain when there is no obvious fracture. The acute injury is usually identified on magnetic resonance imaging (MRI).

PROXIMAL TIBIA

The proximal tibia is divided into lateral and medial plateaus by the intercondylar eminence. The lateral tibial plateau is convex in shape and extends proximally relative to the concave medial plateau (**Figure 22.1**).[3] The iliotibial tract inserts on the anterolateral tibia, the pes anserine inserts on the anteromedial tibia, and the semimembranosus inserts on the posteromedial proximal tibia. Tibial slope, defined as the angle between a line perpendicular to the mid-diaphysis of the tibia and the posterior inclination of the tibial plateaus, is normally $10° ± 3°$ and plays a critical role in anterior tibial translation in both cruciate-intact and cruciate-deficient knees (**Figure 22.1B**).[4-6]

LIGAMENTS AND SOFT TISSUES OF THE KNEE (SEE FIGURE 22.1)

The ligamentous connections in and around the knee are integral in maintaining stability throughout weight bearing and range of motion due to the lack of bony containment of the joint. The main ligaments of the knee joint are the anterior cruciate ligament (ACL), the posterior cruciate ligament (PCL), the lateral (or fibular) collateral ligament (LCL), and the medial collateral ligament (MCL).

The MCL is a broad, flat, membranous ligament that originates on the posterior aspect of the medial femoral condyle

proximally and posterior to the medial femoral epicondyle. It inserts distally on the metaphyseal region of the tibia 4 to 5 cm distal to the joint line deep to the pes anserinus. The MCL provides primary restraint to valgus stress at the knee, varying through the flexion-extension arc of motion.

The LCL originates from the lateral femoral epicondyle posterior and proximal to the popliteus insertion. It inserts on the anterolateral fibular head and is the most anterior structure on the proximal fibula. Its primary function is resisting varus stress, and it becomes increasingly important with joint flexion as resistance by the ACL decreases.

The ACL originates from the medial aspect of the lateral femoral condyle and inserts on the anterior tibia just anterior and between the intercondylar eminences of the tibia. It provides 85% of the stability preventing anterior translation of the tibia relative to the femur, as well inhibiting internal tibial rotation. The ACL is composed of two entities, the anteromedial and posterolateral bundles. When the knee is extended, the posterolateral bundle is tight and the anteromedial bundle is moderately lax. As the knee is flexed, the, femoral attachment of the ACL becomes a more horizontal orientation causing the anteromedial bundle to tighten and the posterolateral bundle to relax.[7]

The PCL originates at the posterior tibial sulcus below the articular surface and inserts on the anterolateral medial femoral condyle. Its main function is to resist straight posterior translation of the tibia relative to the femur, and secondarily, it resists varus/valgus and external rotation of the tibia.

MENISCI

There are medial and lateral cartilaginous menisci (Greek "little moon") that are crescent-shaped in the axial plane. However, they are wedge-shaped in the coronal plane because they are thicker at the periphery. The lateral meniscus is more mobile than the medial meniscus. It is more circular and covers a larger portion of the articular surface compared to the medial meniscus. The menisci are connected anteriorly by the transverse (or intermeniscal) ligament and posteriorly by the coronary ligaments. The meniscofemoral ligament connects the menisci into the substance of the PCL anteriorly by the ligament of Humphrey and posteriorly by the ligament of Wrisberg. The menisci function as shock absorbers, dissipate femoral tibial axial force, and stabilize the knee in a chock-block fashion. The blood supply and healing potential for each meniscus decreases from the periphery toward the center.

FRACTURES OF THE DISTAL FEMUR

INCIDENCE AND MECHANISM

In the United States, distal femur fractures occur at an incidence of 31 fractures per 1 million citizens as of 2006.[8] Distal femur fractures occur in the young and the elderly. In young patients, the fractures occur more commonly in males and result from high-energy mechanisms, and in the elderly, the fractures occur more commonly in women as a result of low-energy mechanisms.[9] These fractures occur as a result of a direct load to a flexed knee.

Soft-tissue injuries commonly occur with distal femur fractures and need to be investigated with every fracture. Ligamentous injuries occur in up to 20%.[10] As with every injury, a thorough neurovascular examination is required for every patient. Missing a vascular or neurological injury can lead to compartment syndrome or even amputation.

CLASSIFICATION

The most commonly used distal femur fracture classification is the AO/OTA classification[11] (**Figure 22.4**). The classification is used for both relaying fracture information and unifying research.

NONOPERATIVE TREATMENT

Due to the poor results of operative management of distal femur fractures in the 1960s, nonoperative treatment with functional cast, bracing, or traction became the main stay.[12] However, as orthopaedic implants and techniques have improved, and the consequences of prolonged immobilization and limited weight bearing have been elucidated, nonoperative treatment is reserved for patients that have an unacceptably high anesthetic risk, extremely low demand, or limited life expectancy.[13]

REHABILITATION (TABLE 22.1)

If nonoperative management is chosen, the fracture is immobilized with a knee-spanning device—knee immobilizer, hinged knee brace, or hinged cast brace.[14] The patient is kept limited or non–weight bearing 6 to 12 weeks or until fracture callus is seen in the metaphysis. If weight bearing or knee range of motion is started too soon, the fracture may displace. It is important to immobilize the knee in full extension to avoid late extensor lag. Range of motion is typically started once pain allows and is typically after 3 weeks from injury.

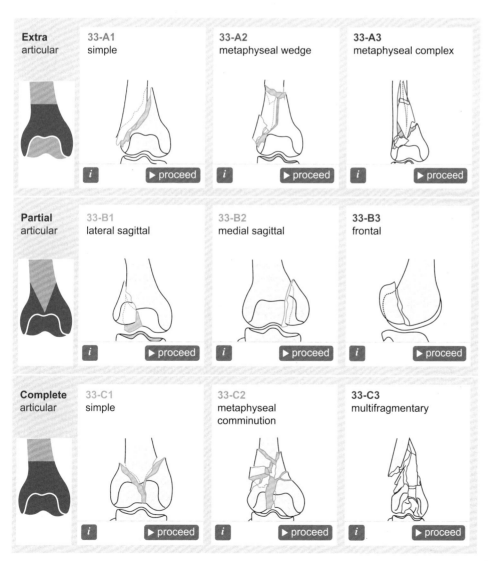

FIGURE 22.4 AO/OTA distal femur fracture classification. (Copyright by AO Foundation, Switzerland; AO Surgery Reference, Available at https://classification.aoeducation.org/?_ga=2.148128247.1926149264.1592835836-993055567.1592835836.)

TABLE 22.1

Day 1 to Week 1

Precautions	Avoid passive range of motion
Range of motion	Full extension
Strength	No strengthening exercises prescribed to the knee
Immobilization	Splint, knee immobilizer, hinged knee brace locked in extension
Functional activities	Non–weight bearing stand/pivot transfers and non–weight bearing ambulation
Weight bearing	None
Radiographs	AP and lateral femur, and knee x-rays if concern for clinical change

2-3 Weeks

Precautions	Avoid passive range of motion
Range of motion	Maintain full extension
Strength (knee)	Isometric exercises to quadriceps in supine position and knee in full extension
Immobilization	Knee immobilizer, hinged knee brace, hinged cast brace locked in extension
Functional activities	Non–weight bearing ambulation and stand/pivot transfers
Weight bearing	None
Radiographs	AP and lateral femur, and knee x-rays

4-8 Weeks

Precautions	Avoid passive range of motion
Range of motion	Gradually advancing active range of motion. Start 0°-30° and advance up to 90° as pain allows
Strength	Isometric exercises to quadriceps and hamstrings
Immobilization	Hinged knee brace or hinged cast brace
Functional activities	Limited weight bearing stand/pivot transfers and non–weight bearing ambulation
Weight bearing	Only advance to partial weight bearing if metaphyseal callus is evident
Radiographs	AP and lateral femur, and knee x-rays

TABLE 22.1   (Continued)

8-12 Weeks

Precautions	No aggressive passive range of motion
Range of motion	Active, active-assistive range of motion; gentle passive range of motion as tolerated
Strength	Isometric and isotonic exercises to quadriceps and hamstrings
Immobilization	Wean out of brace as tolerated
Functional activities	Limited weight bearing ambulation and stand/pivot transfers
Weight bearing	Partial weight bearing and advance as tolerated if metaphyseal callus is evident
Radiographs	AP and lateral femur, and knee x-rays

12-16 Weeks

Precautions	Do not be aggressive in passive range of motion
Range of motion	Active and passive range of motion; emphasize terminal extension to reduce extension lag
Strength	Isometric, isotonic, and isokinetic exercises to quadriceps and hamstrings; add gentle progressive resistive exercises
Immobilization	Wean out of brace as tolerated
Functional activities	Progression to full weight bearing as tolerated during ambulation and transfers
Weight bearing	Weight bearing as tolerated
Radiographs	AP and lateral femur, and knee x-rays

Modified from Hoppenfeld S, Murthy VL. Treatment and Rehabilitation of Fractures. *Philadelphia, PA: Lippincott Williams & Wilkins; 2000.*

PATELLA FRACTURES

INCIDENCE AND MECHANISM

Patella fractures account for approximately 1% of fractures.[2] Patella fractures result from either eccentric contraction of the extensor mechanism or a direct blow. As described in the anatomy section, the fibers of the quadriceps tendon medially and laterally blend with the medial and lateral patellar retinacula. For complete disruption of the extensor mechanism, disruption of both the patella and the retinacula is required. Generally, if the patella is fractured via a direct blow, the retinacula and therefore the extensor mechanism remain intact. Conversely, if the patella fails from tensile force, the retinacula are usually torn and the extensor mechanism is disrupted. In cases of high-energy trauma, such as a fall from height or dashboard injury in motor vehicle collisions, a high degree of suspicion should exist for concomitant injuries such as distal femur or tibial plateau fractures, knee dislocation, and/or ligamentous injury.

CLASSIFICATION

The AO/OTA fracture classification system incorporates the fracture lines and articular involvement[11] (**Figure 22.5**). Although this system may be less commonly used than for other fractures, it is helpful for communication and research.

NONOPERATIVE MANAGEMENT

Nonoperative treatment of patella fractures requires an intact extensor mechanism. Proper evaluation requires the patient to actively extend the knee from a flexed position. Simply maintaining a straight leg raise is insufficient due to the aforementioned retinacular contribution. Hemarthrosis associated with patellar fractures can cause significant pain

that limits physical examination. If the integrity of the extensor mechanism is unclear, hemarthrosis aspiration decreases pain and allows for improved clinical evaluation.

Patella fractures without significant displacement and articular discontinuity less than 2 mm with an intact extensor mechanism may be treated nonoperatively.[2,15] The knee should be immobilized in full extension, but allow for weight bearing as tolerated in extension. Active flexion exercises should be started when pain allows, but limited to 60° for the first 3 weeks and 90° for an additional 3 weeks.[2] Within these limits, flexion should be advanced each week based on pain. Passive range-of-motion exercises should be avoided until complete healing has been achieved. A hinged knee brace is often utilized to limit flexion.

Patients with fractures that would normally be treated operatively, but are either nonambulatory or poor surgical candidates, may also be treated nonoperatively. Brief knee immobilization for pain control is maintained followed by motion as tolerated. Suboptimal knee function should be anticipated, but a hinged knee brace can support the knee in extension when ambulating and allow flexion when seated.[13]

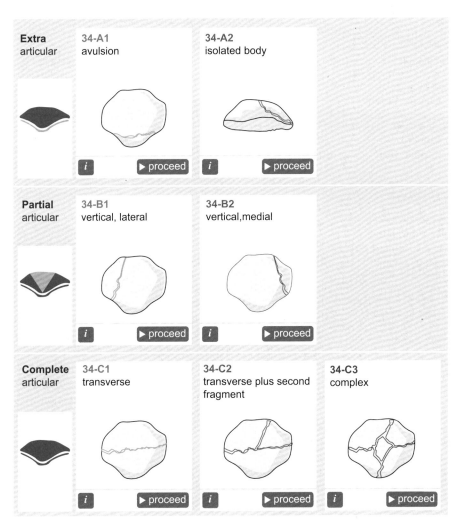

FIGURE 22.5 AO/OTA fracture classification for patella fractures. (Copyright by AO Foundation, Switzerland; AO Surgery Reference, Available at https://classification.aoeducation.org/?_ga=2.148128247.1926149264.1592835836-993055567.1592835836.)

REHABILITATION (TABLE 22.2)

TABLE 22.2

Day 1 to Week 1

Precautions	Avoid passive range of motion
Range of motion	None
Strength	May start isometric quadriceps exercises in brace or splint when pain allows
Immobilization	Knee immobilizer, hinged knee brace, or long leg splint
Functional activities	Weight bearing as tolerated with the knee in full extension if in a brace, non–weight bearing if in a splint
Weight bearing	Same as above
Radiographs	AP and lateral knee x-rays if concerned about displacement

2-3 Weeks

Precautions	Avoid passive range of motion
Range of motion	Active and/or active-assist range of motion up to 30° of flexion as pain allows
Strength	May start isometric quadriceps exercises in brace or splint when pain allows
Immobilization	Convert to hinged knee brace or hinged cast brace
Functional activities	Weight bearing as tolerated with the knee in full extension if in a brace, non–weight bearing if in a splint
Weight bearing	Same as above
Radiographs	AP and lateral knee x-rays to monitor for displacement

4-6 Weeks

Precautions	Avoid passive range of motion
Range of motion	Active and/or active-assist flexion up to 60° as pain allows
Strength	Isometric quadriceps and hamstrings exercises at 6 wk, isotonic exercises to quadriceps with active knee extension: 45°-0° and then from 60°-0°
Immobilization	Hinged knee brace or hinged cast brace

TABLE 22.2   (Continued)

Weight bearing and functional activities	Weight bearing as tolerated; immobilized in full extension when not doing exercises
Radiographs	AP and lateral knee x-rays

7-12 Weeks

Range of motion (knee)	Active and passive range of motion as tolerated; patient may have extension lag secondary to quad weakness and immobilization
Strength (knee)	Progressive resistive exercises to quadriceps and hamstrings with weights as tolerated; isokinetic exercises using Cybex machine (if available); plyometric closed chain exercises
Immobilization	Wean out of brace as tolerated
Weight bearing and functional exercises	Weight bearing as tolerated; open knee brace for range of motion as tolerated with ambulation, and wean out of brace
Radiographs	AP, lateral, and merchant knee x-rays

Modified from Hoppenfeld S, Murthy VL. Treatment and Rehabilitation of Fractures. *Philadelphia, PA: Lippincott Williams & Wilkins; 2000.*

TIBIAL PLATEAU FRACTURES

INCIDENCE AND MECHANISM

Like other fractures about the knee, tibial plateau fractures have a bimodal distribution.[13] In the young population, high-energy mechanisms present more commonly, but in the growing elderly population, low-energy fractures occur in the setting of osteoporosis and obesity.

Tibial plateau fractures are sustained by specific force patterns with varying degrees of knee flexion. Valgus deformity, varus deformity, or combinations of axial compression with varus/valgus influence are the usual culprits.

CLASSIFICATION

The Schatzker classification system for tibial plateau fractures is currently the most frequently used system for tibial plateau fractures[16] (**Figure 22.6**). Types I-III are laterally based fractures and are generally considered lower energy, while types IV-VI are the result of high-energy mechanisms.

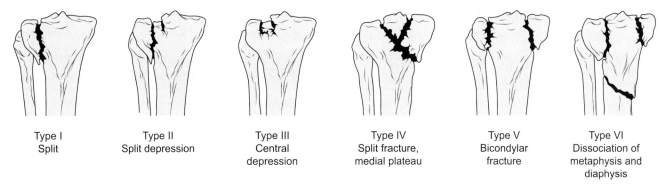

Type I Split	Type II Split depression	Type III Central depression	Type IV Split fracture, medial plateau	Type V Bicondylar fracture	Type VI Dissociation of metaphysis and diaphysis

FIGURE 22.6 Schatzker classification of tibial plateau fractures. (With permission from Zeltser DW, Leopold, SS. Classifications in brief: Schatzker classification of tibial plateau fractures. *Clin Orthop Relat Res.* 2013(471):371-374.)

ASSOCIATED INJURIES

Although the main focus in managing tibial plateau fractures is the osseous anatomy, the associated soft-tissue injury can direct treatment. Due to the shearing and compressive loads required to produce these fractures, collateral and cruciate ligaments, menisci, and cartilage are at considerable risk with up to 99% of the fractures having a soft-tissue injury finding on MRI.[13]

The energy required to fracture the proximal tibia can also lead to compartment syndrome and occurs in about 10% of fractures.[17] The incidence increases as the energy increases and the Schatzker type increases. One should be vigilant in identifying and treating compartment syndrome due to the devastating long-term sequelae. Radiographic findings predictive of compartment syndrome include the relative displacement of the axes of the femur and tibia and widening of the tibial plateau compared to femoral condylar width.[18] These findings should be considered associations, and their absence does not exclude the possibility of compartment syndrome.

NONOPERATIVE MANAGEMENT

Nonoperative management may be considered in tibial plateau fractures that meet specific criteria that include minimally displaced fractures, including those with articular surfaces less than 3 mm, peripheral submeniscal fractures, stable to varus and valgus stress, low-energy fractures with minimal comminution, and fractures in low-demand or poor surgical candidates[19-21] (**Figure 22.7**).

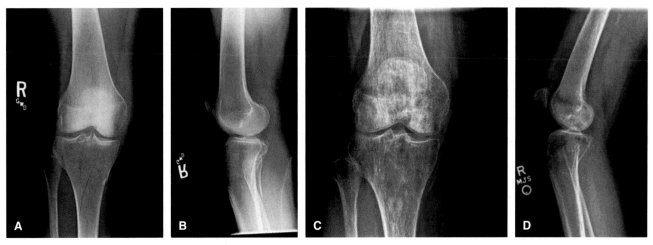

FIGURE 22.7 A 61-year-old s/p ground level fall. Wanted to avoid surgery. AP (**A**) and lateral (**B**) injury films of a Schatzker 6 tibial plateau fracture. Three years postinjury standing AP (**C**) and lateral knee (**D**). She was ambulating with a walker still and recovered from chronic regional pain syndrome. Notice the chronic osteopenia.

REHABILITATION (TABLE 22.3)

TABLE 22.3	
Day 1 to Week 1	
Precautions	No varus or valgus stress on knee; no passive range of motion
Range of motion	None
Strength	None
Immobilization	Long leg splint, well-padded knee immobilizer, or hinged knee brace
Weight bearing and functional activities	25 lb weight bearing stand/pivot transfers and ambulation with crutches/walker
Radiographs	AP and lateral knee, and tibia/fibula x-rays if clinically concerned about displacement
2-3 Weeks	
Precautions	No varus or valgus stress on knee; no passive range of motion
Range of motion	Active, active-assistive flexion/extension up to 30°
Strength	Isometric quadriceps exercises
Immobilization	Convert to hinged knee or cast brace; immobilize in full extension
Weight bearing and functional activities	25 lb weight bearing stand/pivot transfers and ambulation with crutches
Radiographs	AP and lateral knee, and tibia/fibula x-rays
4-6 Weeks	
Precautions	No varus or valgus stress on knee; no passive range of motion
Range of motion	Active and active-assistive range of motion to the knee up to 90°
Strength	Isometric quadriceps exercises
Immobilization	Hinged knee or cast brace; immobilize in full extension
Weight bearing and functional activities	25 lb weight bearing transfers and ambulation with crutches
Radiographs	AP and lateral knee, and tibia/fibula x-rays

TABLE 22.3 (Continued)	
8-12 Weeks	
Precautions	No varus or valgus stress
Range of motion	Active, active-assistive, and passive range of motion to the knee as tolerated
Strength	Isometric and add resistive exercises to the quadriceps and hamstrings as tolerated
Immobilization	Hinged knee brace and allow range of motion as tolerated; wean out of brace as tolerated
Weight bearing and functional activities	Weight bearing as tolerated and wean out of brace
Weight bearing	Weight bearing as tolerated when radiographs metaphysis shows callus
Radiographs	AP and lateral knee, and tibia/fibula x-rays

Modified from Hoppenfeld S, Murthy VL. Treatment and Rehabilitation of Fractures. Philadelphia, PA: Lippincott Williams & Wilkins; 2000.

REFERENCES

1. Browner BD, Jupiter JB, Krettek C, Anderson P. *Skeletal Trauma: Basic Science, Management, and Reconstruction.* 5th ed. Philadelphia, PA: Elsevier/Saunders; 2015.
2. Galla M, Lobenhoffer P. Patella fractures. *Chirurg.* 2005;76(10):987-997. quiz 998-989.
3. Hashemi J, Chandrashekar N, Gill B, et al. The geometry of the tibial plateau and its influence on the biomechanics of the tibiofemoral joint. *J Bone Joint Surg Am.* 2008;90(12):2724-2734.
4. Dejour H, Bonnin M. Tibial translation after anterior cruciate ligament rupture. Two radiological tests compared. *J Bone Joint Surg Br.* 1994;76(5):745-749.
5. Genin P, Weill G, Julliard R. The tibial slope. Proposal for a measurement method. *J Radiol.* 1993;74(1):27-33.
6. Giffin JR, Vogrin TM, Zantop T, Woo SL, Harner CD. Effects of increasing tibial slope on the biomechanics of the knee. *Am J Sports Med.* 2004;32(2):376-382.
7. Petersen W, Zantop T. Anatomy of the anterior cruciate ligament with regard to its two bundles. *Clin Orthop Relat Res.* 2007;454:35-47.
8. Zlowodzki M, Bhandari M, Marek DJ, Cole PA, Kregor PJ. Operative treatment of acute distal femur fractures: systematic review of 2 comparative studies and 45 case series (1989 to 2005). *J Orthop Trauma.* 2006;20(5):366-371.
9. Arneson TJ, Melton LJ III, Lewallen DG, O'Fallon WM. Epidemiology of diaphyseal and distal femoral fractures in Rochester, Minnesota, 1965-1984. *Clin Orthop Relat Res.* 1988;234:188-194.
10. Wenzel HCP, Casey PA, Herbert P, Belin J. Die operative Behandlung der distalen Femurfraktur. *AO Bull.* 1970.

11. Fracture and dislocation compendium. Orthopaedic Trauma Association Committee for Coding and Classification. *J Orthop Trauma.* 1996;10 (suppl 1):v-ix, 1-154.

12. Neer CS II, Grantham SA, Shelton ML. Supracondylar fracture of the adult femur. A study of one hundred and ten cases. *J Bone Joint Surg Am.* 1967;49(4):591-613.

13. Stannard JP, Schmidt AH. *Surgical Treatment of Orthopaedic Trauma.* 2nd ed. New York, NY: Thieme; 2016.

14. Hoppenfeld S, Murthy VL. *Treatment and Rehabilitation of Fractures.* Philadelphia, PA: Lippincott Williams & Wilkins; 2000.

15. Bostrom A. Fracture of the patella. A study of 422 patellar fractures. *Acta Orthop Scand Suppl.* 1972;143:1-80.

16. Schatzker J, McBroom R, Bruce D. The tibial plateau fracture. The Toronto experience 1968–1975. *Clin Orthop Relat Res.* 1979;138:94-104.

17. Crist BD, Della Rocca GJ, Stannard JP. Compartment syndrome surgical management techniques associated with tibial plateau fractures. *J knee Surg.* 2010;23(1):3-7.

18. Ziran BH, Becher SJ. Radiographic predictors of compartment syndrome in tibial plateau fractures. *J Orthop Trauma.* 2013;27(11):612-615.

19. Mills WJ, Nork SE. Open reduction and internal fixation of high-energy tibial plateau fractures. *Orthop Clin North Am.* 2002;33(1):177-198, ix.

20. Stokel EA, Sadasivan KK. Tibial plateau fractures: standardized evaluation of operative results. *Orthopedics.* 1991;14(3):263-270.

21. Brown TD, Anderson DD, Nepola JV, Singerman RJ, Pedersen DR, Brand RA. Contact stress aberrations following imprecise reduction of simple tibial plateau fractures. *J Orthop Res.* 1988;6(6):851-862.

The Ankle

Andrew Dodd
Kelly A. Lefaivre

ANKLE FRACTURES

ANATOMY

The ankle joint is made up of three bones: the tibia, fibula, and talus. Medially, the talus articulates with the medial malleolus, the anteromedial bony prominence of the distal tibia. Superiorly, the talus articulates with the tibial plafond, which is the major weight-bearing surface of the tibia. Laterally, the distal fibula ends in the lateral malleolus, which articulates with the lateral aspect of the talus. The posterior, distal projection of the tibia serves as an attachment point for important ligaments and is termed the posterior malleolus. The majority of load transfer through the ankle joint occurs between the tibial plafond and the talus with only a minor contribution from the talofibular articulation. The distal tibiofibular joint is important to ankle stability and is termed the ankle syndesmosis.

Many important ligaments are necessary for ankle stability. The deltoid ligament (superficial and deep components) anchors the talus to the medial malleolus and is extremely important for normal ankle stability and function. Laterally, the anterior talofibular ligament, calcaneofibular ligament, and posterior talofibular ligaments are the key stabilizers. Four ligaments afford stability of the syndesmosis: the anterior-inferior tibiofibular ligament, interosseous ligament, posterior-inferior tibiofibular ligament, and the transverse-inferior tibiofibular ligament. Injury to the bony or ligamentous stabilizers of the ankle joint can lead to altered biomechanics and joint dysfunction.

EPIDEMIOLOGY

The broad term "ankle fracture" includes fractures of the medial, lateral, and posterior malleolus that do not extend into the tibial plafond. These injuries are common, representing up to 9% of all fractures,[1] making them one of the most common fracture types managed by orthopaedic surgeons.[2] Rates of ankle fractures are increasing, especially in the elderly.[3,4] Fractures of a single malleolus are most common (~2/3), followed by bimalleolar fractures (~1/4), with trimalleolar fractures being least common.[3]

CLASSIFICATION (FIGURE 23.1)

- Weber[5]
  - The Weber classification defines fractures of the fibula by their relationship to the ankle syndesmosis
  - Weber A: infra-syndesmotic (AO type A)
  - Weber B: trans-syndesmotic (AO type B)
  - Weber C: supra-syndesmotic (AO type C)
- AO/OTA[6]
  - The AO/OTA classification also defines the fibula fracture by its relationship to the syndesmosis; however, it includes associated injuries to the medial malleolus, posterior malleolus, and ligaments.
- AO 44-A: infra-syndesmotic
  - 44-A1: isolated fibula fracture
  - 44-A2: bimalleolar fracture
  - 44-A3: trimalleolar fracture
- AO 44-B: trans-syndesmotic
  - 44-B1: isolated fibula fracture
  - 44-B2: bimalleolar fracture (lateral and medial)
  - 44-B3: trimalleolar fracture (lateral, medial, and posterior)
- AO 44-C: supra-syndesmotic
  - 44-C1: simple fibula fracture (with any associated injuries)
  - 44-C2: comminuted fibula fracture (with any associated injuries)
  - 44-C3: proximal fibula fracture (Maisonneuve fracture)

DIAGNOSIS

Patients usually present with the history of a twisting injury to the ankle, with subsequent inability to weight bear.

The Ottawa ankle rules dictate that an ankle x-ray be performed if, after injury, a patient presents with pain in the malleolar area in addition to one of the following[7]:

1. Bone tenderness at the posterior edge or tip of the lateral malleolus.
2. Bone tenderness at the posterior edge or tip of the medial malleolus.
3. Inability to weight bear immediately and in the emergency department.

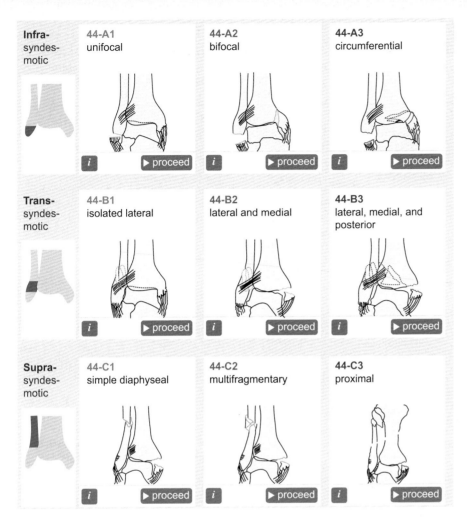

Infra-syndes-motic	44-A1 unifocal	44-A2 bifocal	44-A3 circumferential
Trans-syndes-motic	44-B1 isolated lateral	44-B2 lateral and medial	44-B3 lateral, medial, and posterior
Supra-syndes-motic	44-C1 simple diaphyseal	44-C2 multifragmentary	44-C3 proximal

FIGURE 23.1 AO and Weber classification of ankle fractures. (Permission from Malleolar Segment, Journal of Orthopaedic Trauma, 2018;32(suppl 1), p s65-70. Copyright © 2017 by AO Foundation, Davos, Switzerland; Orthopaedic Trauma Association, IL, US.)

Important radiographic features to note include the level of the fibula fracture and any associated medial or posterior malleolus involvement. Lateral talar shift is evidence of a deltoid ligament injury and can be determined by measuring the medial clear space between the medial malleolus and talus (normal <4 mm)[3]. The relationship between the tibia and fibula at the physeal scar is important in the diagnosis of a syndesmotic ligament disruption. The tibiofibular clear space should be <6 mm on all radiographic views.[3]

TREATMENT

Nonoperative

Nonoperative management of ankle fractures is reserved for nondisplaced or minimally displaced fractures of the fibula (Weber A, B), without evidence of deltoid ligament injury (lateral talar shift) or syndesmosis disruption. Treatment involves immobilization in a below-knee cast until evidence of clinical and radiographic union (approximately 6 weeks).

Operative

Operative management is recommended for displaced fibula fractures (>2 mm), Weber C fibula fractures, bimalleolar or bimalleolar equivalent injuries, trimalleolar injuries, and fractures with associated syndesmosis disruption. Surgical management involves restoration of the normal bony anatomy of the distal fibula and tibia, and anatomic reduction of any intra-articular pathology. The reduction is typically maintained with plate and screw constructs.

POSTTREATMENT

Immediately postoperatively, the affected extremity is placed in a well-padded splint. The patient is instructed to be non–weight bearing on the limb and to maintain elevation to the level of the heart.

At approximately 2 weeks postoperatively, the splint is removed and the surgical sites are examined. If wound healing is adequate, range-of-motion exercises may begin. The patient is placed into a removable cast boot. Typically, patients are instructed to be non–weight bearing for 6 weeks after surgery; however, the treating surgeons may choose to shorten or lengthen that time at their discretion.

At 6 weeks postoperatively, the cast boot is removed and weight bearing begins. Rehabilitation under the supervision of a therapist begins (**Table 23.1**).

TABLE 23.1 Rehabilitation Protocol

	Phase I—Inflammation + Swelling Control (~0-2 wk)	Phase II—Early ROM (~2-6 wk)	Phase III—Strengthening + Proprioception (~6-12 wk)	Phase IV—Return to Activities/Sport (>12 wk)
Weight bearing	NWB	Stable ankle—begin protected WB Unstable ankle—NWB Pilon—NWB Talus—NWB	Stable ankle—FWB Unstable ankle—FWB Pilon—protected WB (>8 wk) Talus—protected WB (>8 wk)	Stable Ankle—FWB Unstable Ankle—FWB Pilon—FWB Talus—FWB
Immobilization	Below-knee plaster splint	Stable ankle—below-knee cast boot (PRN) Unstable ankle—below-knee cast boot Pilon—below-knee cast boot Talus—below-knee cast boot	Stable ankle—none Unstable ankle—wean cast boot Pilon—below-knee cast boot Talus—below-knee cast boot	None
Range of motion	Toe wiggling Knee ROM Hip ROM	Stable ankle—begin WB ROM exercises Unstable ankle—NWB ROM exercises Pilon—NWB ROM exercises Talus—NWB ROM exercises	FWB ROM exercises	FWB ROM exercises
Strengthening	Straight-leg raises	Straight-leg raises	Isotonic strengthening	Isotonic strengthening Plyometrics Sport-specific training
Proprioreception			Gait training Single-leg stance Inversion-eversion boards Mini-trampoline	Gait training Single-leg stance Inversion-eversion boards Mini-trampoline Sport-specific exercises
Modalities	Elevation Cryotherapy	Elevation Cryotherapy Compression stocking Aquatic therapy TENS Ultrasound	Elevation Cryotherapy/heat Compression stocking Aquatic therapy TENS Ultrasound Manual therapy Active-release/massage	Elevation Cryotherapy/heat Compression stocking Aquatic therapy TENS Ultrasound Manual therapy Active-release/massage

FWB, full weight bearing; NWB, non–weight bearing; ROM, range of motion; TENS, transcutaneous electric nerve stimulation; WB, weight bearing.

CASE EXAMPLE

A 21-year-old female inverted her ankle while playing soccer, resulting in a trimalleolar ankle fracture (AO 44-B3) (**Figures 23.2** and **23.3**). Open reduction and internal fixation was performed with all three malleoli being addressed (**Figures 23.4** and **23.5**).

Postoperatively, she was placed in a splint for 2 weeks, followed by a removable cast boot. Range-of-motion exercises began at 2 weeks; however, she was kept non–weight bearing for 6 weeks. Progressive weight bearing began at 6 weeks, and supervised therapy followed the protocol outlined in **Table 23.1**.

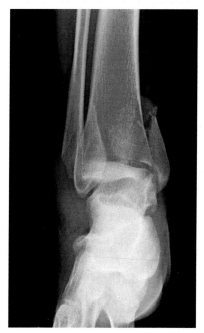

FIGURE 23.2 Anteroposterior (AP) x-ray of trimalleolar ankle fracture.

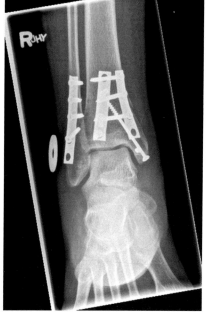

FIGURE 23.4 Postoperative anteroposterior (AP) x-ray of ankle after open reduction and internal fixation of trimalleolar ankle fracture.

PILON FRACTURES

ANATOMY

The tibial plafond is the distal weight-bearing surface of the tibia. The plafond is concave in the anterior-posterior plane and slightly convex in the medial-lateral plane. The distal, lateral tibia contains a concave groove in which the fibula sits, termed the incisura. The anterior and posterior projections of the incisura, named the Chaput and Volkmann tubercles, respectively, are attachment sites for the syndesmotic ligaments.

EPIDEMIOLOGY

Fractures that extend into the tibial plafond are referred to as pilon fractures. Pilon fractures are relatively uncommon, representing less than 1% of all lower extremity fractures.[8]

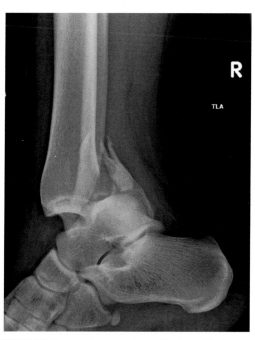

FIGURE 23.3 Lateral x-ray of trimalleolar ankle fracture.

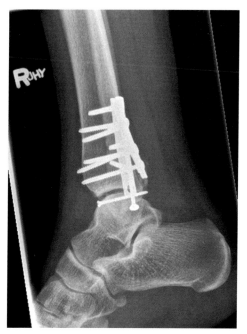

FIGURE 23.5 Postoperative lateral x-ray of ankle after open reduction and internal fixation of trimalleolar ankle fracture.

Typically, these are high-energy injuries that occur in falls from height or motor vehicle collisions.[3] Low-energy variants do exist, particularly in osteoporotic or pathologic bone.[9] Patients who sustain pilon fractures are commonly multiply injured, which can have an impact on recovery and rehabilitation.[8]

CLASSIFICATION (FIGURE 23.6)

- AO/OTA[6]
  - AO 43-B: partial articular injuries (part of articular surface remains attached to metaphysis)
    - 43-B1: split
    - 43-B2: split-depression
    - 43-B3: comminuted
  - AO 43-C: complete articular injuries (articular surface no longer attached to metaphysis)
    - 43-C1: simple articular injury, simple metaphyseal injury
    - 43-C2: simple articular injury, comminuted metaphyseal injury
    - 43-C2: comminuted articular and metaphyseal injuries

DIAGNOSIS

Tibial pilon fractures occur after high-energy trauma, which differentiates them from the more common ankle fractures. Examples include falls from height and motor vehicle collisions. Patients present with significant pain and swelling about the foot and ankle, usually with obvious deformity. Radiographs demonstrate the intra-articular nature of the fracture in the distal tibial plafond. Computed tomography (CT) scans are recommended to aid in preoperative planning.

TREATMENT

Nonoperative

Due to the intra-articular nature of pilon fractures, nonoperative management is rarely undertaken. Nonoperative management may be considered in nondisplaced fractures, or fractures in patients with medical comorbidities that preclude operative intervention. Treatment involves immobilization in a below-knee cast until evidence of clinical and radiographic union (approximately 8-12 weeks).

Operative

Operative management is recommended in most tibial pilon fractures. Unlike in simple ankle fractures, surgery may be delayed by 1 to 2 weeks if significant soft-tissue swelling precludes safe surgery. The goals of surgical intervention include restoration of the length, rotation, and alignment of the distal tibia and fibula, and anatomic reduction of the articular surface. After reduction is obtained, it is maintained with plate and screw constructs.

POSTTREATMENT

Immediately postoperatively, the affected extremity is placed in a well-padded splint. The patient is instructed to be non–weight bearing on the limb and to maintain elevation to the level of the heart.

At approximately 2 weeks postoperatively, the splint is removed and the surgical sites are examined. If wound healing is adequate, range-of-motion exercises may begin. The patient is placed into a removable cast boot. Typically, patients are instructed to be non–weight bearing for a minimum of 8 weeks after surgery. The treating surgeon must decide the appropriate time for discontinuing use of the cast boot and initiation of weight bearing based on the

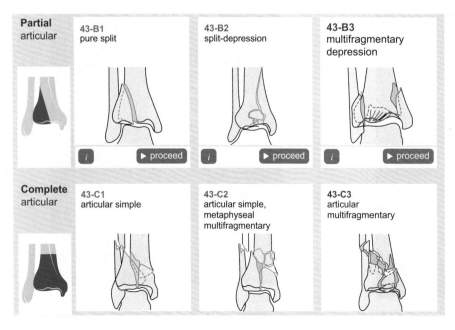

FIGURE 23.6 AO classification of pilon fractures. (Permission from Malleolar Segment, Journal of Orthopaedic Trauma, 2018;32(suppl 1), p s65-70. Copyright © 2017 by AO Foundation, Davos, Switzerland; Orthopaedic Trauma Association, IL, US.)

presence or absence of clinical and radiographic union of the fracture(s). Rehabilitation follows the protocol outlined in **Table 23.1**.

CASE EXAMPLE

A 50-year-old male fell 8 feet from a ladder, landing directly on his right foot, resulting in a comminuted pilon fracture of the right tibia (AO 43-C3) (**Figures 23.7-23.9**). Open reduction and internal fixation was performed (**Figure 23.10**).

Postoperatively, the patient was placed in a well-padded splint to accommodate swelling. Two weeks postoperatively, the splint was removed and exchanged for a cast boot. Range-of-motion exercises commenced. The patient was instructed to be non–weight bearing for 12 weeks due to the comminuted nature of the fracture. Once weight bearing began, a formal supervised therapy followed the protocol outlined in **Table 23.1**.

TALUS FRACTURES

ANATOMY

The talus represents the link between the leg and the foot and is crucial for normal ankle and hindfoot motion. It is made up of the head, neck, body, and lateral and posterior processes (**Figure 23.11**). The majority of the talus is covered in articular cartilage, and it has no direct musculotendinous attachments. The talus articulates with multiple bones including the tibia, fibula, calcaneus, and navicular.

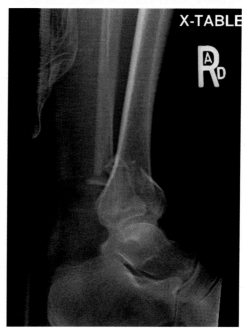

FIGURE 23.8 Lateral x-ray of pilon fracture.

EPIDEMIOLOGY

Fractures of the talus are uncommon and represent less than 1% of all fractures.[10] Talar neck fractures account for approximately half of all talus fractures[10] and, along with fractures of the body, have the most significant consequences. Talar neck fractures occur when an axial load is applied to the plantar aspect of the foot, with the talar body held rigidly between the tibia and calcaneus.[3,11] Fractures of the talar neck and body are typically high-energy injuries, whereas fractures of the processes may be from lower-energy events.[3]

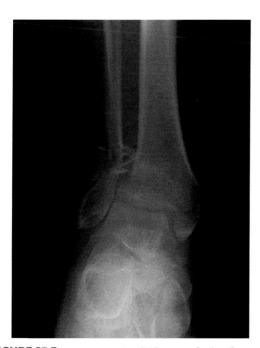

FIGURE 23.7 Anteroposterior (AP) x-ray of pilon fracture.

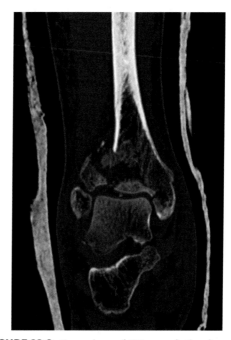

FIGURE 23.9 Coronal cut of CT scan of pilon fracture.

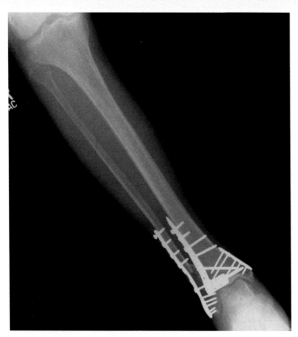

FIGURE 23.10 Postoperative anteroposterior (AP) x-ray after open reduction and internal fixation of pilon fracture.

CLASSIFICATION (FIGURE 23.12)

- Anatomic
  - The anatomic classification divides talus fractures into those of the neck, body, and processes (see **Figure 23.11**)
- Hawkins[12] (see **Figure 23.12**)
  - Hawkins categorized talar neck fractures by the associated joint dislocations

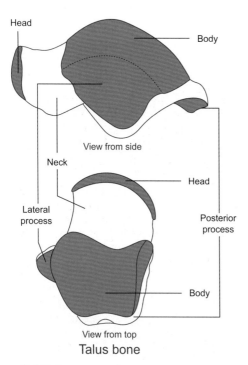

FIGURE 23.11 Surface anatomy of the talus.

- Hawkins I: nondisplaced fracture of the talar neck
- Hawkins II: displaced talar neck fracture, subtalar joint subluxation/dislocation
- Hawkins III: displaced talar neck fracture, subtalar, and ankle joint subluxation/dislocation
- Hawkins IV: displaced talar neck fracture, pantalar dislocation

DIAGNOSIS

Talus fractures are caused by high-energy trauma, such as falls from height and motor vehicle collisions. Patients typically present with foot and ankle pain and swelling, with varying degrees of deformity. Radiographic diagnosis can be challenging, particularly in minimally displaced fractures. For that reason, and to aid with treatment planning, CT scans are recommended for the majority of talus fractures.

TREATMENT

Nonoperative

Nonoperative management of talus fractures is uncommon. Nonoperative management may be considered in nondisplaced fractures, or fractures in patients with medical comorbidities that preclude operative intervention. Treatment involves immobilization in a below-knee cast until evidence of clinical and radiographic union (approximately 8-12 weeks).

Operative

Most fractures of the talus are managed operatively. The talus articulates with the tibia, fibula, calcaneus, and navicular, and residual deformity is poorly tolerated. The goals of surgery are anatomic reduction and stable internal fixation. This is typically accomplished with open reduction and internal fixation with a combination of plates and screws.

POSTTREATMENT

Immediately postoperatively, the affected extremity is placed in a well-padded splint. The patient is instructed to be non–weight bearing on the limb and to maintain elevation to the level of the heart.

At approximately 2 weeks postoperatively, the splint is removed and the surgical sites are examined. If wound healing is adequate, range-of-motion exercises may begin. The patient is placed into a removable cast boot. Typically, patients are instructed to be non–weight bearing for a minimum of 8 weeks after surgery. The treating surgeon must decide the appropriate time for discontinuing use of the cast boot and initiation of weight bearing based on the presence or absence of clinical and radiographic union of the fracture(s). Rehabilitation follows the protocol demonstrated in **Table 23.1**.

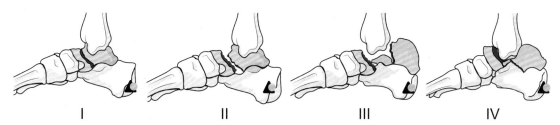

| I | II | III | IV |

FIGURE 23.12 Hawkins classification of talar neck fractures. (Permission from Malleolar Segment, Journal of Orthopaedic Trauma, 2018;32(suppl 1), p s65-70. Copyright © 2017 by AO Foundation, Davos, Switzerland; Orthopaedic Trauma Association, IL, US.)

CASE EXAMPLE

A 25-year-old female fell while rock climbing, falling 10 ft. Assessment revealed a displaced right talar neck fracture (Hawkins II) (**Figures 23.13** and **23.14**). Operative management was undertaken (**Figure 23.15**).

Postoperatively, a well-padded splint was used. Approximately 2 weeks postoperatively, the splint was removed and range-of-motion exercises commenced. A cast boot was used and the patient remained non–weight bearing for 8 weeks, followed by progressive weight bearing. When weight bearing began, formal therapy followed the protocol in **Table 23.1**.

COMMON REHAB PROTOCOLS (SEE TABLE 23.1)

Rehabilitation after foot and ankle injury and surgery proceeds in four stages[13]:

1. Control of inflammation and swelling
2. Regaining range of motion
3. Improving strength and proprioception
4. Return to activities/sport

Protocols are similar for many foot and ankle injuries. Immobilization is undertaken for 2 weeks postoperatively, to allow time for incisions to heal and swelling to decrease. Early range-of-motion exercises are then begun. Early motion may improve ligament and tendon healing, increase blood supply to healing tissues, decrease muscle atrophy, and improve cartilage nutrition.[14] Early motion may also prevent deep vein thrombosis; however, the evidence for this is weak.[15] The clinical research on early versus delayed motion suggests that early motion may improve functional outcomes and lead to an earlier return to work after surgery. Risks of early motion may include a higher superficial infection rate.[15] The surgeon must balance the risks and benefits of early motion on a patient-specific basis.

There is a lack of clinical evidence to guide weight-bearing protocols in the postoperative period. The literature suggests that early weight bearing after surgical treatment of ankle fractures is safe; however, there does not appear to be an effect, positive or negative, on long-term outcomes.[16] There is little guidance in the literature on the effect of early weight bearing on the outcomes of pilon or talus fractures, and most protocols advocate prolonged non–weight bearing

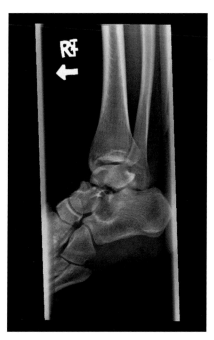

FIGURE 23.13 Lateral x-ray of Hawkins II talar neck fracture.

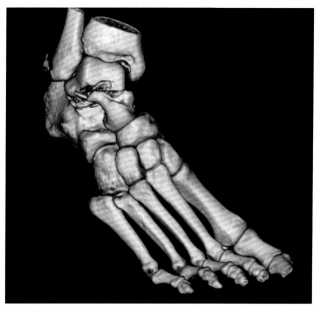

FIGURE 23.14 Three-dimensional CT reconstruction of Hawkins II talar neck fracture.

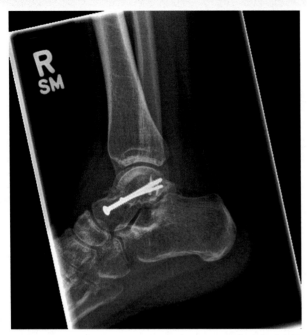

FIGURE 23.15 Postoperative lateral x-ray after open reduction and internal fixation of talar neck fracture.

(2-3 months). The final decision on when a patient is able to weight bear is made by the treating surgeon and is based upon many factors including the stability of fixation, quality of bone, type of injury, patient compliance, and presence or absence of complications.

Strengthening begins when full range of motion has returned (or range of motion has plateaued). Strengthening prior to this may worsen preexisting stiffness.[14] Patients often wish to begin strengthening before range of motion has been maximized and should be guided appropriately.

Proprioception retraining is an important part of recovery after injury and surgery. Trauma to the foot and ankle decreases normal proprioception and predisposes patients to reinjury[17]. Proprioception training can improve function and help avoid future injuries.[14]

The final phase of rehabilitation is patient-specific and depends on the patients' preinjury functional status and their activity goals. In low-demand elderly patients, their goals may be as basic as resuming activities of daily living. Young, active patients more often wish to return to higher-demand activities, and sport-specific rehabilitation is recommended.

SPECIAL CONSIDERATIONS

DIABETIC PATIENTS

Patients with diabetes mellitus who suffer foot and ankle trauma warrant special attention. Diminished sensation, poor vascularity, and impaired immunity contribute to high complication rates following injury, whether managed operatively or nonoperatively.[4] Infection, wound dehiscence, malunion, and nonunion all occur at higher rates than in

healthy patients.[18] All members of the team managing diabetic patients must be aware of these risks and close follow-up is necessary. Rehabilitation is often delayed due to prolonged soft tissue and bony healing. Strict immobilization is recommended until surgical wounds have healed. Weight bearing should be delayed until clinical and radiographic evidence of union is present, which may be upward of 12 weeks for even simple ankle fractures.

DELAYED/NONUNION

Although uncommon in ankle and talus fractures, delayed unions and nonunions are relatively common in pilon fractures.[19] If stable internal fixation has been used, delayed or nonunion should not preclude early range-of-motion exercises. Weight bearing may be delayed until evidence of bony union, at the discretion of the treating surgeon.

SOFT-TISSUE COMPLICATIONS

Soft tissue complications may include open fractures, superficial or deep infection, or wound dehiscence/breakdown. In these situations, healing of the soft tissues becomes the primary concern. Rehabilitation must be delayed to allow for soft tissues to heal. Immobilization is recommended until definitive wound healing and eradication of infection is confirmed. Similarly, weight bearing should be delayed until soft tissues are healed to the satisfaction of the treating surgeon.

FRAGILITY FRACTURES

Fragility fractures are low-energy fractures occurring through areas of poor bone quality. Osteoporosis is a common cause of fragility fractures, and the incidence of these fractures is increasing.[20,21] These fractures often occur in the elderly with multiple medical comorbidities. Surgical management of these fractures is complicated by poor soft-tissue quality, impaired vascularity, and often significant comminution.[20] Traditional implants and fixation techniques are often unreliable in severely osteoporotic bone. Although the goals of treatment should be to promote early motion and weight bearing, this may not be possible. Prolonged immobilization and non–weight bearing may be necessary. For many elderly patients, this means confinement to a wheelchair, as mobilizing with walking aids may not be possible due to weakness and fall risk.

REFERENCES

1. Petrisor BA, Poolman R, Koval K, et al. Management of displaced ankle fractures. *J Orthop Trauma.* 2006;20(7):515-518.
2. vander Griend R, Michelson JD, Bone LB. Instructional Course Lectures, The American Academy of Orthopaedic Surgeons – Fractures of the ankle and the distal part of the tibia. *J Bone Joint Surg Am.* 1996;78(11):1772-1783.
3. Rockwood CA, Bucholz RW, Court-Brown CM, et al. *Rockwood and Green's Fractures in Adults.* 7 ed. Philadelphia, PA: Lippincott Williams & Wilkins; 2010.

4. Michelson JD. Ankle fractures resulting from rotational injuries. *J Am Acad Orthop Surg.* 2003;11(6):403-412.

5. Müller ME, Allgöwer M, Perren SM. *Manual of Internal Fixation: Techniques Recommended by the AO-ASIF Group.* Berlin: Springer; 1991.

6. Marsh JL, Slongo TF, Agel J, et al. Fracture and dislocation classification compendium – 2007: Orthopaedic Trauma Association classification, database and outcomes committee. *J Orthop Trauma.* 2007;21(10 suppl):S1-S133.

7. Stiell IG, McKnight RD, Greenberg GH, et al. Implementation of the Ottawa ankle rules. *J Am Med Assoc.* 1994;271(11):827-832.

8. Browner B, Levine A, Jupiter JB, et al. *Skeletal Trauma.* 4 ed. Philadelphia, PA: Saunders; 2009.

9. Helfet DL, Koval K, Pappas J, et al. Intraarticular "pilon" fracture of the tibia. *Clin Orthop Relat Res.* 1994;298:221-228.

10. Fortin PT, Balazsy JE. Talus fractures: evaluation and treatment. *J Am Acad Orthop Surg.* 2001;9(2):114-127.

11. Peterson L, Goldie IF, Irstam L. Fracture of the neck of the talus: a clinical study. *Acta Orthop Scand.* 1977;48:696-706.

12. Hawkins LG. Fractures of the neck of the talus. *J bone Joint Surg Am.* 1970;52(5):991-1002.

13. English B. Phases of rehabilitation. *Foot Ankle Clin.* 2013;18(2):357-367.

14. Barill ER, Porter DA. *Baxter's The Foot and Ankle in Sport.* 2nd ed. Philadelphia, PA: Elsevier Inc; 2008.

15. Egol KA, Dolan R, Koval KJ, et al. Ankle Fractures. *Orthop Trauma Dir.* 2006;4(4):1-7.

16. Kubiak EN, Beebe MJ, North K, et al. Early weight bearing after lower extremity fractures in adults. *J Am Acad Orthop Surg.* 2013;21(12):727-738.

17. Lephart SM, Pincivero DM, Giraldo JL, et al. The role of proprioception in the management and rehabilitation of athletic injuries. *Am J Sports Med.* 1997;25(1):130-137.

18. Chaudhary SB, Liporace FA, Gandhi A, et al. Complications of ankle fracture in patients with diabetes. *J Am Acad Orthop Surg.* 2008;16(3):159-170.

19. Thordarson DB. Complications after treatment of tibial pilon fractures: prevention and management strategies. *J Am Acad Orthop Surg.* 2000;8(4):253-265.

20. Cornell CN. Internal fracture fixation in patients with osteoporosis. *J Am Acad Orthop Surg.* 2003;11(2):109-119.

21. Ekman EF. The role of the orthopaedic surgeon in minimizing mortality and morbidity associated with fragility fractures. *J Am Acad Orthop Surg.* 2010;18(5):278-285.

24

Tibial Shaft Fractures

Trevor J. Shelton
Laurence Cook
Philip R. Wolinsky

Fractures of the tibial shaft are the most common long bone injury, occurring with a frequency of 17 per 100,000 people per year.[1] Tibial shaft fractures, like other long bone fractures, are more common in young adult males.[2] When tibial fractures occur in a young adult patient, they typically are the result of a high-energy trauma such as a motor vehicle accident. Tibial fractures are more often associated with a ground-level fall in the geriatric population.[1] Osteoporosis is typically a predisposing factor for these patients, especially for the geriatric female population.

The treatment of tibial shaft fractures has undergone significant change over time. The debate between operative versus nonoperative management has been lively since the early 1960s, and continues to this today.[3,4] General criteria for surgical treatment of tibial shaft fractures include coronal angulation exceeding 5°, sagittal angulation greater than 10°, shortening more than 1 cm, displacement greater than 50%, and severe comminution.[4]

ANATOMY

The tibia is the major weight bearing bone of the lower leg and spans the area between the knee and ankle joints. It is triangular in cross section and expands at the proximal and distal portions to form the knee and ankle joints, respectively. Distally, the tibia and the distal fibula make up the ankle mortise. The medial malleolus portion of the tibia articulates with the talus to contribute to the ankle joint. Proximally, the lateral and medial tibial plateaus create the lower articular surface of the knee joint. The proximal fibula does not contribute to the knee joint. A fibrous connective tissue called the interosseous membrane spans the interval between the tibia and fibula shafts.[5] The tibia and fibula are covered by the anterior, lateral, and posterior muscular compartments of the lower leg.

MECHANISMS OF INJURY

Tibial shaft fractures are caused by a variety of injury mechanisms. The first distinction to be made is between a high- and low-energy injury. A high-energy tibial shaft fracture caused by a pedestrian versus auto accident will be treated differently than a lower energy one caused by a ground-level fall. The prognosis and postoperative course will be different for these two injuries as well. This is important when planning a rehabilitation protocol and assessing the likelihood of the patients, return to their preinjury level of function.

The amount of traumatic energy absorbed by the soft tissues and bone, and the amount of damage to those tissues, is higher in a high-energy mechanism tibial shaft fracture than a low-energy mechanism fracture. The complication rate therefore is higher for high-energy injuries as a result of the amount of soft-tissue damage (pain, stiffness, swelling, blood supply damage, nerve damage), bone damage (comminution, displacement), and periosteal stripping (blood supply damage). This creates challenges for the treating clinicians planning a treatment course.

HIGH-ENERGY INJURIES

Motor vehicle accidents produce the highest number of tibial shaft fractures yearly.[1]

Violent trauma such as gunshot wounds and direct blows make up a smaller percentage of high-energy tibial fractures.

LOW-ENERGY INJURIES

Sports-related injuries are common among younger population, with soccer being the most common sport involved with injury.

Geriatric trauma is generally the result of twisting in combination with a ground-level fall.[1]

CLASSIFICATION

Fracture classifications systems have been developed to standardize specific subsets of injuries to give prognostic information/predictions to both patients and surgeons. The most comprehensive classification system for the tibial shaft is the Orthopaedic Trauma Association (OTA) classification (**Figure 24.1**). This is a radiographic classification based on anteroposterior and lateral radiographs. As one progresses through the OTA classification system for tibial shaft fractures, the fracture becomes more complex, and in general, the soft-tissue trauma also increases. This system also helps assigning a treatment algorithm for patients.

Open fractures of the tibial shaft are classified using the Gustilo and Anderson (GA) classification.[6-8] This classification is based upon the amount of soft-tissue and bony injury, a measure of the energy absorbed by the leg at the time of injury. Injuries are classified as GA I, II, or III according to the severity of the injury. As fractures become more complex, they receive a high classification type. The amount of foreign contamination and the mechanism of injury also play important roles in determining a classification type.

Type III injuries were subdivided by Gustilo in 1987 when they acknowledged that subsets of type III open fractures had a worse prognosis than others within the same classification. Type IIIA fractures are those with a large soft-tissue wound (greater than 5 cm) but have adequate soft-tissue coverage. Those that require local or free soft-tissue transfer to cover the exposed bone are assigned type IIIB open fractures. Fractures with such severe injuries that they require vascular repair to revascularize the extremity are classified as type IIIC open fractures.

TREATMENT

NONOPERATIVE TREATMENT

Functional bracing has been described as a method for the treatment of minimally displaced or nondisplaced "stable" tibial shaft fractures. This concept was popularized by Sarmiento who reported on the treatment of 1000 tibial shaft fractures treated with closed methods.[9] Functional bracing or cast management requires frequent follow-up to ensure that displacement or malalignment is detected early.

Nonsurgical treatment is indicated for low-energy, length-stable, minimally displaced fractures of the tibial shaft. There are radiographic criteria that have been found to be predictors of good outcome with nonoperative treatment. These criteria include fractures with less than 50% fracture displacement, less than 10° of fracture angulation in any plane, less than 1 cm of shortening, and less than 10° of rotational malalignment on the injury images.[4] Fractures that do not meet these radiographic criteria have higher rates of failure when treated nonoperatively. Patients treated nonoperatively with functional bracing generally begin with a period of

non–weight bearing for 6 to 8 weeks.[9] Depending on fracture pattern, patient may begin a gradual progressive return to weight bearing in a functional brace at the 6- to 8-week mark. If the fracture pattern is not axially stable, the period of non–weight bearing can be longer than 6 to 8 weeks.

There are risks for nonoperative management that are important when discussing treatment options with a patient and planning a rehabilitation protocol. Shortening and malunion are two fracture complications that can have long-lasting repercussions for the patient. Long leg casting or functional bracing can result in shortening of at least a half an inch in one-third of patients in some series.[10] Malunion, or a healed fracture which falls outside of the radiographic parameters discussed previously, has been reported to occur in up to 50% of patients treated with casting.[2-4,10] In addition to fracture complications, joint stiffness related to soft-tissue trauma is also a problem for any patient treated with a prolonged period of immobilization and non–weight bearing. This can be an added issue that requires additional rehabilitation and may cause prolonged morbidity.

OPERATIVE TREATMENT

Operative treatment of tibial shaft fractures is used for the treatment of unstable fracture patterns. The absolute indications for operative treatments include open fractures, compartment syndrome, and vascular injuries that require repair. Relative indications include patients with multiple injuries, ipsilateral tibia and femur fractures (floating knee), and patterns that have predictors of being "unstable," including no fibula fracture, a fibula fracture at the same level as the tibial fracture, and increasing fracture comminution.[4]

The options for surgical stabilization of tibial fractures include intramedullary nailing, plating, and external fixation. Each option has its own set of indications and associated risks and benefits.

Intramedullary Nailing

Treatment of "unstable" tibial shaft fractures with reamed interlocked nails provide multiple benefits over nonoperative or treatment with traditional open reduction and plating performed using large incisions. Reamed, interlocked nails provide high union rates, low malunion rates, and low infection rates when used for closed fractures.[11] Because the surgical incisions are distant to the area of trauma, it gives the added benefit of not further traumatizing the area of injury with an additional soft-tissue insult. Intramedullary nailing can be used to treat a variety of injuries including proximal and distal third tibial fractures.

Court-Brown et al found that anterior knee pain occurs in 60% of patients who had an intramedullary nail placed using a patella tendon splitting or parapatellar incision.[2] This pain is usually activity related and exacerbated by kneeling, and 80% of patients have improvement in their knee pain after nail removal. The improvement in pain is not always complete. The cause of the pain is unknown. The pain does

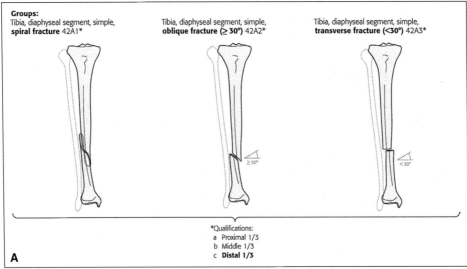

Groups:
Tibia, diaphyseal segment, simple, **spiral fracture** 42A1*

Tibia, diaphyseal segment, simple, **oblique fracture (≥ 30°)** 42A2*

Tibia, diaphyseal segment, simple, **transverse fracture (<30°)** 42A3*

*Qualifications:
a   Proximal 1/3
b   Middle 1/3
c   **Distal 1/3**

A

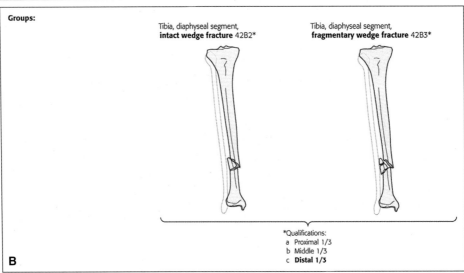

Groups:

Tibia, diaphyseal segment, **intact wedge fracture** 42B2*

Tibia, diaphyseal segment, **fragmentary wedge fracture** 42B3*

*Qualifications:
a   Proximal 1/3
b   Middle 1/3
c   **Distal 1/3**

B

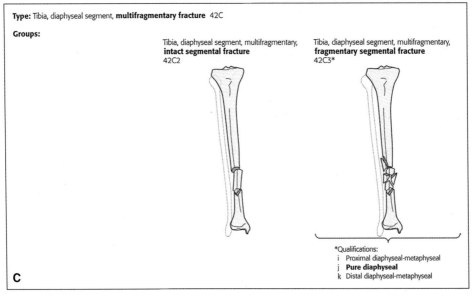

Type: Tibia, diaphyseal segment, **multifragmentary fracture** 42C

Groups:

Tibia, diaphyseal segment, multifragmentary, **intact segmental fracture** 42C2

Tibia, diaphyseal segment, multifragmentary, **fragmentary segmental fracture** 42C3*

*Qualifications:
i   Proximal diaphyseal-metaphyseal
j   **Pure diaphyseal**
k   Distal diaphyseal-metaphyseal

C

FIGURE 24.1 Orthopaedic Trauma Association (OTA) classification for tibial (4) shaft (2) fractures. The letter designation is then given for simple fracture (**A**), wedge fracture (**B**), or multifragmentary fracture (**C**). (Reproduced with permission from Tibia. *J Orthop Trauma.* 2018;32:49-60.)

decrease over time, and pain relief seems to peak between 3 and 8 years. Increasing quadriceps muscle strength did improve pain in patients who had anterior knee pain after a nail insertion.

Plating

Historically, plating of tibial shaft fractures was not successful when performed using large incisions with soft-tissue stripping of the bony fragments. This technique added significant amounts of soft-tissue damage to an area where the soft tissue had already been damaged. This increased the risk of infections, wound complications, and fracture nonunion. The more recent introduction of minimally invasive plating techniques, which are particularly for the treatment of comminuted fractures, has reintroduced plate fixation as a viable option for stabilization of the tibia. The technique of bridge plating can be used to "bridge" the area of comminution using multiple small incisions. This mimics the concept of intramedullary nailing in that it uses small incisions distant to the area of trauma for hardware insertion. The tibia is reduced and instrumented with the aid of fluoroscopy rather than through direct visualization. Plating is still used for patients with open growth plates or fractures that extend into the knee or ankle joint.

External Fixation

External fixation with traditional ½ pin frames was once the treatment of choice for open tibial shaft fractures. In certain parts of the developing world, it is still the standard of care. In the United States, ½ frames are most often used as a temporizing method of stabilization until either the patient and/or the limb can tolerate a definitive procedure. External fixation is not the definitive treatment of choice for most fractures because of the high rate of pin site infections with the prolonged use of external fixation. In addition, malunion rates are higher with the use of external fixation than those treated with intramedullary nailing.

AFTERCARE AND REHABILITATION

Postoperative rehabilitation after a tibial fracture is dependent on the mode of treatment as well as the extent of the soft-tissue and bony injury. Patient's with stable fractures who are treated with weight bearing braces must bear weight early in order to stimulate a healing response. Functional bracing and cast management require attention to detail and close follow-up for optimal results. As swelling subsides, the braces or casts may become loose and no longer restrict the fracture fragments from moving. This can lead to malunion if not recognized early on by the treatment team. Patients with axially unstable fractures treated with bracing or casting are treated with a 4 to 6 week course of non–weight bearing followed by a gradual progressive return to full weight bearing.

Patients with unstable tibial fractures that are treated operatively with an intramedullary nail are typically placed in short leg splints for 5 to 10 days to prevent equinus contracture of the gastroc-soleus muscle complex. If there is more than 50% cortical contact at the fracture sites, patients can begin early weight bearing. Those with greater comminution are kept toe-touch bearing until there is early callus seen on x-ray and their pain has diminished. This generally occurs at the 6- to 8-week mark.

For tibial fracture treated with plating, there is less consensus on early weight bearing. Fractures of the tibial shaft take a much longer time for bony union when compared to other long bones like the femur. The femur has a much more robust muscle mass and therefore blood supply to the bone when compared to the tibia with its less robust blood supply. The risk of hardware failure that may result from the hardware bearing much of the weight until healing begins to take place must be balanced against the benefits of early weight bearing. Because of this idea, patients who receive plating for tibial fracture are kept non–weight bearing for 6 to 8 weeks followed by a gradual progressive weight bearing protocol with the help of a physiatrist.

REFERENCES

1. Larsen P, Elsoe R, Hansen SH, et al. Incidence and epidemiology of tibial shaft fractures. *Injury*. 2015;46:746-750. doi:10.1016/j.injury.2014.12.027.
2. Court-Brown CM, Rimmer S, Prakash U, et al. The epidemiology of open long bone fractures. *Injury*. 1998;29:529-534. doi:10.1016/s0020-1383(98)00125-9.
3. Essilfie A, Sabour A, Hatch GFR, et al. An increasing rate of surgical management of closed tibia fractures in an adolescent population: a national database study. *J Am Acad Orthop Surg*. 2019;27:816-822. doi:10.5435/JAAOS-D-17-00926.
4. Lindsey RW, Blair SR. Closed tibial-shaft fractures: which ones benefit from surgical treatment? *J Am Acad Orthop Surg*. 1996;4:35-43. doi:10.5435/00124635-199601000-00005.
5. Minns RJ, Hunter JA. The mechanical and structural characteristics of the tibio-fibular interosseous membrane. *Acta Orthop Scand*. 1976;47:236-240. doi:10.3109/17453677608989725.
6. Gustilo RB, Anderson JT. Prevention of infection in the treatment of one thousand and twenty-five open fractures of long bones: retrospective and prospective analyses. *J Bone Joint Surg Am*. 1976;58:453-458.
7. Gustilo RB, Mendoza RM, Williams DN. Problems in the management of type III (severe) open fractures: a new classification of type III open fractures. *J Trauma*. 1984;24:742-746. doi:10.1097/00005373-198408000-00009.
8. Kim PH, Leopold SS. In brief: Gustilo-Anderson classification. [corrected]. *Clin Orthop Relat Res*. 2012;470:3270-3274. doi:10.1007/s11999-012-2376-6.
9. Sarmiento A, Gersten LM, Sobol PA, et al. Tibial shaft fractures treated with functional braces. Experience with 780 fractures. *J Bone Joint Surg Br*. 1989;71:602-609.
10. Hooper GJ, Keddell RG, Penny ID. Conservative management or closed nailing for tibial shaft fractures. A randomised prospective trial. *J Bone Joint Surg Br*. 1991;73:83-85.
11. Schemitsch EH, Kowalski MJ, Swiontkowski MF, et al. Comparison of the effect of reamed and unreamed locked intramedullary nailing on blood flow in the callus and strength of union following fracture of the sheep tibia. *J Orthop Res*. 1995;13:382-389. doi:10.1002/jor.1100130312.

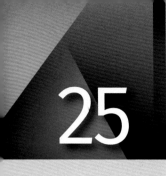

Rehabilitation of the Foot

Dolfi Herscovici Jr
Julia M. Scaduto

The modern foot is a marvelous, evolutionary development. When we changed into an upright being, it became absolutely necessary that the 26 individual bones in each foot, along with its associated muscles, ligament, and tendons, interact biomechanically to provide stability and allow propulsive gait. With signals from the central nervous system, the foot allows us to adjust to walking along different kinds of surfaces, running when we have to, and jumping when the need arises. When fractures of the foot occur, they can present within a wide spectrum of injuries ranging from simple toe fractures to complex mid- and hindfoot injuries. When these bony injuries occur, and unless managed appropriately, they can ultimately affect both stability and the patient's ability to produce a consistent and painless gait. This "altered" gait can lead to difficulties with shoe wear and produce complaints affecting the knee, the hip, and the spine. The decision driving the treatment of these fractures should be based primarily on the injury pattern and not solely on the patient's age. Given the advancements in techniques and implants, this chapter will hopefully provide a rational approach for the physician and healthcare providers tasked with managing and rehabilitating foot fractures in the adult patient.

EMBRYOLOGY, GAIT AND BIOMECHANICS

The surface of the foot plate can be recognized at the fifth embryonic week. However, no toes are visible. By the sixth week, digital rays and interdigital notching are present. Chondrification of the foot bones begins at this time and continues until week 9. By week 7, the toes are well delineated and both feet face each other in a nearly sagittal plane. From weeks 8 to 14, the foot slowly increases in length and then accelerates, at a rate of 3 mm/wk, until week 26 when it slows down slightly until birth. During this time, the fetal foot also narrows gradually. Beginning at the third gestational month, the forefoot (phalanges and metatarsals) begins ossification of the cartilaginous bones in the embryo. Ossification of the hindfoot begins between 3 and 5 months, first with the calcaneus and followed in sequential order by the talus, navicular, cuboid, medial cuneiform, and then the lateral and middle cuneiforms.[1] By the age of 1.0 year in girls and 1.5 years in boys, the foot achieves half its adult dimension. It grows 0.9 cm annually, through the age of 12 years in girls and 14 years in boys. In girls, the mature foot length is reached at 14 years of age. In boys, the foot continues to grow until 16 years of age, eventually becoming, on average, 2.2 cm longer length than the female foot. However, the female foot has been shown to increase in size and width following pregnancy.[1]

Walking upright separates a child from an infant and is usually seen around 12 months of age. There are gradual improvements in flexibility and strength until walking (gait) becomes a rhythmic, cyclical forward progression of the body. Each gait cycle is divided into two phases, stance and swing. The stance phase takes up approximately 60% of the cycle and occurs when any part of the foot contacts the ground. The stance phase influences the weight-bearing alignment of the limb because it is in constant contact with the ground and requires that all joints (and bones) function properly[2] and can be divided into early, mid-, and terminal phases. During the **early stance** phase, the heel strikes the ground producing a force of between 70% and 100% of the total body weight. During heel strike, an eversion of the subtalar joint occurs, which slowly reverses to maximal inversion at the onset of preswing. During the **mid-stance** phase (single-limb stance), the midtarsal joints bear an average pressure of 10% of the total body weight. The calcaneocuboid and talonavicular joints "lock" and "unlock" the midtarsal region that were necessary for heel strike and will also be needed during toe-lift.[3] During this part of stance, a dorsiflexion of the midtarsal joints occurs producing a flattening of the arch. At **terminal stance** (toe-rise), the heel rises off the ground causing the metatarsophalangeal joints to dorsiflex. About one-third of the total body weight is transmitted through the first metatarsal.[4] As the hindfoot is lifted higher, maximum dorsiflexion of the toes is achieved, allowing the foot to roll over the metatarsal heads rather than onto the tips of the toes.

The swing phase takes up the other 40% of the gait cycle and is defined as the part of gait that occurs when the foot does not contact the ground. After the foot is lifted from the ground during this phase, the subtalar joint drifts back to neutral, the arch is restored, and the toes drop toward the line of the metatarsal shafts. Working together, these two phases make up a *stride*, defined as the linear distance from heel-strike to heel-strike of the same foot. A *step* is defined as the distance between successive points of foot-to-floor contact of alternate feet. Having defined these two markers for gait, it is important to realize that there are two *steps* in each *stride*, and the three major articulations that allow *stride* and *step* to occur consist of the subtalar, midtarsal (primarily Chopart joint), and the metatarsophalangeal joints.[2]

EPIDEMIOLOGY

Epidemiologically, fractures in the foot are common injuries. A recent study by Shibuya et al., analyzed the data obtained from the United States National Trauma Data Bank, from 2007 to 2011.[5] They identified a total of 119,278 fractures of the foot, for an average of 23,856 foot fractures per year. In their study, the metatarsal ($n = 35,111$) was found to be the most common location for a fracture of the foot followed in descending order by fractures of the calcaneus (26,158), the talus (22,119), toe phalanges (15,423), the cuboid (7659), the navicular (5627), cuneiforms (4632), and a grouping listed as unspecified foot fractures (2549). In addition, they also discussed the number and percentage of open fractures found with these specific bony injuries. Unfortunately, they did not separate the specific age of patients in their study but rather gave the overall average age and range of all patients to be 43.87 + 19.25 years. In addition, no information about the incidence of these fractures is given, nor is there any statistics on the grade or type of open fractures patients sustained, nor are there any data on the male to female ratio for these injuries (**Table 25.1**).

Currently, the best epidemiological study, looking at bony injuries of the foot, was presented by Court-Brown and Caesar.[6] They reviewed the records of almost 6000 adult patients who presented to Royal Infirmary of Edinburgh during one calendar year, either as an inpatient or outpatient, in whom a diagnosis of a fracture of the foot was made. Separating the bony injuries that occurred in the foot, they also noted that metatarsal fractures were the most common foot fracture seen in adults. These were identified in 6.8% of the adult population, which occurred at an annual rate of 75.4/100,000, and were noted in patients who were at an average age of 42.8 years. In order of decreasing incidence, other fractures were segregated into those of the toe phalanx, seen in 3.6% of adults and occurring at a rate of 39.6/100,000, calcaneal fractures, seen in 1.2% of the adults and occurring in 13.7/100,000, fractures of the midfoot, seen in 0.4% and occurring in 5/100,000, talus fractures, identified in 0.3% and occurring in 3.2/100,000, and one patient who presented with a fracture of the sesamoid (**Table 25.1**). Unfortunately, no information is given as to how many of these fractures presented as open injuries.

In a separate study, Court-Brown et al. evaluated the epidemiology of open foot fractures from 1988 through 2010 at the Royal Infirmary.[7] During the 23 years of the study, they identified a total of 348 open fractures that presented to their institution, giving an incidence of a patient presenting with an open foot fracture to be 2.84/100,000 per year. In their study, the most common open fracture occurred in the phalanges ($n = 223$), followed by the metatarsals (64), the calcaneus (34), the midfoot (13), and the talus (12). They also noted that it was rare that any of these fractures occurred as an isolated injury and that most presented as Gustilo type III injuries[8] (**Table 25.1**).

It should also be noted that although commonly seen, fractures of the foot are also the most commonly missed orthopaedic injuries, especially in polytrauma patients.[9] This often occurs because on presentation the trauma teams are often focusing on life- or limb-threatening problems and give little attention to the foot, unless the patient presents with an open fracture or has an obvious dislocation to the foot. Given the frequency of foot fractures, if the fracture is not identified during the primary survey of the trauma patient, it should hopefully be identified during the secondary survey.

MANAGEMENT AND REHABILITATION OF FOOT FRACTURES

GENERAL OVERVIEW

The goals for the management of any foot fracture should include obtaining a healed fracture with good alignment and stable bony anatomy. This will allow patients to easily fit into a shoe, it avoids the development of any pressure areas on the foot, it allows patients to stand and bear weight for long periods of time, and it avoids complications leading to any loss of limb or function. This comes with the caveat that even though you would like to see all patients return to their previous levels of flexibility and activities, the reality is that not all patients will be able to achieve their preinjury levels of function. Therefore, the treatment of any foot fracture should be directed toward providing stable fixation when necessary, followed by a period of immobilization (usually to allow the incisions to heal), and then allowing the patient to begin the rehabilitation of their injuries (**Table 25.2**).

It is important to understand, however, that for all bony injuries, significant swelling can be expected, and this needs to be addressed before any definitive surgery is performed. This may require splinting the patient (**Figure 25.1**) and performing weekly evaluations until wrinkling of the skin in noted (**Figure 25.2**). The ability to wrinkle the skin usually indicates that the edema has resolved and the patient is ready, if surgery is indicated. Additionally, some injuries produce so much swelling of the foot that the patient develops either hemorrhagic or serous fractures blisters (**Figure 25.3**). The authors' preference is not to puncture or unroof these blisters but to simply dress them with some type

TABLE 25.1 Epidemiology of Foot Fractures

	Mean Age (Years)	Incidence (per 100,000)	Number of Fractures	% Foot Fractures	Male/ Female Ratio	Number of Open Fxs (% Type III)	% Open Fracture
Shibuya et al[5]	43.87 (+19.25)						
Metatarsals		a	35,111	29.5	a	5598	15.9
Calcaneus		a	26,158	21.9	a	5215	19.9
Talus		a	22,119	18.5	a	4141	18.7
Toe phalanx		a	15,423	12.9	a	5100	33.1
Cuboid		a	7659	6.5	a	970	12.76
Navicular		a	5627	4.7	a	880	15.6
Cuneiform		a	4632	3.9	a	808	17.4
Unspecified foot bone		a	2549	2.1	a	505	19.8
Court-Brown and Caesar[6]				**% Total Adult Fxs**			
Metatarsals	42.8	75.4	403	6.8	43/57	a	a
Toe phalanx	35.3	39.6	212	3.6	66/34	a	a
Calcaneus	40.4	13.7	73	1.2	78/22	a	a
Midfoot	36	5	27	0.4	48/52	a	a
Talus	30.5	3.2	17	0.3	82/18	a	a
Sesamoid	58	0.2	1	0.01	100/0	a	a
Court-Brown et al[7]				**% Foot Fractures**			
Phalanges	41.6	1.82		64.2	71/29	223 (20.6)	
Metatarsals	40.8	0.52		18.4	76/24	64 (53.1)	
Calcaneus	38.2	0.29		10.3	77/23	36 (72.2)	
Midfoot	32.1	0.11		3.7	70/30	13 (84.6)	
Talus	29.7	0.07		3.4	82/18	12 (75)	

Fxs, fractures.
[a]No information provided.

of nonadherent petroleum-based dressing (eg, Xeroform® or Adaptic®), reapply the splint, and follow them again at weekly intervals. Once these blisters have re-epithelialized, definitive fixation can then be performed. For both edema and blisters, the patient should understand that it may take 2 to 3 weeks until the problems with the soft-tissue envelope have improved to tolerate surgery. Additionally, should any postoperative soft-tissues concern occur (eg, wound dehiscence, cellulitis or drainage), these may produce a delay in their rehabilitation.

The management for all foot fractures should also be directed toward preventing complications. Due to the need for periods of immobilization, both preoperatively and postoperatively, vigilance should be directed to make certain that the foot and ankle are always *maintained in a neutral position*. This will avoid producing an equinus deformity of the ankle, which will not only affect the patients' ability to rehabilitate their injuries, but it may also may require a surgical correction. Additionally, due to the use of immobilization, there may be concerns about developing a deep vein thrombosis (DVT) and the use of a prophylaxis for these patients. Overall, there is a low incidence of thromboembolism (DVT and pulmonary embolism) relating to foot and ankle trauma.[10] Due to this low incidence, the American College of Chest Physicians Evidence-Based Clinical Practice

TABLE 25.2 Postoperative Management of Foot Fractures

	Week 1	Weeks 2-3	Weeks 3-12	Months 4-5	Month 6
Calcaneus					
Tongue-type, intra-articular, nondisplaced	Well-padded splint or cast-NWB[a]	Short leg NWB cast	Remove any sutures, boot, ROM[b] therapy, NWB	Slowly advance to CWBAT[d]	Unrestricted activity
Talus					
Head, neck, body, lateral process, nondisplaced	Well-padded splint or cast-NWB	Short leg NWB cast	Remove any sutures; **if pins present, recast** until pins are out; boot; ROM therapy; NWB	Slowly advance to CWBAT	Unrestricted activity
Navicular	Well-padded splint or cast-NWB	Short leg NWB cast	Remove any sutures; **if pins present, recast** until pins are out; boot; ROM therapy; NWB; **remove pins week 7-8**	Slowly advance to CWBAT	Unrestricted activity
Cuboid	Well-padded splint or cast-NWB	Short leg NWB cast	Remove any sutures; **if pins present, recast** until pins are out; boot; ROM therapy; NWB; **remove pins week 7-8**	Slowly advance to CWBAT	Unrestricted activity
Cuneiforms	Well-padded splint or cast-NWB	Short leg NWB cast	Remove any sutures; **if pins present, recast** until pins are out; boot; ROM therapy; NWB; **remove pins week 7-8**	Slowly advance to CWBAT	Unrestricted activity
Metatarsals	Cast-NWB (if painful or surgery) or shoe-WBAT[c]	Cast-NWB (if painful or surgery) or shoe-WBAT	Remove any sutures; **if pins present, recast** until pins are out; boot; ROM therapy; NWB; **remove pins week 7-8**	Slowly advance to CWBAT	Unrestricted activity
Phalanges	Cast-NWB (if painful or surgery) or shoe-WBAT	Cast-NWB (if painful or surgery) or shoe-WBAT	Remove any sutures; **if pins present, recast** until pins are out; boot; ROM therapy; **remove pins week 6, then WBAT**	Unrestricted activity	

[a]Non–weight-bearing (NWB).
[b]Range of motion (ROM) and strengthening.
[c]Weight-bearing as tolerated (WBAT).
[d]Controlled WBAT (CWBAT). While wearing boot, this is obtained by having the patient press foot down onto a scale. Week 1 to 2, 25 % body weight applied to foot; week 3 to 4, 50% week 5 to 6, 75% after week 6, WBAT.

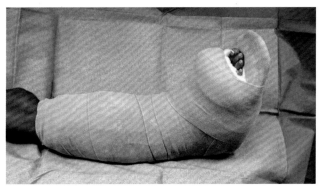

FIGURE 25.1 A typical postoperative splint; cotton batting is used for compression, and plaster splints are placed around the leg, to immobilize the foot and ankle.

Guidelines suggest no prophylaxis be used in patients with isolated lower leg injuries requiring lower leg immobilization.[11] Given this information, the authors' preference is to avoid the use of DVT prophylaxis when managing patients with fractures of the foot.

Lastly, two other issues that patients frequently have questions about include implant removal and the use of nonsteroidals during the healing phase of the fractures. In the former, the authors' preference is to not remove any implants unless they become an irritant. Patients are told that they may choose to have the implant(s) removed but that the authors' preference is not to take them out sooner than after a minimum of 12 months. The reason for delaying removal, if there are no complications related to the implants themselves (eg, loosening or failure of fixation), is that the

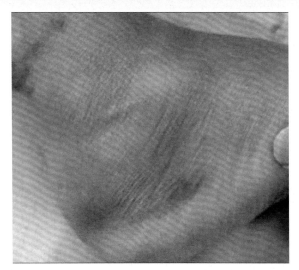

FIGURE 25.2 Clinical appearance of the lateral border of the hindfoot in a patient with a calcaneal fracture. Note the wrinkling of the skin, which occurred at 3 weeks post-injury.

implant contacting the surface of the bone may damage the blood supply to that area, producing some bony necrosis. This will result in remodeling (removal and replacement, ie, creeping substitution) that removes the dead bone and results in a temporary period of porosis, usually beginning 2 to 3 months after the onset of necrosis.[12] After 12 months, the fractures should have healed, the entire bone will have been completely revascularized, and implant removal can then be performed without a concern of producing a secondary fracture through the area of porotic bone.

The second issue concerns the use of a nonsteroidal anti-inflammatory drug (NSAID), especially during the healing phase of the fracture. The NSAID is attractive for use in fractures because it helps control swelling and decreases the need for opioids. However, there is strong evidence that conventional NSAIDs impair bone healing, prolong healing time, decrease the mechanical properties of bone, such as strength, and cause a deterioration in the quality of newly

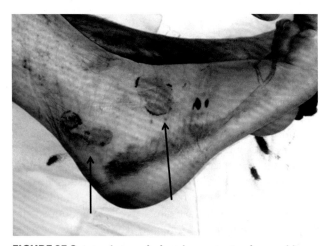

FIGURE 25.3 Lateral view of a foot demonstrating fracture blisters (arrows) that are almost completely healed, indicating that the patient is ready for surgery. (robert_ostrum@med.unc.edu.)

formed bone.[13] It does this by interfering with the production of certain types of prostaglandins (PGs), which in turn inhibits the function of cyclooxygenase (COX) isozymes. These isozymes produce PGs necessary for normal cell activity (COX-1) and those that are involved in the inflammatory response (COX-2). This leads to a loss of PG production that are necessary at the site of the fracture, which then affects the proper blood flow for the entire bone healing cascade.[13] In fact, a recent study showed that patients given NSAIDs, those with type-I or type-II diabetes, or patients that had been involved in a motor vehicle accident were the three most common group of patients demonstrating high odds of developing fracture-healing complications, when compared to a control group of similarly managed fractures.[14] This has been identified regardless as to whether patients had long or short (less than 90 days) histories of NSAID use.[15] With concern for the issues affecting fracture healing, it is the authors' preference to avoid the use of any NSAID during the first 90 days of postfracture management.

CALCANEUS FRACTURES

Calcaneus fractures represent 2% of all fractures. Anatomically, the calcaneus has four articular surfaces, two processes, and a large posterior area of bone, known as the tuberosity. The tuberosity is the site of attachment for the Achilles tendon, plantar fascia, and the short adductors and abductors of the forefoot. Of its four articular surfaces, three lie superiorly (anterior, middle, and posterior facets) and articulate with the talus while the fourth is distal and articulates with the cuboid. The two processes are anterior, near the cuboid, and medial (sustentaculum tali), which supports the talar neck and part of talar body. The arterial supply to the calcaneus is through the branches of the medial and lateral calcaneal arteries (branches of the posterior tibial and peroneal arteries), lateral and medial plantar arteries, and arteries of the sinus tarsi and the tarsal canal and directly from perforating arteries of the peroneal artery.

Biomechanically, the subtalar joint of the calcaneus allows flexion, extension, abduction, and adduction. At the calcaneocuboid joint, it contributes to supination and pronation, as part of the transverse tarsal, or Chopart joint. When a varus malunion occurs, it produces a flexed, supinated, and rigidly adducted forefoot that restricts eversion. Immobility of the calcaneocuboid joint produces less disability but can also contribute to mobility problems of the subtalar or talonavicular joints.[16]

Radiographically, lateral x-rays of the foot are used to measure the amount of intra-articular displacement, described using Böhler angle and the crucial angle of Gissane (**Figure 25.4**). Böhler angle, normally 20° to 40°, describes collapse (impaction) of the posterior facet, when the angle is described as either flat (zero) or with a negative value. The crucial angle of Gissane supports the lateral process of the talus and also describes a fracture of the posterior facet when the angle is described as being increased.

Historically, lateral plain radiographs have been used to describe fracture patterns, based on its relationship to posterior facet. Computed tomography (CT) scans have

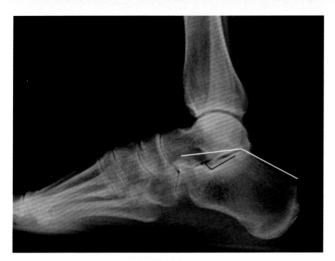

FIGURE 25.4 Lateral x-ray of the foot demonstrating Böhler angle (yellow line) and the angle of Gissane (red line).

significantly improved our ability to evaluate and understand intra-articular displacement of calcaneal fractures. Using CT scans has led to the development of classifications, consisting of four patterns (types I-IV) based on the coronal CT scan. Type I are described as nondisplaced fractures. Type II has two posterior facet fragments with three subtypes (A, B, and C). Type III has three posterior facet fragments, with a centrally depressed segment, and the same three subtypes as type II. Type IV describes a comminuted posterior facet with four or more fragments. However, there is little intra- or interobserver agreement as to the subtype patterns. Recently, the Orthopaedic Trauma Association (OTA) compendium has come forward with a much simpler classification in which it has divided *all calcaneal fractures* into types A, B, and C. Type A describes fractures of the anterior process, sustentaculum tali or the tuberosity with further subdivision into noncomminuted (type 1) or comminuted (type 2) patterns. Type B describes nonarticular body fractures and classifies them into those with or without comminution. Type C describes fractures involving the posterior facet and divides them into nondisplaced, two-part fractures, three-part fractures, or those with four or more parts.[17]

Fracture Patterns

Nondisplaced Fractures

If the decision is made to offer the patient a nonoperative treatment, it should be reserved for the nondisplaced fracture. Other factors for using nonoperative care should include significant medical comorbidities that preclude any surgical intervention, chronic steroid dependency, bed- or wheelchair-bound patients, patients who present with significant peripheral vascular disease, neuropathic patients, those with a substantial smoking history that would affect overall healing, or as a staged approach to allow the soft-tissue envelope to improve to safely allow surgery to be performed. The nonoperative treatment of these fractures usually involves placing the patient into a non–weight-bearing cast for 3 weeks. The patient is kept non–weight-bearing for the first 12 weeks and is then advanced to full weight-bearing over

the next 6 weeks. The return to unrestricted activity is usually allowed at 5 months. For management see **Table 25.2**.

Tuberosity (Tongue-Type) Fractures

Most of these are extra-articular fractures, but some can have a small remnant of posterior facet. Because of the potential for skin necrosis at the Achilles region, these fractures often require emergent, or at the minimum, urgent care (**Figure 25.5**). Fixation can be performed using either a

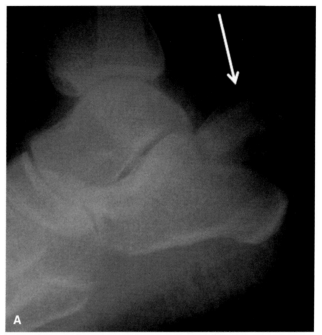

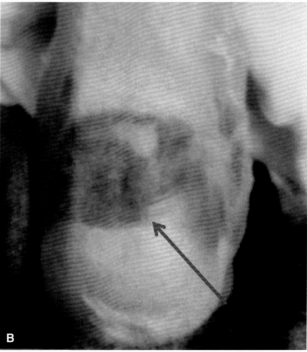

FIGURE 25.5 A, Lateral view of the heel demonstrating a patient who sustained a displaced tongue-type fracture of the calcaneus (arrow). **B**, Clinical appearance of the patient who was referred for treatment at 36 hours after the injury. Note the ecchymosis and potential skin necrosis that has occurred (arrow) on the skin.

formal open approach, a minimally invasive approach, or through a percutaneous, paratendinous technique. Due to pull of the Achilles tendon, if the tuberosity fracture cannot be reduced, a lengthening of the Achilles tendon or the use of gastrocnemius recession (Strayer) technique is often necessary to allow a reduction of the fracture (**Figure 25.6**). For postoperative care see **Table 25.2**.

Articular Fractures

The goals for these fractures are to reconstruct the height, narrow the width, reconstruct the length, correct the deformity of the tuberosity, and reduce the joint (**Figure 25.7**). Although there has been some recent discussion in managing these injuries, using percutaneous or limited approaches, most of these fractures are usually approached via a lateral, extensile approach (**Figure 25.8**). Once the height, length, width, varus deformity, and the articular surface have been provisionally reduced, definitive fixation can then be accomplished using 3.5-, 2.7-, or 2.0-mm screws, combined with low-profile, preformed, locked calcaneal plates. A variation of the articular fracture is an isolated fracture of the sustentaculum tali. When displaced, the authors' preference is to use an open technique medially, in which lag screws are used to compress the fracture and miniplates are used as a buttress or neutralization type of fixation, in order to avoid malalignment at the subtalar joint (**Figure 25.9**). For postoperative care see **Table 25.2**.

Rehabilitation Protocols for Calcaneal Fractures

Regardless whether patients have been treated operatively or nonoperatively, all patients are treated with immobilization, in a cast or splint, for the first 3 weeks. This period of time will allow the soft-tissue envelope to improve, if treated nonoperatively, or allow the surgical incisions to heal. In patients with tuberosity fractures, in which surgery to the Achilles or gastrocnemius has been performed, the authors' preference is to splint the foot into a mild plantar flexed position, with

the patient recasted and slowly dorsiflexed every 2 weeks until a neutral position of the ankle has been achieved. This may take 4 to 6 weeks.

Unless the patient has a nondisplaced extra-articular calcaneal fracture, the authors' preference is for all calcaneal fractures to maintain non–weight-bearing for the first 12 weeks. For those with extra-articular nondisplaced fractures, weight-bearing is begun at 8 weeks. After the splint or cast has been permanently removed, usually at the 3 week mark, patients are placed into a compression stocking, given a removable hinged boot, and sent to physical therapy for range of motion and flexibility exercises. After either 8 or 12 weeks, the patients are slowly advanced to full weight-bearing over the subsequent 6 weeks, and therapy should also include strengthening exercises. Unrestricted activity is allowed at 4 months, for nondisplaced fractures, and at 5 months for all other patients. For management and postoperative care, see **Table 25.2**.

As the calcaneus contributes to motion as part of the subtalar joint, the goal is to obtain similar motion to the non-injured, contralateral extremity. This motion at this joint usually has a *maximum range of motion being* 50° (30° inversion and 20° eversion).[18] Clinically, a practical average range of motion, which will easily allow activities of daily to be performed, is 25° to 30° of inversion and 5° to 10° of eversion. However, as part of the talocalcaneonavicular joint, it also contributes to eversion and inversion of the whole foot, and this motion has been measured for a total *range of motion of* 90° (30° eversion and 60° inversion).[19]

Special Considerations
Age

In the elderly, internal fixation of calcaneal fractures has demonstrated healing rates, complications, and outcomes equivalent to those of younger patients.[20,21] The only difference has been an increase in the development of posttraumatic

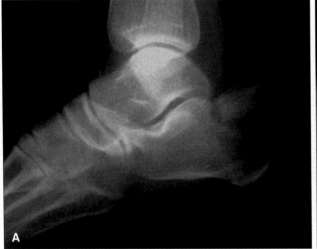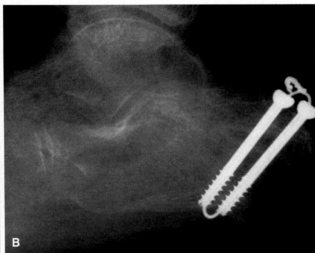

FIGURE 25.6 A, Lateral x-ray of a foot demonstrating a displaced tongue-type fracture. **B**, X-ray demonstrating fixation of the fracture using percutaneous placed screws.

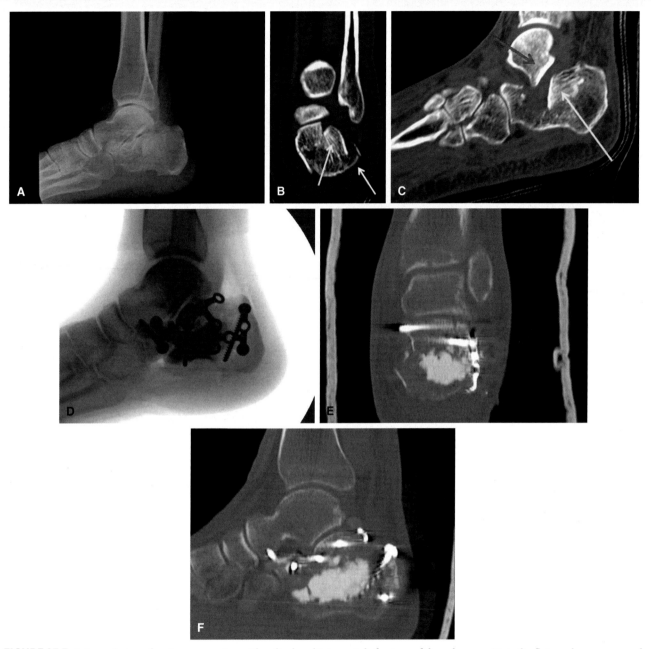

FIGURE 25.7 **A**, Lateral view of patient presenting with a displaced intra-article fracture of the calcaneus. Note the flattened appearance of the calcaneus. **B**, Coronal computed tomography (CT) scan demonstrating the impaction with a lateral wall that has been pushed out (white arrow) and lateral third of the joint pushed plantarly (yellow arrow). **C**, Sagittal CT scan demonstrating a 90° rotation that has occurred to the lateral third of the joint (yellow arrow). The joint should be facing the talus (red arrow). **D**, Lateral view post-fixation of the fracture with plates and screws. **E**, Postoperative coronal CT scan demonstrating reduction of the joint. **F**, Sagittal CT scan demonstrating the reduction that has been achieved.

arthritis of the subtalar joint of the elderly, which has been attributed to some preexisting arthritis.[21] Today's generation of elderly are healthier, more mobile, and much more active than previous generations, with great numbers exceeding the national guidelines of moderate activity for at least 30 minutes per day.[22] Although some literature has demonstrated some bias against offering fixation to the elderly,[23] the decision driving treatment should be based primarily on the injury pattern and not solely on the patient's age.

Nonoperative Care

Displaced intra-articular fractures represent almost 75% of all calcaneal fractures. Fixation is demanding, the soft-tissue envelope is vulnerable, the calcaneus has a complex anatomy, and these injuries are known to have high rates of complications with and without surgery. Even with recent advancements, however, the management is still controversial and nonoperative approaches have been proposed.[23]

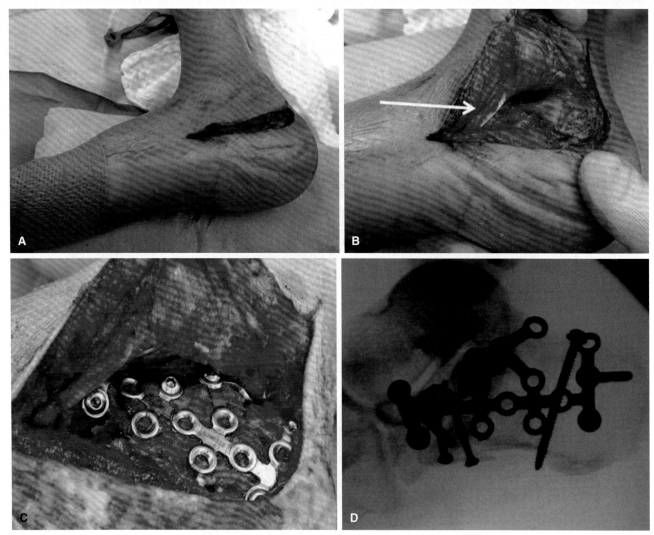

FIGURE 25.8 A, Clinical view of the surgical incision on the lateral border of the heel. **B,** The dissection is performed subperiosteally and is elevated as a full-thickness fasciocutaneous flap deep to the peroneal (arrow) tendons. **C,** The plate has been placed on the lateral border of the calcaneus to maintain the fixation. **D,** Lateral radiograph of the fixation.

If nonoperative treatment is used for displaced intra-articular fractures, poor outcomes with significant complications can occur, resulting in a difficult salvage of these injuries. In these patients, the tuberosity displaces laterally and superiorly, producing a malunited varus or valgus hindfoot. The calcaneus widens, leading to the development of painful bony exostoses, calcaneofibular impingement, and problems with shoe wear. Continued impaction decreases the height of the calcaneus and leads to a talar declination and the potential for anterior impingement of the tibiotalar joint. This is in addition to the development of posttraumatic arthritis in the subtalar, lateral ankle, and calcaneocuboid joints (**Figure 25.10**). These bony abnormalities can lead to impingement, entrapment, or dislocation of the peroneal tendons and the posterior tibial and sural nerves. It can also result in pressure necrosis to the skin, necessitating free tissue transfers or even result in an amputation in a nonsalvageable extremity.

Surgical Complications

Good to excellent outcomes can be expected in nondisplaced fractures or those with adequate reductions and fixation. However, posttraumatic arthritis of the subtalar joint can still occur. In tuberosity fractures, failure of fixation or a malreduction of the fragment can occur, producing a flattened heel or an elevated fragment. Other complications can include entrapments or lacerations of the Achilles tendon or the sural nerve resulting from the fixation that was used during the management of the fracture.

For articular fractures managed with internal fixation, healing rates have approached 97%. The most common soft-tissue complications consist of dehiscence and wound edge necrosis, which occurs in 2% of all closed fractures and commonly occurs at the apex of the incision. Although deep infections can occur, most wounds can often be managed with nonoperative approaches. Other soft-tissue complications include damage to the sural nerve, scarring of the tarsal

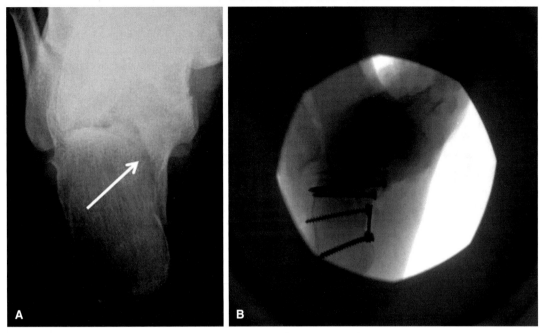

FIGURE 25.9 A, Harris view of the calcaneus demonstrating a large fracture of the sustentaculum tali (arrow). **B**, Intraoperative Harris view demonstrating the fixation of the calcaneus.

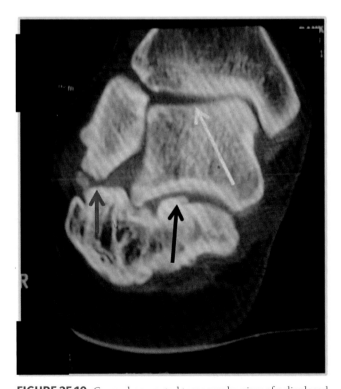

FIGURE 25.10 Coronal computed tomography view of a displaced calcaneal fracture treated nonoperatively. Note the malaligned subtalar joint (black arrow), the lateral half of the joint that has been pushed laterally causing malalignment of the fibula (red arrow), which has ultimately produced a malalignment of the ankle joint (yellow arrow).

tunnel, and nonspecific heel pain. Bony complications consist of malreductions and the development of arthritis, similar to those identified with the nonoperative management of displaced fractures.

In fractures of the sustentaculum tali, nonoperative care of displaced fractures can lead to malalignment or collapse of the subtalar joint. For fractures managed surgically, open reductions can damage or produce impingement to the posterior tibial, the flexor hallucis longus, and flexor digitorum longus tendons.

TALUS FRACTURES

The talus is an interesting bone because it has no tendinous attachments and has more than 60% of its surface covered with articular cartilage. It is divided into a head, neck, and body and articulates superiorly with the tibia, laterally with the fibular, inferiorly with the calcaneus, and distally with the navicular. The extraosseous blood supply arises from the dorsalis pedis, peroneal, and posterior tibial arteries, with the latter two giving rise to the arteries of the tarsal sinus and the tarsal canal. There are also intraosseous arteries that supply blood to the head, neck, the posterior talar tubercle, and the medial talar body. The artery of the tarsal canal supplies most of the body while the artery of the dorsal pedis helps supply the head and neck.

Biomechanically, the talus links motion from the leg to the foot, allowing gait to proceed from heel strike to toe lift. At the talocrural (ankle) joint, it allows dorsiflexion and plantar flexion. At the syndesmosis, it produces external rotation of the fibula (during dorsiflexion) and internal rotation (during plantar flexion). At the subtalar joint, it contributes to flexion-abduction and extension-adduction of the hindfoot. Lastly, it contributes to pronation and supination at the midfoot, as part of the transverse tarsal (Chopart) joint. Therefore, malalignment can compromise motion of the ankle, subtalar, and transverse tarsal joints.

The radiographic evaluation is obtained using plain radiographic views consisting of anteroposterior, mortise, and lateral views of the ankle. At times, specialized (Canale) views are used to evaluate the neck of the talus, but more often, CT scans are utilized to determine the damage that has occurred to the articular surfaces and in identifying the fracture patterns. This is extremely important in helping to decide whether a fracture can be treated nonoperatively.

Fractures are classified as those occurring to the talar neck, body, head, lateral, and posterior processes or those producing an osteochondral injury. Historically, talar neck fractures have been classified as presenting with four different patterns, using Hawkins classification with the Canale-Kelly modification.[24,25] For neck fractures, a type I denotes a nondisplaced fracture, type II describes a displaced fracture producing subluxation of the subtalar joint, a type III describes a neck fracture that has produced subluxation or dislocations of both the subtalar and tibiotalar joints,[24] and type IV describes a type III fracture that presents with an associated talonavicular dislocation.[25]

Classifications for fractures of the body are not as commonly recognized and none has gained acceptance because classifications often combine descriptions of both the neck and body fractures. However, to differentiate whether one is dealing with a neck or a body fracture, Inokuchi et al. stated that fracture lines exiting anterior to the lateral process were considered to be neck fractures while those exiting posterior to the lateral process are to be classified as a talar body fracture.[26] Body fractures can also be described as osteochondral injury, presenting as a coronal or sagittal shear, a fracture of the posterior tubercle or the lateral process, or presenting as a crush fracture.

The OTA compendium[17] has classified all talus fractures into three *simple* groups: A, B, and C. Group A describes fractures involving the lateral or posterior processes, the talar head, or those producing an avulsion fracture. Group B divides talar neck fractures into three patterns: nondisplaced, displaced with subluxation of the subtalar joint, or displaced with subluxation of both the subtalar and tibiotalar joints. The latter two are also subdivided into noncomminuted, comminuted, or those involving the talar head. Group C divides body fractures into dome fractures, those affecting the subtalar joint, and those involving both the subtalar and tibiotalar joints. All three types of group C fractures are also subdivided into noncomminuted and comminuted patterns.

Fracture Patterns

Nondisplaced Fractures

Nondisplaced fractures are uncommon injuries. Any fracture demonstrating more than 1 mm of displacement is diagnosed as being displaced. This is more often made using CT scans and/or magnetic resonance imaging (MRI) scans, which can confirm whether a patient can be treated nonoperatively.

The authors' preferred method for the nonoperative treatment of these fractures is to place the patient into a below-knee, non–weight-bearing cast for 6 weeks. The patient is re-x-rayed every 2 to 3 weeks, to make sure that there has been no displacement, and after 6 weeks, the patient is placed into a removable boot and begins therapy. The patient is kept non–weight-bearing for the first 12 weeks. For management, see **Table 25.2**.

Talar Neck Fractures

Most displaced fractures are managed through a dual-incision approach. The *anterolateral incision* begins distally between the bases of the third and fourth metatarsals and extends toward Chaput tubercle of the tibia. The superficial peroneal nerve is protected as it crosses the field (**Figure 25.11**) just below the skin, and the extensor retinaculum is identified and divided exposing the extensor tendons. The *medial incision* extends from the medial malleolus toward the tuberosity of the navicular and is made just dorsal to the posterior tibial tendon. Working through both incisions allows visualization of the fracture to determine whether an anatomic reduction has been obtained. Posterior and percutaneous approaches are rarely indicated because they do not allow for adequate visualization. As far as fracture-dislocations, the authors' preference is to reduce as soon as possible in order to avoid any necrosis to the underlying soft tissues.

Unless there is comminution, compression techniques are often used to manage these injuries. The goal is to place at least two screws across the fracture. Kirschner (K-wires) pins are only used for provisional fixation or to act as temporary fixation, providing fixation when there is instability identified at the subtalar or talonavicular joint. If comminution is present, compression techniques are avoided, since it produces shortening not only of the neck but also the medial column of the foot. For these fracture patterns, transfixion (nonlag technique) screws or minifragment plates are used in order to maintain length of the talar neck (**Figure 25.12**). Intraoperative fluoroscopy is often used to judge whether an appropriate reduction and length of the talus have been achieved. If there is any instability with any of the adjacent joints, K-wires are placed across those joints to maintain alignment. For postoperative care, see **Table 25.2**.

Talar Body Fractures

Body fractures can present with a sagittal, coronal, or horizontal pattern. To improve exposure, osteotomies of the medial or lateral malleoli may be necessary. Most fractures can be managed using either 2.7- or 3.5-mm screws, which are countersunk and placed perpendicular to the fracture

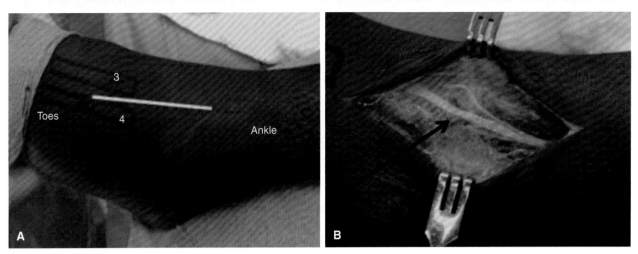

FIGURE 25.11 A, Clinical image demonstrating the surgical incision that is performed for fixation of a talar neck fracture. The incision is started between the third and fourth metatarsals and is extended toward Chaput tubercle on the tibial plafond. **B**, Immediately deep to the skin lies the superficial peroneal nerve (arrow).

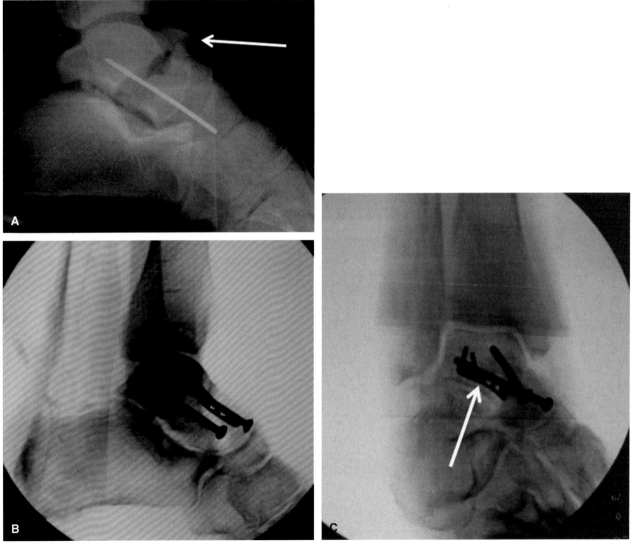

FIGURE 25.12 A, Lateral x-ray of the hindfoot demonstrating a comminuted (arrow) fracture of the talar neck. **B**, Intraoperative lateral view of the hindfoot demonstrating fixation of the talus. **C**, Canale view demonstrating the plate (arrow) that has been used to help maintain the length of the talar neck.

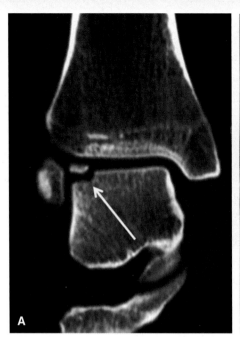
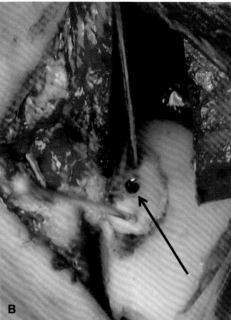

FIGURE 25.13 A, Coronal computed tomography scan demonstrating an osteochondral fracture of the lateral dome of the talus (arrow). **B**, Intraoperative image demonstrating fixation using a screw that has been countersunk below the level of the articular cartilage (arrow).

line. If an adjacent osteochondral fragment is present, the use of a poly-L-lactic acid (PLLA) pin or a small headless screw can also be used (**Figure 25.13**). Due to the articulation with the tibia, it is important that all implants be placed below the articular surface. If adjacent joint instability is detected, temporary K-wires are often placed across the joint to provide stability. For postoperative, care see **Table 25.2**.

Lateral Process Fractures
Lateral process fractures are often overlooked and account for 24% of all body fractures. The injury often results from acute ankle dorsiflexion combined with inversion of the foot and is known by the eponym snowboarder's or skateboarder's fracture. A large, displaced fracture can produce chronic ankle instability and problems with the subtalar joint. The fracture is often approached with an incision placed across the sinus tarsi (Ollier approach). To improve visualization, distraction of the joint is often necessary. If the fragment is a single, large piece, fixation is obtained using one or two 2.0-mm screws. If there is any comminuted present, a minifragment plate is often used to buttress the fracture (**Figure 25.14**). For postoperative care, see **Table 25.2**.

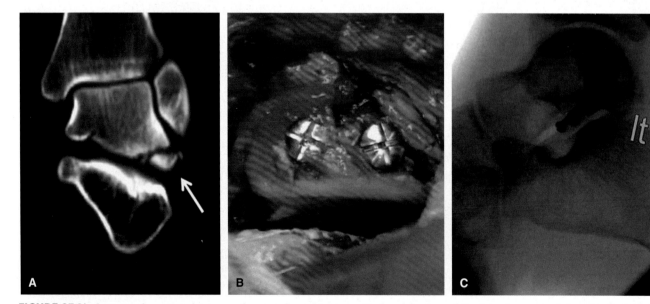

FIGURE 25.14 A, Coronal computed tomography scan demonstrating a displaced fracture of the lateral process of the talus (arrow). **B**, Intraoperative view demonstrating the fixation that has been achieved using two small screws. **C**, Lateral radiograph demonstrating the fixation of the lateral process.

Talar Head Fractures

Displaced fractures can be approached dorsally, medially, anterolaterally, or, if necessary, through two incisions. Fixation is achieved with countersunk 2.4- or 2.0-mm regular or headless screws that can be augmented with the use of PLLA pins, for smaller osteochondral lesions. If fixation is deemed inadequate, the addition of a temporary transarticular pin, placed across the talonavicular joint, will increase stability. If impaction is identified, disimpaction and bone grafting may be needed to restore medial column stability. If excision is contemplated, the goal is to retain at least 70% of the head. If joint instability is noted, the talonavicular joint is pinned using K-wires. For postoperative care, see **Table 25.2**.

Rehabilitation Protocols for Talar Fractures

All patients are treated with immobilization, in a cast or splint, for the first 3 weeks to allow the soft-tissue envelope to improve and the surgical incisions to heal. After the splint or cast has been permanently removed, the patient is placed into a compression stocking and a boot and is sent to therapy for range of motion and strengthening exercises therapy. Unless the patient has a nondisplaced fracture, the authors' preference is for all talus fractures to maintain non–weight-bearing for the first 12 weeks. After these 3 weeks, patients are placed into a removable boot, given compression stockings, and sent to therapy for flexibility and range of motion exercises. K-wires are pulled after 7 to 8 weeks. After 12 weeks, the patients are slowly advanced to full weight-bearing over the subsequent 6 weeks, and therapy now includes strengthening exercises. Unrestricted activity is allowed at 4 months, for nondisplaced fractures, and at 5 months for all other patients. For postoperative care, see **Table 25.2**.

As part of the subtalar joint, the expected *maximum range of motion is 50°* (30° inversion and 20° eversion).[18] Similarly, since it also contributes to eversion and inversion of the foot, as part of talocalcaneonavicular joint, the goal is to obtain a *range of motion of 90°* (30° eversion or supination and 60° inversion or pronation).[19]

Special Considerations

Age

In the elderly patient, a nonoperative approach is likely to occur. The suspected reasons for this approach are that these are small bones, patients are of lower physical demand, the injuries are on the cusp as to whether surgery is indicated, and there is often a subjective feeling that they will "do well" with casting. The indications for surgery for these injuries, however, should be the same regardless of the patient's age, and managing elderly patients similar to nonelderly patients have shown similar outcomes.[27] Therefore, the patient's age should not influence outcomes, but comminution and dislocations or subluxation of the joint, managed nonoperatively, will affect outcomes.

Timing of Surgery

No difference exists as to whether fractures were treated before or after 6 hours. However, fracture-dislocations are urgently reduced, in order to avoid necrosis of the adjacent soft tissues. Despite an anatomic reduction, however, outcomes have demonstrated that at an average of 3 years, some patients may still develop significant functional impairments, especially for talar neck fractures.[28]

Malunions

Delayed unions or nonunions are relatively uncommon, with a reported incidence occurring between 4% and 13%. However, malunions of talar fractures occur more frequently. For patients presenting with talar neck fractures, malunions are often seen with inadequate fixation. This produces a shortened talar neck, which leads to an adducted deformity of the forefoot. Malunions may also result due to a missed fracture or from a loss of the surgical reduction. In fractures of the talar body, a malunion usually results from inadequate visualization or poor reduction techniques, frequently seen after using closed or percutaneous methods (**Figure 25.15**). Poor reductions or failure of fixation directly affects the development of posttraumatic arthritis in both the ankle and subtalar joints. For fractures of the lateral process, outcomes are directly attributed to inadequately treated or missed injuries. The complications associated with lateral process fractures consist of chronic lateral ankle instability, nonunions, and a potential impingement of the ankle at the talofibular joint. Lastly, nonunions of talar head fractures are exceedingly rare, but malunions occur due to inadequate reductions or if displaced fractures are managed nonoperatively. This can lead to the development of talonavicular arthrosis.

Avascular Necrosis

Avascular necrosis (AVN) of the talus has received the most attention in the literature, often because it is the most devastating outcome for these injuries. Fractures or fracture-dislocations are often associated with disruptions of the intraosseous and extraosseous blood supply, which leads to healing problems and ultimately produces avascular areas of the talus. Historically, AVN for talar neck fractures has been reported to approach 60% to 100% of all patients. However, recent studies, utilizing modern reduction techniques, have

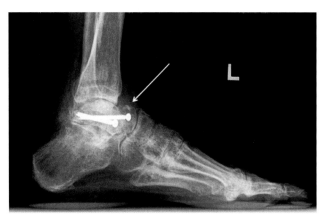

FIGURE 25.15 Lateral view of the foot demonstrating dorsiflexion malreduction of the talar head and neck (arrow).

reported an incidence of 36% to 40%.[27,29] For talar body fractures, the incidence has been reported in 35% to 40% of patients, usually noted in those presenting with open fractures, those with significant comminution, or those associated talar neck fractures.[30] AVN of the talar head is uncommon but can occur in about 10% of all cases, usually as a result of malalignment of the fracture.

Posttraumatic Arthritis

The most common complication, for any kind of talar fracture, is the development of posttraumatic arthritis. Displaced fractures treated nonoperatively run the highest risk of developing posttraumatic arthrosis. Historically, the incidence has been reported to approach 90% for the ankle and 50% for the subtalar joint. However, recent literature has shown an incidence of 65% for ankle joints and 35% for the subtalar joint.[28,30] Additionally, other studies have reported that 60% to 100% of patients with talus fractures will eventually develop some arthritis in the ankle, subtalar, or talonavicular joint.[17,27] However, the degree of arthritis is variable. For fractures of the lateral process and the talar head, the development of arthritis is usually seen in the subtalar or talonavicular joints.

MIDFOOT FRACTURES

The midfoot extends from the talonavicular-calcaneocuboid (midtarsal or Chopart) joint to the tarsometatarsal (Lisfranc) joint and consists of the navicular, cuboid, and the three cuneiforms. Evaluating motion of the midfoot has demonstrated that with isolation of specific joints, an average of 26° (range 2.3-33.8) of supination-pronation has been identified at Chopart joint with an average of 4.3° (range 0.2-9.9) at the naviculocuneiform joints. For dorsiflexion-plantar flexion, the average motion identified at Chopart joint is 9.3° (range 0.2-14.9) with an average of 4.3° (range 0.7-7.2) at the naviculocuneiform joints.[31]

NAVICULAR FRACTURES

The navicular is horseshoe shaped with a proximal concavity articulating with the talar head and a distal kidney shape articulating with the cuneiforms. It provides for the calcaneonavicular portion of the bifurcate ligament and has the posterior tibial tendon insert onto its prominent tuberosity, before reaching the cuneiforms and cuboid. Dorsally it is supplied by the dorsalis pedis, and plantarly by a medial plantar branch of the posterior tibial artery, and the tuberosity is supplied by a network of vessels. Biomechanically, the navicular is the keystone for the medial longitudinal arch of the foot. If motion of the subtalar joint is affected, it also limits motion at the talonavicular joint.[16]

Historically, four types of fractures have been identified: cortical avulsion or dorsal lip fractures, stress fractures, fractures of the tuberosity, and fractures of the body. Body fractures are the most severe and often present with other foot injuries. The OTA compendium has proposed a *simple*

approach toward the classification of fractures of the navicular. They have divided all navicular fractures into one of two types: A, without comminution, and B, with comminution.[17]

Nonoperative Treatment

Nonoperative care should be considered only for nondisplaced body fractures, cortical avulsions, or minimally displaced tuberosity fractures. Fragments involving greater than or equal to 20% of the articular surface, those with a greater than 1 mm step-off, or fractures producing talonavicular or naviculocuneiform instability or subluxation should be treated surgically. The authors' preference for the conservative management of these injuries consists of a non–weight-bearing cast for 4 weeks with the patient kept non–weight-bearing for the first 12 weeks. For management, see **Table 25.2**.

Tuberosity and Body Fractures

Surgical management is divided into excisions and fixation. Excision of fragments is directed toward cortical avulsions or small tuberosity fractures that will not affect the stability of the midfoot, while fixation is directed toward body fractures. In large tuberosity fractures, with at least 5 mm of displacement, early fixation rather than excision should be performed in order to avoid a progressive planovalgus deformity (**Figure 25.16**). If fixation is tenuous, a transarticular fixation, extended toward the cuneiforms, using either screws or K-wires is used. Total excision of the navicular is usually avoided because it produces shortening of the medial column and malrotation of the forefoot. For postoperative care, see **Table 25.2**.

CUBOID FRACTURES

The cuboid is a pyramidal-shaped bone with its base located medially and its apex laterally. Distally it articulates with the fourth and fifth metatarsals, proximally with the calcaneus, medially with the lateral cuneiform, and posteromedially with the navicular. Its blood supply is from a plantar arterial rete, from the lateral and medial plantar arteries, and a contribution from the dorsal arterial rete. Biomechanically, it is a spacer to the lateral column of the foot, with a loss of length producing a flatfoot deformity. With the talonavicular joint, it "locks" and "unlocks" the midtarsal region necessary for heel strike and toe-lift.[3] Immobility (fusion) across the calcaneocuboid joint does not produce much disability to either the subtalar to talonavicular joints.[16]

Historical eponyms, such as a "nutcracker fracture," have been used to describe injuries that compress the cuboid between the calcaneus and the metatarsals, but there are no accepted classifications. Currently, fractures are described as extra-articular or avulsion and intra-articular or compression. Extra-articular fractures are the most common. They occur on the lateral aspect of the foot and do not disrupt the lateral column of the foot. Intra-articular fractures involve the entire body of the cuboid or may just involve the articular surface of the tarsometatarsal joint, leading to shortening or dorsal subluxation of the lateral column. The OTA compendium has

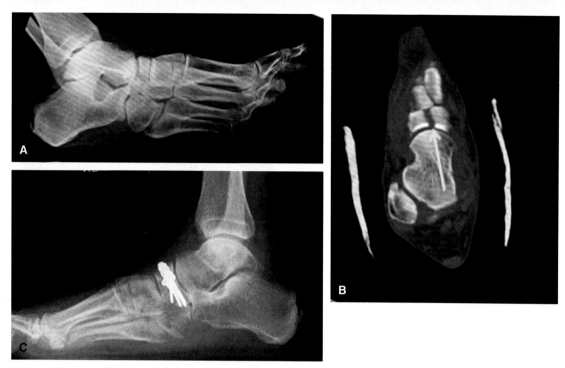

FIGURE 25.16 A, Oblique x-ray of foot demonstrating a displaced (arrow) navicular fracture. **B**, Axial computed tomography scan demonstrating the displacement between the fragments (arrow). **C**, Postoperative lateral view of the foot demonstrating the fixation of the navicular fracture.

proposed a *simple* approach toward classifying cuboid fractures. All fractures have been divided into two patterns: type A, without comminution, and type B, with comminution.[17]

Nonoperative Treatment

Most cuboid fractures present as closed injuries, often with no or minimal displacement. Fractures with little or no articular involvement or those without changes to the morphology of the cuboid can be treated conservatively. This consists of a non–weight-bearing cast for 3 to 4 weeks followed by the use of a boot. The patient is allowed to weight bear once they have the boot and can progress to full weight-bearing as tolerated. For management, see **Table 25.2**.

Operative Treatment

Isolated injuries are rare and are often seen in conjunction with injuries occurring to the tarsometatarsal (TMT) joints. Fractures presenting with a depressed articular fragment, comminution producing shortening of the lateral column, or any injuries producing any dislocations, subluxations, or tenting of the skin are usually managed surgically. As with other midfoot injuries, if fixation is tenuous, an external fixator or transarticular pin fixation across the calcaneus or metatarsals is often used to provide additional stability (**Figure 25.17**). For postoperative care, see **Table 25.2**.

CUNEIFORM FRACTURES

The medial, middle, and lateral cuneiforms are wedge-shaped bones helping to form the transverse arch of the foot. They are supplied by the dorsal arterial rete. Biomechanically,

they provide stability to the medial column of the foot and contribute to the motion of the transverse arch. They allow for compressive forces on the convex (dorsal) side of the foot and tensile forces on the concave (plantar) side. They

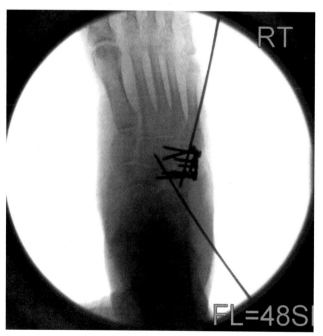

FIGURE 25.17 Anteroposterior (AP) view of the foot demonstrating fixation of a cuboid fracture. Due to periarticular instability, Kirschner wires (K-wires) have also been placed across the calcaneocuboid and fifth tarsometatarsal joints to maintain the alignment of the hindfoot.

also contribute to a small amount of pronation-supination and dorsiflexion-plantar flexion through the tarsometatarsal joints.

Injuries are the result of direct trauma and are described as fractures to the medial, middle, or lateral cuneiforms. Their most common presentation is either as an avulsion or as a nondisplaced fracture. Most fractures are identified as a component of the tarsometatarsal (Lisfranc) joint. The OTA compendium has proposed a *simple* approach in classifying and describing all fractures as those involving the medial, middle, or lateral cuneiform and dividing them into type A, without comminution, and type B, with comminution.[17]

Nonoperative Treatment

The authors' preference for nondisplaced or avulsion fractures is a non–weight-bearing cast for 4 weeks followed by a walking boot for an additional 4 to 6 weeks. For management, see **Table 25.2**.

Operative Treatment

Displaced fractures should be evaluated for midtarsal instability. This can be obtained through the use of CT scans, weight-bearing films, if tolerated by the patient, or through intraoperative stress films. If instability is identified, fixation consists of using a method of transarticular fixation to the other cuneiforms, the metatarsals, or the navicular using plates, screws, or pins, sometimes in combinations, to maintain stability and length across the midfoot. For postoperative care, see **Table 25.2**.

REHABILITATION PROTOCOLS FOR MIDFOOT FRACTURES

All patients are treated with immobilization, in a cast or splint, for the first 3 weeks to allow the soft-tissue envelope to improve and the surgical incisions to heal. After the splint or cast has been permanently removed, the patient is placed into a compression stocking and boot and is sent to therapy for range of motion and strengthening exercises therapy. As with other fractures of the foot and unless the patient has a nondisplaced fracture, the authors' preference is for all midfoot fractures to maintain non–weight-bearing for the first 12 weeks. After the first 3 weeks, the patient is placed into removable boot, given compression stockings, and sent to physical therapy for flexibility and range of motion exercises. After 12 weeks, patients are slowly advanced to full weight-bearing over the subsequent 6 weeks and with therapy to include the addition of strengthening exercises. Unrestricted activity is allowed at 4 months, for nondisplaced fractures, and at 5 months for all other patients. For management and postoperative care, see **Table 25.2**.

As part of Chopart and Lisfranc joints, a *maximum range of motion of 50° (30° supination and 20° pronation)* is the goal.[18] However, more motion is possible since Chopart joint is also part of the talocalcaneonavicular complex. Combining Chopart and Lisfranc joints can allow a *maximum of 90° (60°*

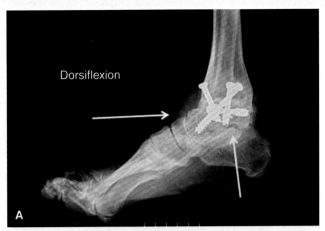

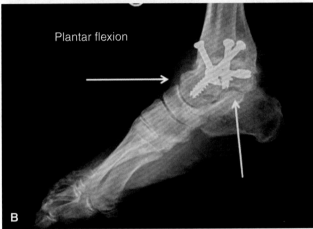

FIGURE 25.18 A, Patient status post ankle arthrodesis demonstrating dorsiflexion of Chopart joint with elevation at the talonavicular joint (white arrow) and narrowing of the subtalar (yellow arrow) joint. **B**, During plantar flexion, Chopart joint demonstrates plantar flexion of the talonavicular (white arrow) joint and widening of the subtalar (yellow arrow) joint.

of supination or inversion and 30° of pronation or eversion).[19] To obtain these measurements, the examiner should hold the leg, at the level of the malleoli, with one hand, and then rotate the entire foot into supination and pronation. Although dorsiflexion and plantar flexion may also be identified at Chopart joint, it may be very difficult to measure this motion but can often be identified using fluoroscopy or with passive manipulation under standard lateral radiographs (**Figure 25.18**).

SPECIAL CONSIDERATIONS

Age

As with other injuries in the foot, the patient's age should not influence outcomes. The things that will ultimately affect outcomes are the presence of comminution, dislocations, or subluxation of the joint(s). Valid reasons for avoiding surgery in the elderly can include bed- or wheelchair-bound patients, patients with severe vascular problems that prevent any surgery from being performed, patients presenting with severe medical problems that preclude any surgical intervention, or patient/family refusal to have any surgery performed. If the patient does not fall into these categories, then the indications for surgery should be based on the injuries not on the patient's age. Managing elderly patients and nonelderly patients in an identical manner has shown similar outcomes.[27]

Malunions and Nonunions

Complications increase with the conservative care of displaced fractures, and outcomes are dependent on the adequacy of the reduction and residual joint instability. For displaced fractures treated nonoperatively, the prognosis is poor. Those with anatomic reductions result in better outcome scores, a decrease in subjective complaints, and a gait without significant abnormality.[32] Malunions are often due to malreductions at the time of fixation, inadequate fixation, early removal of implants, or weight-bearing before adequate healing has occurred. This combination produces loosening of the implants or screw breakage, which leads to a failure in the fixation. For the cuboid, the majority of complications and long-term sequelae are often due to nonoperative care leading to intra-articular incongruity, residual lateral column shortening, and forefoot abduction, with a progressive planovalgus deformity. For the navicular and cuneiforms, the nonoperative care of displaced fractures leads to shortening of the medial column, forefoot adduction, and a progressive planovarus deformity.

Nonunions of are fairly uncommon in the cuboid or cuneiforms but have been reported in the navicular. These are often seen after the management of severely comminuted navicular body fractures, usually identified in the central part of the bone.[33] In cases of any identified malunions or nonunions of the midfoot, reconstruction of the bones, with or without an arthrodesis, is the treatment of choice. When an arthrodesis is used, it not only decreases the motion of that specific joint but can also decrease motion to other areas of the mid- and hindfoot.[16]

Posttraumatic Arthritis

This is probably the most common complication associated with these injuries. For the navicular, posttraumatic arthritis, at the talonavicular joint, can be minimized if at least 60% of the articular surface has been restored.[33] For the cuneiforms, the most common cause of arthritis is often due to a failure to diagnose an injury; however, a 25% incidence has been reported for surgically managed Lisfranc injuries.[34] At the cuboid, isolated injuries producing an impaction that are treated nonoperatively can develop arthritis. More commonly, there is often a component of a crush injury of the cuboid leading to a shortening of the lateral column with the development of posttraumatic arthritis either at the calcaneocuboid, at the 4 to 5 tarsometatarsal joints, or both. This becomes more problematic at the tarsometatarsal joints because it decreases the ability for it to act as a shock absorber for dorsiflexion and plantar flexion of the lateral column.[35] Salvage often consists of an arthrodesis of the affected joints which can also affect other joints of the foot.[16]

Avascular Necrosis

For the navicular, a partial or complete AVN rate of 29% has been reported, especially with body fractures.[34,36] However, it is important to differentiate posttraumatic AVN from those patients presenting with the Mueller Weiss syndrome. For patients presenting with posttraumatic AVN, the lateral third of the bone is most commonly affected, causing a medial shift of the forefoot and a progressive hindfoot varus. Radiographs usually demonstrate the talar head articulating with the lateral cuneiform. A patient presenting with the Mueller Weiss syndrome refers to the spontaneous development of AVN. This is seen more often in women and usually presents with a radiographic appearance of a comma-shaped deformity of the navicular, producing medial protrusion of the talar head and perinavicular osteoarthritis. As a differentiating point, in children, AVN of the navicular is referred to Köhler disease and is usually seen between 4 and 6 years of age. There is little to no literature reporting AVN of the cuboid or cuneiforms.

Implant Irritability

Due to the subcutaneous nature of these bones, prominences due to the implants, or sometimes due to the additional development of bony spurs, can produce some discomfort, especially with shoe wear. This may require removal of the implants and spurs to improve symptoms.

FOREFOOT FRACTURES

Overall, the forefoot contains 21 bones consisting of the metatarsals, phalanges, and the two sesamoids, which extend proximally from the tarsometatarsal (Lisfranc) joint to the tips of the toes.

METATARSAL FRACTURES

The bases of the metatarsals articulate with the cuboid and cuneiforms and help form the transverse arch of the foot, with the apex occurring at the base of the second metatarsal. The first metatarsal is broader than the lesser four but is shorter than the second and the third metatarsals. It is important to recognize that all metatarsals are plantar flexed distally, so that all the metatarsal heads are located in the same horizontal plane at ground level. The first dorsal and plantar metatarsal arteries, along with a superficial branch from the medial plantar artery, supply the first metatarsal while metatarsals 2 to 4 obtain their blood supply from a nutrient artery, formed by the dorsal and lateral plantar arteries. Although the fifth metatarsal also obtains its supply from dorsal and plantar metatarsal arteries, the tuberosity is supplied by two additional arteries producing a radiate pattern.

Biomechanically, the first three metatarsals contribute to the medial column of the foot, the fourth and fifth to the lateral column. About one-third of the body weight is transmitted through the first metatarsal. The second and third tarsometatarsal joints bear forces that are two to three times the force across the first or fourth/fifth tarsometatarsal joints, while the third bears the most force at all loads and foot positions. The first, fourth, and fifth tarsometatarsal joints have a more active role in foot position than at a neutral position.[4]

Fractures are classified as occurring in the head, shaft, or the base but can also be described as injuries to the proximal, middle, or distal thirds. Additionally, fractures to the fifth metatarsal have also been classified as a styloid or avulsion (zone I) fracture, tuberosity or diaphyseal-metaphyseal region (type II) fracture, or diaphyseal (type III) fracture.[37] The OTA compendium has classified metatarsal fractures into three patterns. Type I are simple (transverse, oblique, or spiral) noncomminuted diaphyseal fractures or any nonarticular fracture (with or without comminution) of the proximal or distal ends. Type II are comminuted diaphyseal fractures presenting with a wedge of bone (spiral, bending, or comminuted) or any partial articular fracture of the proximal or distal ends. The articular injuries are subclassified as avulsion or partial split, depression, or split/depression fractures. Type III are comminuted diaphyseal fractures (segmental or complex comminuted) or complete comminution of the proximal or distal articular surfaces. The articular fractures are further subclassified, as simple articular patterns, simple articular with a comminuted metaphyseal patterns, or a comminuted articular and metaphyseal pattern.[17]

Nonoperative Treatment

Fractures of the metatarsals are common injuries that may lead to disability if treated poorly. Injuries result either from a direct blow, a twisting type of injury, or may present as a stress fracture. Isolated or multiple fractures,

presenting without any displacement or deformity, can be treated conservatively. If the pain is mild or moderate, they can be placed immediately into a postoperative shoe or a boot and allowed to weight bear as tolerated. Displaced styloid avulsions, at base of the fifth metatarsal, or displaced fractures 1.5 cm distal to the styloid (Jones fracture) can also be treated conservatively with a shoe or a boot. In patients presenting with severe pain that prevents immediate weight-bearing, the authors' preference is to place the patient into a non–weight-bearing cast, for 3 to 4 weeks, followed by a shoe or boot. For management, see **Table 25.2**.

Operative Treatment

Metatarsal fractures presenting with shortening, angular deformities, or changes to the weight distribution of the metatarsal heads require fixation. Fractures to the neck and shaft are often managed with an open reduction using a K-wire (**Figure 25.19**). For displaced fractures of the first metatarsal, plates and screws may be necessary in order to maintain length and rotation. For patients who present with comminuted metatarsal fractures, especially when they occur at the base, plates and screws are often used to span the TMT joint and maintain length until adequate healing has occurred. For postoperative management, see **Table 25.2**.

FRACTURES OF THE PHALANGES

The lesser toes each have three phalanges while only two phalanges are present in the great toe, and since the proximal phalanges are the longest, they are most often injured.

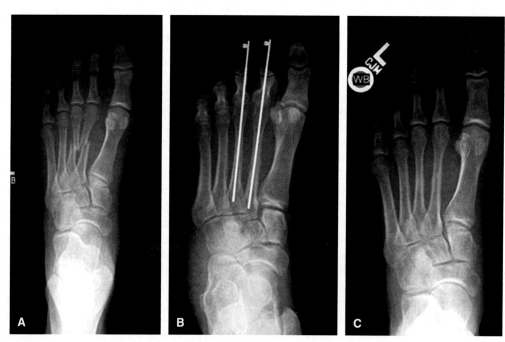

FIGURE 25.19 A, Displaced midshaft fractures of the second and third metatarsals. **B**, Fractures were managed using intramedullary Kirschner wire (K-wire) fixation. **C**, Appearance of the foot at 3 months post-fixation.

The proximal phalanges obtain their blood supply from the dorsal digital arteries, the middle phalanges through plantar and dorsal digital arteries, and the distal phalanges via a plantar supply. Biomechanically, the toes contact the ground during 75% of the stance phase. During heel-rise, the generated force is through an oblique axis from the second through the fifth metatarsophalangeal joints. This is increased by forces from a transverse axis of the first and second metatarsophalangeal joints. Push-off is increased as the transverse axis moves toward the tips of the great toe and second toes, with toes 3 to 5 contributing to a roll-over of the foot.[1]

Historically, fractures have been classified as injuries occurring in proximal, middle, or distal thirds of the phalanx or by describing fractures seen in the proximal or distal articular surfaces. The OTA compendium has classified phalangeal fractures into three types. Type A fractures are simple (transverse, oblique, or spiral) noncommunicated diaphyseal fractures or nonarticular fractures (with or without comminution) of the proximal or distal ends. Type B describes comminuted diaphyseal fractures presenting with wedge of bone (spiral, bending, or comminuted) or partial articular fractures of the proximal or distal ends. The articular fractures are subclassified as avulsion or partial split, depression, or split/depression fractures. Type C describes comminuted diaphyseal fractures (segmental or complex comminuted) or articular fractures with complete comminution of the proximal or distal articular ends. The articular fractures are subclassified as simple articular, simple articular/comminuted metaphyseal, or comminuted articular and metaphyseal fractures. In addition, modifiers describe specific toes. A "T" denotes the great toe and is further delineated as 1-proximal or 2-distal phalanx (eg, T2 describes distal phalanx fracture). An "N" is used for the second toe, "M" for the middle toe, "R" for the ring toe, and "L" for the little toe. The lesser toes are further subclassified 1-proximal, 2-middle, or 3-distal phalanges.[17]

Nonoperative Treatment

Fractures of the lesser toes are often treated with buddy taping it to an adjacent noninjured toe and then placing the patient into a hard-sole shoe. Fractures with some deformity can also be managed nonoperatively, but angular deformities may need to be corrected in order to prevent the development of painful plantar pressures. Immediate weight-bearing in a protective shoe is allowed, and good outcomes can be expected as long as the general alignment is satisfactory. For management, see **Table 25.2**.

Operative Treatment

The primary indication for surgery is a displaced fracture of the proximal phalanx of the great toe, which includes fracture dislocations, displacement of the distal condyles, shaft fractures producing a bayoneting deformity, or angular deformities that may lead to shoe wear problems or a painful gait (**Figure 25.20**). Most often, a simple

pinning is used to manage these fractures, but those presenting with comminution comminuted fractures may need plates and screws. For postoperative care, see **Table 25.2**.

REHABILITATION PROTOCOLS FOR FRACTURES OF THE FOREFOOT

Depending on the fracture pattern, location of the injury, and the patients level of pain, these injuries can be treated either with immobilization, in a cast or splint, for the first 3 weeks, to allow the soft-tissue envelope and the surgical incisions to heal or they may be placed into a stiff-soled shoe and allowed immediate weight-bearing as tolerated. For patients treated nonoperatively, the authors' preference is for all patients with forefoot fractures to be placed into an elastic wrap (Ace wrap), a stiff-soled shoe, and allowed weight-bearing as tolerated. The only addition used for toe fractures is that the injured toe is taped to an adjacent noninjured toe for the first 4 weeks. If the patient has severe pain that prevents them from immediate weight-bearing, the authors' preference is to place the patient into a non–weight-bearing cast for 3 to 4 weeks and then into an elastic wrap, a shoe, and allowed to weight bear as tolerated.

For patients managed surgically, the authors' preference is for the patients to maintain non–weight-bearing for the first 12 weeks, for metatarsal fractures, and 8 weeks for toe fractures. This is done in order to avoid loosening of any implants or bending and breaking any pins that were used during fixation. During this time period, the patient is often immobilized in a cast until the pins are removed, usually at 6 to 8 weeks. After the pins are removed, the patient is placed into removable boot, given a compression stocking, and sent to physical therapy for flexibility and range of motion exercises. It is uncommon that nonoperatively treated patients require any formal rehabilitation. For nonoperatively managed patients, unrestricted activity is allowed after 3 months. For surgically managed metatarsal fractures, these are slowly advanced to full weight-bearing over the subsequent 6 weeks with unrestricted activity allowed at 5 months. For operatively managed phalangeal fractures, unrestricted activity is allowed at 4 months. For management and postoperative care, see **Table 25.2**.

The three joints in the forefoot that need to be rehabilitated consist of the tarsometatarsal, metatarsophalangeal (MTP), and interphalangeal (IP) joints. At the tarsometatarsal joints, the *maximum range of expected motion is* 50° (20° of supination and 30° of pronation).[18] This motion is evaluated by placing the ankle at neutral, holding the heel and hindfoot with one hand, and then placing the forefoot into pronation and supination with the other hand.

At the MTP of the great toe, the *maximum range of expected motion is* 80° (50° of dorsiflexion and 30° of plantar flexion)[18] but has also been recorded with *a maximum range of motion of* 115° (70° of dorsiflexion and 45° of plantar flexion).[19] For MTP joints 2 through 5, the *maximum ranges of expected*

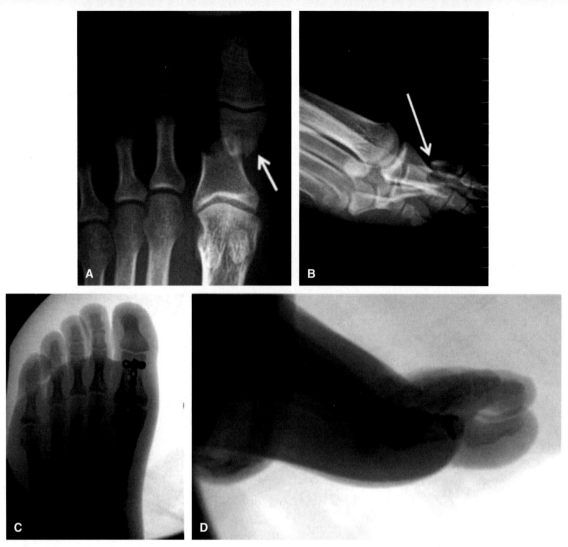

FIGURE 25.20 A, Anteroposterior (AP) x-ray demonstrating a displaced fracture of the proximal phalanx of the great toe (arrow). **B**, Lateral view demonstrating that some overlap or bayoneting (arrow) of the fracture has occurred due to the pull by the extensor tendon. **C**, AP view of the foot demonstrating fixation of the phalanx. **D**, Lateral view of the fixation demonstrating improved alignment of the phalanx.

motion are as follows: *for the second*, 70° (40 dorsiflexion, 30 plantar flexion); *for the third*, 50° (30° dorsiflexion, 20° plantar flexion); *for the fourth*, 30° (20° of dorsiflexion, 10° of plantar flexion); and *for the fifth*, 20° (10° of dorsiflexion, 10° plantar flexion).[16] To accurately measure the MTP and IP joints, it may require that the examiner place the foot onto a hard end plate or board, ending just proximal to the joint(s) being measured.

At the IP joint of the great toe, the *maximum range of expected motion is 30°* (zero degrees of dorsiflexion, because there is no extension, and 30° of plantar flexion).[18] However, other authors have reported a *maximum range of expected motion 80°* (zero degrees dorsiflexion and 80° plantar flexion).[19] For the lesser toes, at the level of the proximal IP joints, the *maximum range of expected motion is 35°* (zero for dorsiflexion and 35° for plantar flexion). At the distal IP joints, the *maximum range of expected motion is 90°* (30° of dorsiflexion and 60° of plantar flexion).[19] Measurement of

the IP joints may be more difficult to obtain unless the foot is also stabilized with a hard plate or board, similar to the method used for measuring the MTP joints.

SPECIAL CONSIDERATIONS

Age

The current elderly are healthier, more mobile, and much more active than previous generations, and as noted for the care of other foot fractures, managing elderly patients in a manner similar to nonelderly patients have shown comparable outcomes.[27] Withholding treatments, due to the expectations that the elderly will not do as well as nonelderly patients comes with the understanding that withholding treatment can produce avoidable complications, result in significant disabilities to the foot, create chronic pain conditions and lead to socio-economic burdens to patients, their families and to payer systems. The decision driving

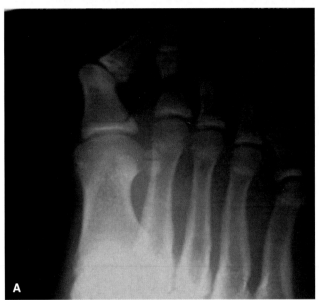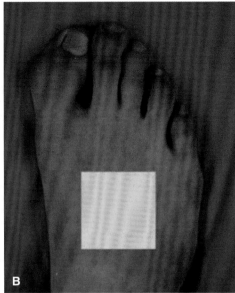

FIGURE 25.21 A, Anteroposterior (AP) x-ray demonstrating malalignment of the great toe due to a displaced fracture of the proximal phalanx managed nonoperatively. **B**, Clinical appearance of the malaligned great toe.

treatment should be based primarily on the injury pattern and not solely on the patient's age. Therefore, it does not appear that age should be used as any contraindication to managing fractures of the forefoot.

Malunions and Nonunions

Nonunions are rare but are often due to loss of reduction, breakage of implants, early removal of implants, or allowing weight-bearing before adequate healing has occurred. For the metatarsals, malunions are more common than nonunions. These malunions are usually identified in the sagittal plane and can be noted during physical examination either with a dorsal prominence and a lack of "presence" of the metatarsal head on the plantar surface, or as a plantar malunion producing a prominent plantar head. These malunions often occur when dorsally or plantarly displaced fractures are treated nonoperatively. The result is that these malunions often produce pain, cause patients to develop painful plantar calluses, produces the mechanical changes in the foot, results in the development of transfer lesions, and leads to disabilities and difficulty with shoe wear.

When malunions occur in the phalanges, symptoms are directly related the amount of anatomic distortion and any pressure that is applied to adjacent toes or to any irritation that occurs from shoe wear. Patients often present with pain and the development of calluses. The most serious type of phalangeal malunion usually occurs in the proximal phalanx of the great toe, often producing a bayonet or angular deformity (**Figure 25.21**). It should be noted that for the metatarsals and the phalanges, the presence of some residual deformity does not often produce much disability. However, when normal weight bearing alignment has been restored, good outcomes can be expected.

Arthritis

Any intra-articular fracture of the phalanges or the metatarsals increases the risk of developing posttraumatic arthritis. In the metatarsals, these are uncommon. A more likely scenario, for the development of arthritis secondary to a metatarsal fracture, is in patients who present with an injury to the TMT joints. However, even in patients with an anatomic reduction of the TMT joint, some arthritis can be expected.[34] Patients identified with nonanatomic reductions of the TMT joints can expect to have higher levels of pain, gait abnormalities, difficulties with shoe wear, more posttraumatic arthritis, and significantly lower outcome scores. Metatarsophalangeal joint stiffness, from either from injuries to the bases of the phalanges or the heads of the metatarsals, has also been reported.

In the phalanges, joint stiffness and posttraumatic arthritis usually result from displaced articular fractures. However, unlike finger movement in the hand, interphalangeal joint motion in the toe is really not an important function. The only time that the arthritis in the toes produces any dysfunction is when it causes some kind of angular deformity of the toe, affecting shoe wear. The exception is posttraumatic arthritis in the interphalangeal joint of the great toe. For these patients, surgery, in the form of an arthrodesis, may be needed to control pain.

REFERENCES

1. Sarrafian SK, Kelikian AS. Development of the foot and ankle. In: Sarrafian SK, ed. *Sarrafian's Anatomy of the Foot and Ankle*. 2nd ed. Philadelphia, PA: Wolters Kluwer/Lippincott Williams & Wilkins; 2011.
2. Perry J. Ankle foot complex. In: Perry J, ed. *Gait Analysis. Normal and Pathological Function*. New York, NY: Slack, Inc; 1992:51-87.
3. Leland RH, Marymont JV, Trevino SG, Varner KE, Noble PC. Calcaneocuboid stability: a clinical and anatomic study. *Foot Ankle Int*. 2001;22:880-884.

4. Likin RC, Degnore LT, Pienkowski D. Contact mechanics of normal tarsometatarsal joints. *J Bone Joint Surg Am.* 2001;83:520-528.

5. Shibuya N, Davis ML, Jupiter DC. Epidemiology of foot and ankle fractures in the United States: an analysis of the National Trauma Data Bank (2007 to 2011). *J Foot Ankle Surg.* 2014;53:606-608.

6. Court-Brown CM, Caesar B. Epidemiology of adult fractures: a review. *Injury.* 2006;37:691-697.

7. Court-Brown CM, Honeyman C, Bugler K, McQueen M. The spectrum of open fractures of the foot in adults. *Foot Ankle Int.* 2013;34:323-328.

8. Gustilo RB, Mendoza RM, Williams DM. Problems in the management of type III (severe) open fractures: a new classification of type III open fractures. *J Trauma.* 1984;24:742-746.

9. Wei CJ, Tsai WC, Tiu CM, Wu HT, Chiou HJ, Chang CY. Systematic analysis of missed extremity fractures in emergency radiology. *Acta Radiol.* 2006;47:710-717.

10. Shibuya N, Frost CH, Campbell JD, Davis ML, Jupiter DC. Incidence of acute deep vein thrombosis and pulmonary embolism in foot and ankle trauma: analysis of the National Trauma Data Bank. *J Foot Ankle Surg.* 2012;51:63-68.

11. Falck-Ytter Y, Francis CW, Johanson NA, et al. Prevention of VTE in orthopedic surgery patients. Antithrombotic therapy and prevention of thrombosis, 9th edition: American college of chest physicians evidence-based clinical practice guidelines. *Chest.* 2012;141(2 suppl):e278S-e325S.

12. Perren SM. Evolution of the internal fixation of long bone fractures. The scientific basis of biological internal fixation: choosing a new balance between stability and biology. *J Bone Joint Surg Br.* 2002;84:1093-1110.

13. Boursinos LA, Karachalios T, Poultsides L, Malizos KN. Do steroids, conventional non-steroidal anti-inflammatory drugs and selective Cox-2 inhibitors adversely affect fracture healing? *J Musculoskelet Neuronal Interact.* 2009;9:44-52.

14. Hernandez RH, Do TP, Critchlow CW, Dent RE, Jick SS. Patient-related risk factors for fracture-healing complications in the United Kingdom General Practice Research Database. *Acta Orthop.* 2012;83:653-660.

15. Geusens P, Emans PJ, De Jong JJA, van den Bergh J. NSAIDS and fracture healing. *Curr Opin Rheumatol.* 2013;25:524-531.

16. Astion DJ, Deland JT, Otis JC, Kenneally S. Motion of the hindfoot after simulated arthrodesis. *J Bone Joint Surg Am.* 1997;79:241-246.

17. Marsh JL, Slongo TF, Agel J, et al. Fracture and Dislocation Compendium-2007. Orthopaedic Trauma Association Classification, Database and Outcomes Committee. *J Orthop Trauma,* 2007;21(10 suppl):S90-S102, S125-S128.

18. Gerhardt JJ, Cocchiarella L, Lea RD. Measuring Joints in the Lower Extremities. In: Gerhardt JJ, Cocchiarella L, Lea RD, eds. *The Practical Guide to Range of Motion Assessment.* 1st ed. American Medical Association; 2002:96-104.

19. Ryf C, Weymann A. Joint measurments. In: Ryf C, Weymann A, eds. *Range of Motion-AO Neutral-0 Method.* Stuttgart, New York: Thieme; 1999:E35-E37.

20. Herscovici D Jr, Widmaier J, Scaduto JM, Sanders RW, Walling A. Operative treatment of calcaneal fractures in elderly patients. *J Bone Joint Surg Am.* 2005;87:1260-1264.

21. Gaskill T, Schweitzer K, Nunley J. Comparison of surgical outcomes of intra-articular calcaneal fractures by age. *J Bone Joint Surg Am.* 2010;92:2884-2889.

22. Paterson DH, Jones GR, Rice CL. Ageing and physical activity: evidence to develop exercise recommendations for older adults. *Can J Public Health.* 2007;98:S69-S108.

23. Buckley RE, Tough S, McCormack R, et al. Operative compared with nonoperative treatment of displaced intraarticular calcaneal fractures: a prospective, randomized, controlled multicenter study. *J Bone Joint Surg Am.* 2002;84:1733-1744.

24. Hawkins LG. Fractures of the neck of the talus. *J Bone Joint Surg Am.* 1970;52:991-1002.

25. Canale ST, Kelly FB. Fractures of the neck of the talus: long-term evaluation of seventy-one cases. *J Bone Joint Surg Am.* 1978;60:143-156.

26. Inokuchi S, Ogawa K, Usami N. Classification of fractures of the talus: clear differentiation between neck and body fractures. *Foot Ankle Int.* 1996;17:748-750.

27. Herscovici D Jr, Scaduto JM. Management of high-energy foot and ankle injuries in the geriatric population. *Geriatr Orthop Surg Rehabil.* 2012;3:33-44.

28. Vallier HA, Reichard SG, Boyd AJ, Moore TA. A new look at the Hawkins classification for talar neck fractures: which features of injury and treatment are predictive of osteonecrosis? *J Bone Joint Surg Am.* 2014;96:192-197.

29. Lindvall E, Haidukewych G, DiPasquale T, Herscovici D Jr, Sanders R. Open reduction and stable fixation of isolated, displace talar neck and body fractures. *J Bone Joint Surg Am.* 2004;86:2229-2234.

30. Vallier HA, Nork SE, Benirschke SK, Sangeorzan BJ. Surgical treatment of talar body fractures. *J Bone Joint Surg Am.* 2003;85:1716-1724.

31. Ouzounian TJ, Shereff MJ. In vitro determination of midfoot motion. *Foot Ankle.* 1989;10:140-146.

32. Teng AL, Pinzur MS, Lomasney L, Mohoney L, Harvey R. Functional outcome following anatomic restoration of tarso-metatarsal fracture dislocation. *Foot Ankle Int.* 2002;23:922-926.

33. Sangeorzan BJ, Bernirscke SK, Mosca V, Mayo KA, Hansen ST. Displaced intra-articular fractures of the tarsal navicular. *J Bone Joint Surg Am* 1989;71:1504-1510.

34. Kuo RS, Tejwani NC, DiGiovanni CW, et al. Outcome after open reduction and internal fixation of Lisfranc joint injuries. *J Bone Joint Surg Am.* 2000;82:1609-1618.

35. Mihalich RM, Early JS. Management of cuboid crush injuries. *Foot Ankle Clin N Am.* 2006;11:121-126.

36. Herscovici D Jr, Sanders R. Fractures of the tarsal navicular. *Foot Ankle Clin N Am.* 1999;4:587-601.

37. Dameron TB Jr. Fractures of the proximal fifth metatarsal: selection the best treatment option. *J Am Acad Orthop Surg.* 1995;3:110-114.

Index

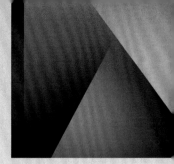

Note: Page numbers followed by 'f' indicate figures and 't' indicate tables.